The Nurse's Liability for Malpractice

A PROGRAMMED COURSE

The Nurse's Liability for Malpractice

A PROGRAMMED COURSE

Eli P. Bernzweig, J.D.
Member of the New York Bar

SIXTH EDITION

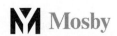 Mosby

St. Louis Baltimore Boston Carlsbad Chicago Naples New York Philadelphia Portland
London Madrid Mexico City Singapore Sydney Tokyo Toronto Wiesbaden

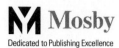

Dedicated to Publishing Excellence

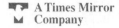 A Times Mirror
Company

Publisher: Nancy L. Coon
Executive Editor: N. Darlene Como
Assistant Editor: Barbara M. Carroll
Project Manager: Dana Peick
Senior Production Editor: Catherine Albright
Designer: Amy Buxton
Manufacturing Manager: Betty Richmond

"This publication is designed to provide accurate and authoritative information in regard to the subject matter covered. It is sold with the understanding that the publisher is not engaged in rendering legal, accounting, or other professional service. If legal advice or other expert assistance is required, the services of a competent professional person should be sought." From a Declaration of Principles jointly adopted by a Committee of the American Bar Association and a Committee of Publishers and Associations.

SIXTH EDITION

Printed in the United States of America
Composition by Shepherd, Inc.
Printing and Binding by R.R. Donnelly & Sons

Mosby
11830 Westline Industrial Drive
St. Louis, Missouri 63146

Library of Congress Cataloging-in-Publication Data
Bernzweig, Eli P.
   The nurse's liability for malpractice : a programmed course / Eli
P. Bernzweig. — 6th ed.
     p. cm.
   Includes bibliographical references and index.
   ISBN 0-8151-0702-1
   1. Nurses—Malpractice—United States—Programmed instruction.
I. Title.
KF2915.N83B4   1995
346.7303'32—dc20   95-30160
[347.306332]   CIP

96 97 98 99 00 / 9 8 7 6 5 4 3 2 1

ABOUT THE AUTHOR

Eli P. Bernzweig is a consultant and writer on professional liability issues and for many years has been recognized as one of the nation's top authorities on medical malpractice. During his 20-year tenure as a government attorney, he was chief legal advisor to the United States Public Health Service hospital system, where he was responsible for reviewing all malpractice claims asserted against the Public Health Service and advising the government with respect thereto. From 1971 through 1973, he served as Executive Director of the H.E.W. Secretary's Commission on Medical Malpractice, the first national body to explore the basic causes and consequences of the growing malpractice problem.

In addition to his government service, Bernzweig has been a vice president of one of the country's major medical malpractice insurers and vice president of one of the world's largest professional liability insurance brokers. In both instances, his responsibilities involved the creation and development of risk management and loss control programs for professionals—first for health care professionals, and later for legal professionals. Over the years, his expertise in the field of professional liability has also led to the development of risk management programs for financial professionals and securities brokerage firms.

Bernzweig has his law degree from Rutgers Law School and is a member of the New York and U.S. Supreme Court bars. He is the author of four books and numerous articles on health care and professional liability issues, and has been a regular contributor to *RN* Magazine and other publications on the legal liability of nurses.

In loving memory of

Abraham and Fannie Bernzweig

Abraham David and Sarah Axelrad Ribner

Isaac L. Ribner

PREFACE

As this is written, the debate on major health care reform continues to rage. Along with a host of other important issues, one of the key reforms being debated both in Congress and throughout the nation is whether basic health care coverage should be a fundamental right for all Americans. To the extent that issue ultimately is decided in the affirmative, even if on a phased-in basis, many more providers of primary health care will be needed than are currently available. Primary care—the type of care required by most Americans—currently is provided by physicians and nurse practitioners (NPs). Both categories are in short supply at the moment but can be expected to increase in numbers if and when health care reform becomes a legislative reality. Nurses with the appropriate education and training are well-positioned to provide primary care, as well as preventive health services, home care and long-term care and are logical choices for providing these basic health services under a comprehensive national health insurance scheme.

If health care reform does in fact propel more nurses into the roles described, they will have to accept stricter legal accountability along with their greater professional recognition. But legal accountability is not limited to nurses in advanced practice; it is a recognized fact of life for every practicing nurse, whether a RN employed as a staff nurse in a hospital, a Certified Nurse-Midwife in independent practice, or a LPN providing care in a long-term care facility or a patient's home. There is little doubt that the ever-present fear of involvement in a malpractice suit—a fear that is not without substance in the current malpractice litigation environment—makes it essential for nurses in all practice settings to be as familiar as possible with the legal guidelines that govern their patient care responsibilities. Although it is seldom fully appreciated, there is a vital relationship between a nurse's knowledge of legal principles and the nurse's daily professional conduct. The nurse who learns how to avoid unnecessary legal risks will not only avoid unwanted malpractice suits, but in the process will be providing a higher quality of patient care.

When this text was first published, some 25 years ago, the author made it clear that its objective was a very selective one: to teach professional and practical nurses at both the student and graduate level what law regulates their routine patient care activities, what nursing conduct might give rise to malpractice suits, and what they can do to lessen the chances of being sued for malpractice. This book does not address, nor was it designed to address, the ever-increasing number of ethical problems facing today's nurses in such areas as the right to die, euthanasia, organ transplantation, "big ticket" research and innovative medical procedures, AIDS, abortion and reproductive technology, and genetic engineering and screening. For this the author makes no apology. While not minimizing the importance of those issues to practicing nurses, dealing with the moral dilemmas and resolving the ethical conflicts in health care is simply too complex and extensive to be included in a basic text on malpractice liability.

The current edition, as was the case with earlier editions, is predicated on the theory that more can and should be done by all medical and nursing personnel to minimize the possibilities of errors or complications in treatment that may lead to litigation. Toward that end, this sixth edition contains several entirely new features designed to alert nurses to some of the practical ways to avoid risky situations in providing patient care. It includes, for example, graphics containing special tips on how to prevent medication errors, how to deal with suicidal patients, how to protect patients from falls, how to deal with questionable physicians' orders, and so forth. For learning-reinforcement purposes, this edition also includes four new tables and two boxed charts depicting specific legal concepts, doctrines, or procedures that are of direct practical concern to all nurses.

A number of topics have been added or substantially expanded, including other important sources of law, patients' rights, the expanded role of nurses, the doctrine of hospital corporate liability, health care reform and managed care, the nurse's criminal liability, the patient's contributory negligence and/or assumption of risk, when to follow or not follow physicians' orders, DNR orders, monitoring and observation problems, communication breakdowns, nurse-specialists in emergency care, the problem of the impaired nurse, short-staffing problems, informed consent, disciplinary action against nurses, special problems in home health care, effectiveness of consent given by a minor parent, and the malpractice litigation process. All programmed text legal material has been updated to conform to the latest statutes and court cases. All Selected References at the end of each Part have been updated and substantially expanded. Finally, the Glossary and Index have been expanded and new Test Questions have been included.

More than ever, the ability of the modern nurse to function effectively requires something beyond the mere acquisition of basic nursing knowledge and skills. Fundamental concern for the patient's safety—always a prime focus of nurses—calls for a heightened awareness of the legal parameters within which they are expected to fulfill their customary nursing duties. This programmed course is geared to meeting that objective, and it is hoped that nurses who complete this material will be better prepared to serve their patients as well as to protect themselves against the legal hazards in modern nursing practice.

Eli P. Bernzweig

INTRODUCTION

This self-instructional course is intended to teach nurses in understandable terms about their legal liability for acts of malpractice. Some nurses may have only the vaguest idea what the terms *liability* and *malpractice* even mean, but by the time this course is completed, the learner will not only know what these words mean but will begin to appreciate the fact that many of the routine nursing functions performed each day have important legal consequences.

Knowledge precedes meaningful action, and nurses who know the legal consequences of daily patient care activities will soon begin to think and act preventively; that is, they will consciously conduct themselves in a manner designed to prevent unwanted suits from ever arising. This conscious behavior on the part of the nurse will save the embarrassment, loss of prestige, and worry that accompany every lawsuit, and it is bound to result in better patient care.

Throughout this course (except where specifically indicated) no attempt has been made to distinguish between the liability of the registered nurse, the practical nurse, and the nursing student since the courts themselves have generally made little distinction in this respect. In the final analysis, the same body of legal principles is equally applicable to all classes of nurses. This fact emphasizes the need for all nurses to become familiar with the information taught in this course.

Statement of Behavioral Objectives

The purpose of this program is not to make lawyers out of nurses or even to teach nurses how to solve specific legal problems. That role is best played by the medicolegal specialist, and the intelligent nurse will always consult such a person when in need of legal advice concerning a particular aspect of this complex field of law. The prime objective of this course is to give the learner a grounding in the fundamental principles of malpractice law and then to show how these fundamental principles are applied in specific fact situations. On completion of the program, the learner should be able to do the following:

1. Analyze a fact situation involving a particular aspect of nursing care, identify the principles of malpractice law that apply, and determine with reasonable certainty the legal consequences (if any) for her or him in the given situation.

2. Determine his or her malpractice-liability potential in carrying out various types of nursing functions and make appropriate changes in behavior to assure not only conformity with the applicable legal standards of care but higher quality care for all his or her patients.

3. Identify patients who are more likely to be suit-prone and take the steps necessary in caring for such patients to forestall the possibility of later malpractice claims.

4. Employ the terminology of malpractice law in a meaningful way when discussing specific legal problems with nursing supervisors, hospital administrators, lawyers, or others.

How to Proceed

A programmed course builds a structure of information in systematically arranged steps, each of which is referred to as a *frame* This particular program utilizes the multiple-choice type of frame, which requires the learner to check the correct response or responses to each question. Programmed instruction is an active teaching process, which requires active responding on the part of the learner. *Checking the appropriate box or boxes, therefore, is a vital and necessary part of the program.* The choice made should be compared with the correct response set at the bottom of the page. The learner should not look at the answer until he or she has indicated what the appropriate response should be. It may be helpful to cover the answer with the provided mask while reading the text.

The questions presented throughout the program are not intended to be deceptive or unusually difficult. The purpose is to teach, not to confuse or confound. The learner who reads carefully and pays close attention to the instructional material should get correct responses to the questions posed in all or nearly all the frames.

Test questions that appear at the end of the program may be used both for pretest and posttest purposes.

CONTENTS

Part 5   REGULATION OF NURSING AND SCOPE OF NURSING PRACTICE

Part 6   PROVING THE NURSE'S LIABILITY

Part 7   PRINCIPLES OF MALPRACTICE CLAIMS PREVENTION

PART ONE

GENERAL PRINCIPLES

TYPES AND SOURCES OF LAW

1-1   Throughout this course we will have occasion to refer to the words "law," "common law," "civil law," and "statutory law," so it is important for you to have a reasonably clear understanding of the meaning of these words and the distinctions between them.

The word "law" has many different meanings and is used in many different ways, depending upon the subject under discussion. For example, we refer to physical laws (such as the law of gravity), economic laws (such as Gresham's law), and psychological laws (such as the law of operant conditioning), and although all these have an effect on human beings in one way or another, none of them has any *legal significance.*

"Law," in the sense we will be using the term in this course, refers to those rules made by humans that regulate social conduct in a formally prescribed and legally binding manner.

Without knowing the exact context in which the word "law" was being used, a person ☐ could   ☐ could not   be sure of the specific sense in which the word was intended.

1-2   Human beings are affected by various types of laws. We will be discussing in this course only those types of laws that

☐ determine human behavior and psychological motivation

☐ regulate human social conduct in a legally binding manner

☐ determine and influence physical environment

1-1   *could not*   **1-2**   *regulate human social conduct in a legally binding manner*

1-3   Check each of the laws listed below that has legal significance in the sense that it regulates human social conduct in a legally binding manner.

☐   law of gravity

☐   law of diminishing returns

☐   Indiana Nurse Practice Act

☐   Federal Drug Abuse Control Act

☐   Murphy's Law

☐   Florida Motor Vehicle Code

☐   law of economic cycles

1-4   Laws that regulate human social conduct are derived from two principal sources. One source of law finds expression in formal legislative enactments, generally referred to as "statutes." When law is formally expressed in a statute, we refer to it as statutory law. A law passed by Congress or a state or a provincial legislative body would be an example of statutory law.

The *distinguishing* feature of statutory law is that it

☐   regulates human social conduct

☐   is one of two basic kinds of law

☐   is derived from formal legislative enactments

1-3 ☐ *If you are not sure of the dis-*
        ☐ *tinction between laws that do*
        ☑ *and laws that do not regulate*
        ☑ *human social conduct, turn to*
        ☐ *p. 9, Note A.*
        ☑
        ☐

1-4 *is derived from formal legisla-tive enactments*

The other two items are also features, but neither of them is the distinguishing feature of statutory law.

NOTE: While all statutes are the result of formal legislative enactments, a statute enacted by the legislative body of one jurisdiction would have no legal effect outside that jurisdiction. Thus, the Nursing Practice Act of the Province of Ontario would not apply to nurses in the State of New York or the Province of Manitoba.

1-5   Legislative bodies cannot possibly enact statutes to cover all types of human conduct, and thus there are gaps in the law that must be filled in another way. The second principal source of law that regulates human social conduct is expressed in juridical decisions that interpret legal issues raised in disputes taken to court. This judge-made law is referred to either as common law or decisional law, to distinguish it from the more formal type of law expressed in legislative enactments. Although common law and statutory law are derived from different sources, they are both of equal importance and legal effect.

How does common law (decisional law) differ from statutory law?

☐ Common law is not the result of a legislative enactment.

☐ Decisional law is less binding than statutory law.

☐ Statutory law does not have the legal effect of decisional law.

1-6   Statutory law and decisional law have the following feature in common (select one):

☐ They both represent the formal expression of law by a legislative (lawmaking) body.

☐ They both regulate the conduct of human beings in a legally binding manner.

☐ They both result from legal disputes between individuals.

1-5   *Common law is not the result of a legislative enactment.*

1-6   ☐ *Only statutory law has to be*
☑ *enacted by a legislative body,*
☐ *and only decisional law is derived from court decisions. However, they both regulate human social conduct.*

1-7 As mentioned before, both statutory law and common law (or decisional law) are of equal importance and legal effect, and it is possible for both types of law to be involved in a single lawsuit.

Consider the following example:

■ In a malpractice suit filed against a licensed practical nurse, the complaining party introduces into evidence the state Practical Nursing Practice Act. The complainant does this to prove that the nurse attempted (unsuccessfully) to perform a function that should have been performed only by a registered nurse (RN). After carefully reading the act, the trial judge rules that the nurse was legally permitted to perform the particular nursing function and that the only question to be resolved by the jury is whether the nurse performed it in a safe and proper manner.

The Practical Nursing Practice Act in this case is an example of
☐   common law   ☐   statutory law   because

☐   it was introduced into evidence in a court of law

☐   it represents a specific legislative enactment or statute applicable in that jurisdiction

---

1-8 The trial judge's ruling in this case is an example of
☐   decisional law   ☐   statutory law   because

☐   it relates to a specific legislative enactment

☐   it laid down a legal principle that will be binding on other courts in future similar cases

---

1-9 A statute that deals with a particular aspect of nursing practice, such as the administration of narcotic drugs, would have

☐   greater legal effect than

☐   the same legal effect as

☐   less legal effect than

a judicial decision dealing with the identical subject matter.

1-7 *statutory law*	1-8 *decisional law*	1-9 *the same legal effect as*
it represents a specific legislative enactment . . .	*it laid down a legal principle that will be binding on other courts . . .*	*If you selected the wrong answer, turn to p. 9, Note B.*

OTHER IMPORTANT SOURCES OF LAW

While the two principal types of law we will be dealing with in this course are statutory enactments and judge-made or decisional law, there are other types and sources of law that also affect our daily activities, not only as nurses but as ordinary citizens. The highest form of law in the United States is the United States Constitution—the basic organic law that guarantees to people certain fundamental rights and liberties and defines the relationship between governmental authority and individual freedoms. The Constitution also defines the functions as well as the powers and limits of the three branches of government: the executive, legislative, and judicial. Constitutional law is the branch of law that is derived from interpretations of the Constitution by the U.S. Supreme Court, usually in the form of lengthy written opinions, whose interpretations represent the highest law of the land. Occasionally, Supreme Court decisions will directly affect the activities of nurses—such as rulings on state abortion laws, federal laws affording immunity from malpractice suits to federally employed nurses, and health care matters affecting patients being treated under various federally funded medical care programs. For the most part, however, Supreme Court decisions deal with significant legal issues that affect the public as a whole.

Under the U.S. Constitution, all powers not granted explicitly to the federal government are retained by the states. The inherent police power of the states includes the authority to enact reasonable laws necessary to preserve public order, health, safety, welfare, and morals. State governments also have enacted constitutions that set forth the fundamental rights and freedoms of their citizens, and in some cases give even greater rights to their citizens than those afforded by the U.S. Constitution. However, state constitutions cannot eliminate or otherwise limit rights granted under the U.S. Constitution.

Another category of law that affects the activities of nurses is administrative law. It would be virtually impossible for a state legislature, in enacting a law designed to regulate a specific area of activity, to include in the legislation all the myriad details for implementing the regulatory process. The legislature normally delegates authority to an administrative agency that has expertise in a particular area of law to promulgate regulations necessary to implement the statute. The general term used to refer to the process of enacting regulations in this manner is "administrative law"; it is important to note that once they are adopted in accordance with a specific rule-making process, these regulations have the same force and effect as any other law. By way of example, state nurse practice acts customarily authorize the state board of nursing (or its equivalent) to promulgate specific regulations governing the practice of nursing, including admission standards, educational standards, the right to grant, suspend, or revoke licenses, and occasionally even some patient care standards.

Neither constitutional law nor administrative law will be covered as separate categories in this course. Our purpose here is solely to make the student aware of these additional sources and types of law. We return now to the course itself.

1-10 Now that you know the kind of law we will be talking about in this course and its two principal sources, let us see where the particular branch of law known as malpractice law fits into the picture. To do this, we must first understand how the entire body of statutory and common law is classified. Although the law is classified in many different ways, for our purposes it is sufficient if we distinguish between two major classifications: criminal law and civil law.

Criminal law deals solely with conduct that is considered an offense against the general public because it is detrimental to the welfare of society as a whole. In marked contrast to civil law, criminal law seeks to punish, deter, and rehabilitate those who violate criminal statutes. Criminal conduct includes such public offenses as murder, robbery, burglary, embezzlement, and assault.

Which of the following *best* expresses the nature and purpose of criminal law?

- ☐ Criminal law deals with unlawful conduct that is considered offensive to society as a whole.

- ☐ Criminal law deals with unlawful conduct by individuals that is usually violent in nature.

- ☐ Criminal law deals with unlawful conduct by individuals who deserve to be punished.

1-10 *Criminal law deals with unlawful conduct that is considered offensive to society as a whole.*

EXPLANATORY NOTES

Note A (from Frame 1-3)

All the laws that are listed have *some* effect on human beings, but not all of them *regulate* the conduct or behavior of human beings in a formal, legal manner. To illustrate, the law of gravity clearly affects all of us in that it describes a uniformly consistent relationship involving the attraction downward toward the center of the earth of all objects on earth; however, this is not the kind of law that guides us in our social conduct as members of society. The key, then, to the type of law or laws we will be talking about in this course is the word "regulate." Unless a particular law *regulates* our social conduct in a formal, legal manner, it is not the type of law with which we will be concerned.

Proceed to Frame 1-4.

Note B (from Frame 1-9)

The correct answer is that a statute that deals with a particular aspect of nursing practice would have the *same* legal effect as a judicial decision that deals with the same subject matter. The particular source of law has no bearing on the importance or legal effect of either type of law. Thus, the trial judge's decision in a nursing malpractice suit concerning a particular nursing function would be just as binding and controlling with respect to the nursing function in question as a statute that announces a specific rule or standard of conduct applicable to that same nursing function.

The key points to remember are: (1) Both statutory law and common law (or decisional law) regulate human social conduct in a formal manner, and (2) both have the same legal significance.

Proceed to Frame 1-10.

1-11 Although we ordinarily associate criminal conduct with violent behavior, this need not be the case. As long as the conduct is expressly prohibited under the common law or by a specific statute, it is considered a crime. And even though the prohibited act is directed against a particular person or the person's property (with or without his or her knowledge), legally it is viewed as an offense against society as a whole.

Indicate whether the following statements are true or false:

True	False	
☐	☐	All violent behavior is considered to be criminal conduct.
☐	☐	Some acts may be considered crimes even though perpetrated entirely without the knowledge of the victim.
☐	☐	To be considered a crime, a person's conduct must be directed against a specific person or entity.

1-12 Criminal actions cannot be prosecuted by private citizens, since they are considered offenses against the general public. Accordingly, they are prosecuted by the controlling government authority (federal, state, or provincial), and if found guilty, the accused may be punished by being fined, imprisoned, or both.

■ A and B are neighbors who do not like each other. One day, in a heated argument over the placement of a boundary fence, A attacks and seriously wounds B with a kitchen knife.

Since A and B know each other and since no one else was involved in the incident, A's conduct would be considered noncriminal.

True ☐ False ☐

1-13 In the previous example, who could institute a criminal action against A?

☐ only B

☐ B or B's spouse

☐ only the controlling governmental authority

☐ any offended onlooker

1-11 True False
☐ ☑
☑ ☐
☐ ☑

1-12 False

Assaulting another person with a deadly weapon is considered a criminal act in all civilized societies.

1-13 ☐ ☐ ☑ ☐ *If the correct answer seems confusing to you, turn to p. 19, Note A.*

1-14 If A is found guilty in a criminal action arising out of the incident described in Frame 1-12, which of the following would be the likely consequence thereof?

☐   A will be fined, sentenced to prison, or placed on probation.

☐   A will be required to pay all B's medical expenses arising from the inflicted wounds.

☐   A will have to publicly apologize to B for such violent conduct.

1-15 The second major class of law, civil law, is concerned with the legal rights and duties of private persons (or combinations of persons, such as corporations). It is in contrast with criminal law, which is concerned solely with public rights and public authority to punish for unlawful conduct. Thus, the unsuccessful party in a civil suit is usually required to pay a sum of money to the successful party in the suit, but is not imprisoned or fined, as in a criminal case.

In what significant respect does civil law differ from criminal law?

☐   Civil law is concerned with conduct that is unlawful but not violent.

☐   Civil law is concerned with conduct that violates the rights of all members of society.

☐   Civil law is concerned with the legal rights and relationships that exist between private persons.

1-14   *A will be fined, sentenced to prison, or placed on probation.*

1-15   *Civil law is concerned with the legal rights and relationships that exist between private persons.*

1-16   Which two of the following statements correctly describe the characteristics of civil law?

☐   The successful party in a civil suit is usually awarded a sum of money.

☐   Civil law does not deal with public offenses or conduct that is deemed detrimental to society as a whole.

☐   Civil law deals only with financial rights and interests of private persons.

1-17   Although criminal law is concerned only with the public interest and civil law is concerned only with private interests, *both* classes of law frequently involve the interpretation of statutes.

Keeping in mind the differences in the legal interests concerned, indicate which of the following excerpts from statutes relate to criminal law and which relate to civil law.

Criminal	*Civil*	
☐	☐	"It shall be unlawful for any person to practice any of the healing arts in this state without first having obtained a license from the State Board of Regents."
☐	☐	"If either party to a contract agrees thereto by reason of fraud, there is no legal agreement and said contract shall be unenforceable in this state."
☐	☐	"No will shall be admitted to probate in this state unless the instrument shows on its face that it has been duly witnessed by at least two persons."
☐	☐	"It shall be unlawful for any licensed physician or nurse to fail to report the existence of a contagious or communicable disease to the local health authorities immediately upon discovery."

NOTE: It should be noted that in the course of a trial a judge is sometimes called on to interpret the applicability or effect of a particular statute, but this does not make such interpretation by the judge the equivalent of a statutory enactment. It is just another aspect of decisional or common law. If this is not quite clear, you may wish to review Frames 1-5 through 1-9 at this point.

1-16	☑	*If you checked the 3d box, turn*	**1-17**	*Criminal*	*Civil*
	☑	*to p. 19, Note B.*		☑	☐
	☐			☐	☑
				☐	☑
				☑	☐

POINTS TO REMEMBER

1. While many types of laws affect human beings, not all of them have legal significance.

2. In this course the term "law" refers to those rules made by humans that regulate social conduct in a formal and legally binding manner.

3. Law is derived from legislative enactments (statutory law) and from judicial decisions (referred to as common law or decisional law).

4. Both statutory and common law are of equal importance and legal effect.

5. Criminal law and civil law are two of the major classifications of law.

6. Criminal law deals with offenses against society as a whole, and criminal actions are accordingly brought by the appropriate governmental authorities.

7. Criminal conduct may be associated with violent behavior, but this is not always the case. To be criminal, the conduct need only be an offense against society prohibited under the common law or, as is usually the case, by statute.

8. If found guilty, the accused in a criminal action is punished.

9. Civil law deals with private legal rights and interests, and the unsuccessful party in a civil action is usually (but not always) required to pay money to the successful party.

CRIMINAL CONDUCT AND NURSING PRACTICE

We have just pointed out that criminal law is one of the two major classifications of law, and that criminal acts are those deemed offenses against society as a whole. Although the focus of this course is the nurse's liability for malpractice—which is strictly a civil law issue—it may be useful to discuss briefly how particular nursing activities or conduct may bring the nurse into contact with the criminal law and the criminal justice system. This is a matter of growing importance, because the number of criminal prosecutions brought against health care providers appears to be increasing, and greater numbers of nurses are being called to testify as witnesses in criminal proceedings involving various aspects of patient care.

Federal criminal law is created entirely by federal statute, while state criminal laws are usually a combination of specific criminal statutes and state common law—although most states have codified their common law crimes and incorporated them into their criminal statutes. Federal criminal statutes generally relate to matters over which the states have no jurisdiction, such as interstate transportation of stolen goods, crimes committed on federal property (hospitals, parks, government office buildings), fraudulent use of the mail or fraudulent interstate business practices, and so forth. State criminal statutes, on the other hand, generally relate to those crimes that existed in common law—such as murder, manslaughter, robbery, burglary, rape, larceny— but may, of course, include other acts the state legislature has chosen to define as crimes. Finally, some acts may be considered crimes under both federal and state laws (e.g., the possession of controlled narcotic substances with the intent to sell or traffic them).

Criminal actions against a nurse can vary from relatively minor offenses called misdemeanors to major crimes called felonies. Misdemeanors are generally defined as all criminal offenses other than those clearly set forth as felonies, and many jurisdictions distinguish between the two by defining a felony as any crime punishable by death or imprisonment in the state penitentiary for more than a year; a misdemeanor is any crime punishable by fine, imprisonment in a local jail, or both. Misdemeanor crimes would include, for example, the illegal practice of medicine, the failure to report elder or child abuse, theft of property, and falsification of medical records. Criminal conduct amounting to a felony would include murder, manslaughter, rape, robbery, arson, larceny, aggravated assault, mayhem, and so forth. It goes without saying that a nurse may be arrested, tried, and convicted if there is evidence of personal involvement in any of these major categories of criminal conduct, whether or not related to his or her professional nursing duties.

There are, however, some nursing activities that by nature pose a significantly greater risk of criminal prosecution, particularly if serious bodily harm or death results. Some examples would include removing life-support systems, carrying out no-code orders, administering high doses of pain-killing drugs to terminally ill patients (euthanasia), and stealing narcotic drugs.

In most states a nurse can be prosecuted for conduct amounting to what is referred to as criminal negligence—or involuntary manslaughter, if death results—in which there has been a failure to act when there is a duty to act, and such inaction is deemed deliberate or reckless indifference to protecting the life of a patient. An example would be observing a physician or fellow nurse providing patient care while impaired by drugs or alcohol. In this situation, depending on the law of the state in question, the nurse's failure to act could result in a charge of either criminal negligence or aiding, abetting, or covering up the criminal conduct of another. Revocation of the nurse's license is another common consequence of such criminal conduct.

Under the criminal law in all states, the accused person's mental state—specifically, his or her *intent* to commit the act in question—is usually considered critical and must be proved before there can be a finding of guilt. In the case of alleged criminal negligence, however, the element of intent can be inferred when it is shown that the nurse knew the consequences of failing to act, thus demonstrating a reckless indifference to the patient's welfare.

The frames that immediately follow touch on the effect of a nurse's violation of specific statutes pertaining to patient care, which may, in some circumstances, result in the nurse's criminal prosecution and liability. The student should note that there are some (relatively few) criminal statutes that impose strict liability, which means that guilt is established without regard to the violator's subjective intent or mental state. We review some of these special situations later in this part.

Finally, Part Four of this course covers the entire subject of intentional torts in depth, including some (such as assault and battery) that may lead to criminal and civil liability.

1-18   As just discussed, some nursing activities, if performed in an unlawful manner, can constitute criminal conduct, with attendant criminal law consequences.

Consider the following situation:

■ State S has a statute that provides: "Only a physician or dentist may prescribe, administer, and dispense narcotic drugs, or he may cause the same to be administered by a nurse or intern under his direction and supervision. . . . Violation of this statute is made a crime, punishable by fine or imprisonment, or both."

Doctor D orders Nurse N to administer a specific quantity of a pain-killing narcotic drug to a patient, and Nurse N administers the drug as directed. Later that evening the patient again complains of severe pain. Nurse N is unable to reach the doctor. Nurse N then obtains and administers a second dose of the narcotic drug, which relieves the patient's pain immediately.

What is the legal effect of Nurse N's conduct?

☐   Nurse N can be held criminally liable for violating the state's narcotic drug statute.

☐   Nurse N can be sued for money damages in a civil suit brought by the patient.

☐   Nurse N's conduct is of no legal effect since no harm resulted to the patient.

☐   No effect, since Nurse N was following the doctor's original orders.

1-18   ☑
        ☐
        ☐
        ☐

1-19 Nurse N violated the state statute by

☐ administering a narcotic drug to a patient

☐ failing to call a second physician for advice

☐ prescribing a narcotic drug for a patient

1-20 Based on the given example, which of the following conclusions is the most accurate?

☐ Nurses will be held criminally liable whenever they administer narcotic drugs to patients outside a prescribing doctor's presence.

☐ Nurses cannot be held criminally liable for prescribing narcotic drugs if a doctor gives them permission to do so.

☐ Nurses may be held criminally liable whenever they prescribe narcotic drugs.

1-19 *prescribing a narcotic drug*   **1-20** ☐   *If you checked the 2d box, turn*
          for a patient   ☐   *to p. 20, Note C.*
                                                        ☑

1-21 State and federal laws mandating the reporting of suspected child abuse (including child neglect and sexual exploitation) are directly applicable to nurses as well as to other health care practitioners. Under most of the state laws, the *good faith* reporting of such cases to the proper authorities—meaning the nurse has reasonable cause to believe the child's injuries were not accidental—will protect the nurse against liability in any lawsuit that might be brought by the person(s) accused claiming defamation of character or invasion of privacy. On the other hand, these laws make the *failure* to report such cases the basis for imposing criminal penalties, including fines and jail sentences.

Which of the following statements *best* expresses the nurse's criminal liability under child abuse reporting laws?

☐ A nurse can be held criminally liable for failure to report all cases of suspected child abuse that are based on reasonable cause and belief.

☐ A nurse can avoid being held criminally liable under the child abuse statute only if the nurse reports every instance of serious injury or trauma to a child.

☐ A nurse cannot be held criminally liable for failing to report any suspected child abuse case in which the nurse is not certain who is responsible for abusing the child.

1-22 Based on the foregoing, it is clear that a nurse   ☐ can   ☐ cannot   be held criminally liable both for taking action and for failing to take action under a particular statute.

1-21 ☑ *Child abuse statutes do not*
      ☐ *require reporting of all trauma*
      ☐ *to children, only trauma that is*
          suspected to have been caused
          by child abuse.

1-22 *can*

1-23 It is important that you understand the relationship of criminal law to nursing activities. We return now, however, to the prime subject of this course, the nurse's liability for malpractice, which falls within the general classification of civil law.

As a general proposition, the nurse's legal liability for malpractice is more important than the nurse's liability for criminal acts.

True   *False*

☐   ☐

1-24 We have thus far discussed:

1. What we mean by "law"

2. Two basic sources of law

3. Two major classifications of law

Now we will get more specific and see just how malpractice law is related to other kinds of law. Civil law, which deals with the legal rights and relationships existing between private persons, includes many different categories, each dealing with a different subject matter.

The general category of civil law with which we are concerned is called the law of torts. A "tort" is a legal wrong committed by one person against the person or property of another. To compensate for such a private legal wrong, the law permits the harmed person to bring a civil action (a lawsuit) against the wrongdoer to recover a sum of money.

Civil law consists of

☐ a single, comprehensive body of law

☐ two fundamental categories of law

☐ many different categories of law

1-23 *False*

If you are at all uncertain about this point, turn to p. 20, Note D.

1-24 *many different categories of law*

EXPLANATORY NOTES

Note A (from Frame 1-13)

Criminal actions are legal processes that can be initiated only by the controlling governmental authority. This does not mean that the victim of a criminal act (such as B in the given example) will not be *involved* in the criminal prosecution. In fact, B undoubtedly will be the principal witness for the state (or province). It should be noted that the fact that B cannot institute a *criminal* action against A does not affect B's right to institute a *civil* action arising out of the incident. This point is discussed more fully later in Part 1.

Proceed to Frame 1-14.

Note B (from Frame 1-16)

While it is true that civil law is concerned with private legal interests and that payment of a sum of money is the *usual* way in which these private legal interests are vindicated, there are other private legal interests that do not involve an award of money. Examples are the granting of a divorce, the granting of an injunction or restraining order against some specific type of offensive conduct, and a declaratory judgment establishing the ownership of property. Accordingly, one cannot categorically state that *all* civil actions involve purely financial rights and interests of private persons.

Proceed to Frame 1-17.

EXPLANATORY NOTES

Note C (from Frame 1-20)

Getting the doctor's permission to perform an unlawful act (prescribing a narcotic drug) will not help the nurse escape criminal liability. It will simply make the doctor an accessory to the crime. Because the administering of narcotic drugs is a common nursing function, all nurses should become thoroughly familiar with the pertinent statutes governing their use in the state or province in which they practice. These statutes must be followed *strictly* if criminal consequences are to be avoided.

Proceed to Frame 1-21.

Note D (from Frame 1-23)

Many aspects of criminal law are of special interest and importance to practicing nurses. Since their criminal liability can conceivably result in a fine or imprisonment, as well as the loss of their license to practice, it would be foolish to say that their criminal liability is less important than their civil liability. However, the subject of criminal law is so extensive that it really warrants a separate study in itself. For that reason, *and that reason alone,* we will not be discussing the nurse's criminal liability in more detail.

Proceed to Frame 1-24.

1-25   The particular branch of civil law that deals with private legal wrongs (i.e., wrongs committed by and against private persons or entities) is called

☐   the law of torts

☐   the law of private interests

☐   the law of compensation

1-26   A tort may be either an *intentional* wrong, such as assault, battery, false imprisonment, libel, or invasion of privacy, or an *unintentional* wrong, such as negligence. The one thing all torts have in common, however, is that the person or persons who have been wronged have the legal right to institute a civil action (i.e., a lawsuit) against the person or legal entity who caused the wrong.

Which of the following statements is correct?

☐   Private legal wrongs (torts) may result from conduct that the wrongdoer never intended.

☐   All private legal wrongs (torts) arise out of intentional willful behavior.

☐   An intentional private legal wrong (tort) will subject the wrongdoer to a criminal action.

1-27   Which of the following involves unintentional conduct?

☐   false imprisonment

☐   invasion of privacy

☐   negligence

1-25 ☑   **1-26** ☑   **1-27** *negligence*
       ☐   ☐
       ☐   ☐

1-28 A tort action can be brought by

☐ a single individual only

☐ one or more private persons

☐ local government units only

1-29 The common element of all torts is that they deal with

☐ intentional conduct

☐ private wrongs

☐ unintentional conduct

1-30 Some *intentional* torts represent antisocial behavior of a sort that is also punishable under criminal law. Examples are the torts of assault and battery. If A assaults B and is brought to trial on a charge of *criminal* assault, B would still be legally entitled to bring a civil action against A for the tort of *civil* assault.

Which of the following statements accurately summarizes the foregoing?

☐ An act that constitutes a tort may also constitute a crime.

☐ An act must be either a tort or a crime, but cannot be both.

☐ An assaulted person can bring both a tort action and a criminal action against the wrongdoer.

NOTE: From this point on, all references to torts will be limited to their civil-law aspect only. We will discuss intentional torts later in the course.

1-28 *one or more pri-vate persons*   **1-29** *private wrongs*   **1-30** ☑ *If you would like fur-*
☐ *ther clarification of*
☐ *this point, turn to p.*
27, Note A.

1-31 There are many types of torts, but the one that relates most directly to the basic subject of this course is the tort of negligence. Negligence law is a broad field of law that includes many types of harmful conduct in carrying out one's legal responsibilities to others. It encompasses the area commonly referred to as malpractice law and includes the harmful conduct of physicians, dentists, nurses, pharmacists, engineers, lawyers, architects, and other professionally trained persons.

The law of negligence is a subcategory of

☐ the law of contracts

☐ the law of torts

☐ the law of malpractice

1-32 The circles below symbolically represent the fields of tort law, negligence law, and malpractice law. Place the letter of each circle in the box beside the field of law it represents.

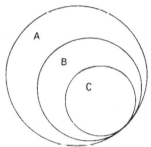

☐ Tort law

☐ Malpractice law

☐ Negligence law

1-33   Malpractice law is concerned with

    ☐   all types of harmful conduct

    ☐   the harmful conduct of all professional persons

    ☐   the harmful conduct of professional medical personnel only

---

CONCEPT OF NEGLIGENCE

1-34   Now that you have some idea of the general relationship between tort law, negligence law, and malpractice law, let us analyze the concept of negligence in more detail.

According to law *every* person is always responsible for behaving in a reasonable and prudent manner, whether a layperson or a professional and whether engaged in the simplest or most complex type of activity. When persons fail to conduct themselves in this required manner and thereby do harm to others, we say they are legally "negligent."

Insofar as the law is concerned, persons are expected to conduct themselves in a reasonable and prudent manner

    ☐   at all times

    ☐   only when engaged in professional activities

    ☐   only when performing simple functions

    ☐   only if they are professional persons

1-33   *the harmful conduct of all*   **1-34**   *at all times*
professional persons

1-35 Persons are expected to conduct themselves in this manner

☐ whether they are professionals or laypersons

☐ only if they are professionals

☐ only if they are laypersons

1-36 The law characterizes a person who fails to act in a reasonable and prudent manner as being

☐ imprudent

☐ unreasonable

☐ negligent

1-37 A person whose negligence causes harm or injury to the person or property of another may be legally required to pay a sum of money to that person. This type of remedy, as you will recall, is what distinguishes civil law from criminal law.

The law provides that if injury results to a person because of negligent conduct on the part of another, the one whose negligence caused the injury

☐ can avoid liability by showing that he or she is a professional

☐ may be required to pay a sum of money to the injured person

☐ more than likely will be subject to a criminal action

1-35 *whether they are professionals or laypersons*	1-36 *negligent*	1-37 *may be required to pay a sum of money to the injured person*

1-38 In general, the term "negligence" as used in malpractice law has the same meaning as the term "carelessness." Thus, conduct that is careless is usually negligent. However, a person might be held negligent in the eyes of the law even if he or she acts carefully *from a personal point of view.* Here is a simple illustration: If a nurse attempts a nursing procedure for which he has had no prior training and does it as carefully as he knows how, his conduct may nevertheless be deemed negligent if, *judged by objective standards,* his conduct was careless and caused harm to the patient. To begin with, he should not have attempted the procedure at all without previous training or experience. The fact that he was as careful as possible, in his subjective opinion, is considered immaterial from the legal standpoint.

Indicate whether the following statements are true or false:

True	*False*	
☐	☐	In malpractice law the terms negligence and carelessness generally have the same meaning.
☐	☐	A nurse who fails to meet the required standard of care in a given situation may be deemed legally negligent even though he acts as carefully as he knows how.
☐	☐	When a nurse's carelessness in carrying out his professional duties causes a harm to his patient, the nurse probably will be found legally negligent.
☐	☐	Harm resulting from the performance of an act that is beyond a nurse's training and experience may be the basis for holding the nurse legally negligent.

1-38	*True*	*False*	
	☑	☐	*If you missed any of these, see*
	☑	☐	*p. 27, Note B.*
	☑	☐	
	☑	☐	

EXPLANATORY NOTES

Note A (from Frame 1-30)

Many find this concept somewhat difficult to understand, so a little further explanation may be helpful. To begin with, a tort is usually defined as a wrongful act done by one person causing injury to another for which the injured party may demand legal redress (usually money damages) in a civil suit. A *wrongful* act under tort law, however, does not necessarily mean an act that is morally wrong or intentionally harmful. Thus, a man erroneously believing himself to be the owner of certain real property may be sued by the true landowner for the tort of trespass without regard to any question of morality or harmful intent involved.

On the other hand, *some* wrongful acts that fall into the category of tortious conduct, thereby permitting civil suits for damages, are simultaneously considered violations of public rights (i.e., crimes) since they strike at the very being of society. In the case of assault, the private legal right violated is the right of every individual that one's bodily safety shall be respected; and for the wrong done to this legal right, the sufferer is entitled to legal damages. The act of violence is likewise viewed as a menace to the safety of society in general and will therefore be punished by the state. It is not such a far-fetched idea, after all, for one and the same act to constitute both a tort and a crime.

Proceed to Frame 1-31.

Note B (from Frame 1-38)

This is not an easy concept to grasp, so do not feel disappointed if you missed one or more of these true-false choices. The point being made is that a nurse's *careful* conduct may still be *legally negligent* if what the nurse does (even though with great care) is not what other prudent nurses would have done in the same circumstances. This statement assumes, of course, that some harm results from the nurse's act, for without any harm resulting, no legal wrong (tort) has been committed. In the overwhelming majority of cases, careful conduct will *not* give rise to a charge of negligence. The exceptional situation was outlined in Frame 1-38 only to show how the rule might apply to an act of nursing practice.

Proceed to Frame 1-39.

CONCEPT OF MALPRACTICE

1-39 The word "liability" appears in the title of this book, and you will see the words "liable" and "liability" used repeatedly throughout the course. Since these words have a specific, technical meaning in the law, now would be a good time to make their legal meaning as clear as possible.

When we say that an individual is *legally liable* to another person because of negligent conduct, we mean the individual can be held *legally responsible* for the harm caused the other person. "Liability" thus refers to the state of being held legally liable. In a malpractice action (as in most other civil actions) liability is assessed in monetary terms, commonly referred to as either "money damages" or simply "damages."

Which one of the following comes *closest* to the meaning of the phrase "legal liability"?

☐ legal indebtedness

☐ legal impediment

☐ legal responsibility

☐ legal damages

1-40

■ P, a former patient, sues Nurse N in a malpractice action in which P claims N's negligent conduct caused him serious injury. Nurse N is found legally liable for the harm caused P.

What is the *most likely* legal effect this ruling will have on Nurse N?

☐ Nurse N's license to practice as a nurse will be revoked.

☐ Nurse N will be obligated to reimburse P for the financial loss P sustained as a result of his injuries.

☐ Nurse N will have to stand trial on a criminal charge for the harm she caused P.

1-39 *Legal responsi-*   **1-40** ☐ *If you checked the 1st or 3d*
         bility   ☑ *box, turn to p. 33, Note A.*
                                          ☐

1-41   As you have already learned, according to law all persons are held legally responsible for conducting themselves in a reasonable and prudent manner, and can be held legally liable for failure to act as other reasonably prudent persons would act in the same or similar situation.

Negligence is the general term that embraces the negligent (careless and harmful) conduct of all types of persons, while *malpractice* is the specific term used in referring to the negligent conduct of persons with specialized professional education and training who are engaged in occupations requiring the employment of highly technical skills.

Indicate whether the following statements are true or false:

True	*False*	
☐	☐	Not every act of negligence can be classified as an act of malpractice, but every act of malpractice involves some type of negligent conduct.
☐	☐	Malpractice and negligence are totally unrelated concepts.
☐	☐	Negligent conduct may or may not be considered malpractice depending on the background of the individual in question.
☐	☐	A layperson who committed a negligent act could not be held liable for malpractice.

1-41	*True*	*False*
	☑	☐
	☐	☑
	☑	☐
	☑	☐

1-42   Assume that each of the following persons failed to act in a reasonable and prudent manner in carrying out some aspect of his or her normal work duties. Which of them could be held liable for malpractice, and which of them could be held liable only for negligence?

Malpractice	Negligence	
☐	☐	Veterinarian
☐	☐	Ambulance driver
☐	☐	Pharmacist
☐	☐	Medical secretary
☐	☐	Public health nurse
☐	☐	Licensed practical nurse (LPN)

1-43   A negligent act committed by a professional person constitutes malpractice only if it involves negligence in the carrying out of his or her professional duties.

■ While driving his automobile into the hospital parking lot, Doctor D fails to exercise caution and accidentally strikes and injures P, a man on crutches, who happens to be Doctor D's own patient.

    Assuming a lawsuit is filed against Doctor D by patient P, which of the following is true?

☐   Doctor D can be held liable for negligence, but not for malpractice.

☐   Doctor can be held liable only for malpractice.

☐   Doctor D can be held liable both for negligence and for malpractice.

1-42	Malpractice	Negligence	**1-43**	Doctor D can be held liable for negligence, but not for malpractice.
	☑	☐		
	☐	☑		
	☑	☐		
	☐	☑		
	☑	☐		
	☑	☐		

1-44   Under appropriate circumstances, even a layperson could be held liable for malpractice.

	True	*False*
	☐	☐

1-45   Since the concept of malpractice is limited to those situations in which persons with specialized professional training are negligent in carrying out some phase of their professional duties, in which of the following instances might the person in question be held liable for malpractice?

☐   A consulting engineer miscalculates the tensile strength of certain structural materials, resulting in the collapse of a building.

☐   A hospital orderly negligently mops a hallway, causing a patient on crutches to slip and fall on a wet spot and thereby sustain further serious injury.

☐   A nurse-anesthetist's negligence in administering an anesthetic agent during a surgical procedure causes the patient's face to be seriously burned.

☐   A lawyer's negligence in failing to file suit on behalf of a client before a certain date results in the client's claim being barred by the statute of limitations.

☐   A medical ward nurse negligently mishandles a patient's dentures and they cannot be found.

NOTE: "Medical malpractice" is the broad, general term used to describe acts constituting negligence on the part of *all* categories of professional medical personnel when they are carrying out some aspect of medical care and treatment. However, when the health professional is someone other than a physician, more specific terminology is commonly used. When the person involved is a nurse, it is called "nursing malpractice," and when it is a pharmacist, it is called "pharmacy malpractice." In all malpractice cases, however, the legal standards of care reflect the distinction between ordinary negligence and professional malpractice. This point is covered more fully later in Part 1.

1-44   *False*   **1-45**   ☑
                                                         ☐
            Negligence, but not malprac-   ☑
            tice.   ☑
                                                         ☐

1-46 Which of the following types of negligent conduct would fall within the broad category of medical malpractice?

☐ A physician injures a patient with a sharp instrument while conducting a routine physical examination.

☐ A hospital pharmacist erroneously dispenses a drug in a form that is double the strength ordered by the physician, causing harm to the patient.

☐ A nurse knocks over an IV stand in a patient's room. The stand strikes the ankle of the patient's husband, causing a serious fracture.

☐ An intern neglects to check a patient's chart, which clearly shows a hypersensitivity to penicillin. The intern prescribes the drug for the patient, who suffers a severe reaction.

1-47 You have now been exposed to a whole series of terms and concepts that are related to the course you are studying. These words and concepts, and their meanings, are listed below in random order. Match the letter of each word or concept with its meaning.

A. Negligence   The state of being held legally responsible to   ☐
                         another for some harm caused that person.

B. Nursing malpractice   Negligent conduct by professional medical personnel   ☐

C. Malpractice   A legal wrong committed against the person or   ☐
                         property of another

D. Legal liability   Failure to act in a reasonable and prudent manner   ☐

E. Medical malpractice   Negligent conduct in the performance of profes-   ☐
                         sional duties

F. Tort   Negligent conduct by a nurse in the performance of   ☐
                         professional duties.

1-46 ☑ *If you checked the 3d box, turn*   **1-47** D
          ☑ *to p. 33, Note B.*   E
          ☐   F
          ☑   A
                                                                C
                                                                B   ← *Turn to p. 34, Note C, For*
                                                                        amplification.

EXPLANATORY NOTES

Note A (from Frame 1-40)

Negligent conduct—or malpractice—on the part of a nurse rarely involves the willful intent to harm another, but if such intent *could* be shown, the nurse could be guilty of criminal behavior. In such event, the nurse's license to practice might well be revoked upon conviction for the crime in question.

At this point, the reader may wish to review the Note on pages 14 and /15, Criminal Conduct and Nursing Practice, which discusses, among other things, the requirement of *willful intent* before a nurse can be held criminally liable.

Proceed to Frame 1-41.

Note B (from Frame 1-46)

The nurse who knocked over the IV stand in the third example undoubtedly would be held liable for the harm caused the patient's husband, but for ordinary *negligence* rather than *malpractice.* The nurse was legally required to exercise reasonable care to see that no harm would come to the patient's husband (or any other visitor, for that matter), and failure to do so would constitute negligence. "Malpractice" is a term used only when referring to negligent conduct on the part of professional persons in carrying out their professional duties on behalf of someone to whom they owe a special duty of care, such as a nurse's duty to a patient. (This latter point is covered more fully in the material that immediately follows.)

Turning the situation around, if the stand had fallen on the patient, the nurse *could* be held liable for malpractice since (1) the safety and welfare of the patient is one of the nurse's fundamental responsibilities and (2) the proper positioning of an IV stand is a function the nurse would normally be expected to perform with care to assure the patient's safety and welfare.

Proceed to Frame 1-47.

EXPLANATORY NOTES

Note C (from Frame 1-47)

One of the benefits of characterizing the legal action against a nurse as "nursing malpractice" (i.e., *professional negligence*, as opposed to *ordinary negligence*) is that it brings the nurse within the protection of the time limits for filing a malpractice claim under state law. In most states, the limitations period (called the statute of limitations) for bringing a malpractice suit against a health professional is much shorter than the statutory period for bringing an ordinary negligence action. Commonly, the statutory period for bringing malpractice claims is 1 year, while in most states ordinary negligence claims can be filed as long as 3 years after the alleged occurrence. The applicable time period varies by jurisdiction. Moreover, because of the practical difficulties faced by patients in determining exactly when a medically induced injury occurred, many states have engrafted exceptions to their malpractice statutes of limitations. These rulings hold that the limitations period does not begin to run until the injured person discovers or reasonably should have discovered the injury in question. Finally, the fact that the injured person is a minor or is otherwise under a legal disability (e.g., legally incompetent) usually will extend the period within which a malpractice action may be brought in most states.

Proceed to Frame 1-48.

POINTS TO REMEMBER

1. Tort law is that branch of civil law that deals with legal wrongs committed by one person or legal entity against the person or property of another.

2. Torts (legal wrongs) may be intentional or unintentional.

3. Negligence is an unintentional tort that involves harm resulting from the failure of persons to conduct themselves in a reasonable and prudent manner.

4. Negligence and carelessness are not synonymous. One can be careful and yet be considered legally negligent for failure to act as other reasonably prudent persons would have acted in the particular circumstances.

5. Malpractice refers to the negligent acts of persons with specialized professional training and education, such as registered nurses, licensed practical or vocational nurses, nurse practitioners, physicians' assistants, and other professionally trained and licensed health care providers.

6. An act constituting malpractice necessarily reflects negligence, but not all negligent acts constitute malpractice.

7. When persons are held legally responsible for their negligent conduct, we say they are legally liable.

8. A person held legally liable in a civil suit for harm caused another is required to pay money damages to the latter.

9. Medical malpractice is the broad, general term that refers to the negligent acts of all categories of health professionals when carrying out their patient care responsibilities.

10. Nursing malpractice is the more specific term used when referring to the negligent acts of nurses when carrying out their patient care responsibilities.

> **NOTE:**   When an act of nursing malpractice occurs, the law holds the nurse legally liable to the patient because of the particular legal relationship that exists between them—the nurse-patient relationship. In the material that follows we will see how this relationship is created and some of the legal consequences thereof.

THE NURSE-PATIENT RELATIONSHIP

1-48   The nurse-patient relationship is a legal status that is created the moment a nurse actually provides nursing care to another person. This relationship is important because of the legal duties and responsibilities that are attached. Once a nurse-patient relationship is established, the nurse legally owes a *special duty of care* to the patient that is greater than the *general duty of care* the nurse owes to other persons generally. As we shall see a little later, it is the failure to meet this special duty of care owed to their patients that forms the heart of all malpractice suits against nurses.

An act of nursing malpractice will give rise to legal liability only if a
☐ sociological   ☐ legal   ☐ moral   relationship exists between the parties.

1-49   The particular legal status or relationship in question is called the
☐ nurse-patient   ☐ nurse-litigant   ☐ nurse-liability   relationship.

1-48 *legal*   **1-49** *nurse-patient*

1-50 Which of the following statements correctly explains the difference between the nurse's legal responsibilities to one who is his or her patient and to the public generally?

☐ Because of their professional training, nurses owe a greater duty of care than others to members of the general public as well as to their patients.

☐ A nurse's legal duty to care to his or her patient is neither greater nor lesser than his or her legal duty of care to members of the general public.

☐ As ordinary citizens, nurses owe members of the general public a general duty of care, but as nurses they owe their patients a greater duty of care.

1-51 What must the nurse and the patient do or say to create the nurse-patient relationship? No special words, agreement, or contract is required. The only thing that *is* required is the actual providing of nursing services to an individual with that person's acquiescence or implied consent thereto.* The fact that the recipient (the patient) may not have verbally requested such services has no bearing on the legal effect or consequences of the nurse's actions.

The essence of the nurse-patient relationship is

☐ an express verbal or written agreement to provide nursing care to an individual

☐ the actual furnishing of nursing care to an individual

☐ the establishment of a good therapeutic relationship with an individual

---

*NOTE: An adult who is not *in extremis* and is otherwise competent may always refuse medical or nursing treatment. The subject of consent to treatment is covered in detail in Part 4 of this course.

1-50 *As ordinary citizens, nurses owe members of the general public . . .*

1-51 *the actual furnishing of nursing care to an individual*

1-52 The patient's verbal agreement to enter into a nurse-patient relationship
☐ is ☐ is not necessary.

1-53 Could a nurse-patient relationship be established with an unconscious person?

Yes   **No**
☐   ☐

1-54 The manner in which nurses are employed, by whom they are employed, or whether they are technically employed at all is of no legal significance with respect to their legal liability for malpractice. Insofar as the law is concerned, the crucial factor is whether a nurse-patient relationship exists.

Typically, general-duty nurses do not enter into a series of contracts to provide nursing care to selected persons but enter into single contracts of employment with a hospital, an industrial firm, a public health department, a school, or the like. The important thing to note is that, although their contracts may be with particular employers, *the law holds them legally responsible to all persons for whom they actually provide nursing services.*

From the standpoint of legal liability for nursing malpractice, the manner in which a nurse's professional services are engaged ☐ is ☐ is not a matter of legal significance.

1-55 The legal consequences of a nurse's performance of nursing services are primarily based on

☐ formal legal arrangements made with specific patients

☐ the manner in which the nurse renders those services

☐ the nature of the nurse's specific nursing assignments

1-52 *is not*   **1-53** *Yes*   **1-54** *is not*   **1-55** *the manner in which the nurse renders those services*

1-56

■ The nurse for an industrial firm is informed of an injury to an employee of a neighboring firm that has no nurse. The nurse rushes next door to give the necessary emergency care but negligently injures the employee while in the process.

Under these circumstances which of the following is true?

☐   The nurse can be held liable for malpractice because the act of giving emergency care created a nurse-patient relationship.

☐   The nurse cannot be held liable for malpractice but only for negligence because no nurse-patient relationship could have been created with an employee of a firm by whom the nurse was not employed.

☐   The nurse cannot be held liable for malpractice because the giving of emergency care does not create a nurse-patient relationship.

1-57

■ A former hospital patient sues a hospital nurse for malpractice that occurred while he was a patient at the hospital. Before he is permitted to offer proof of the nurse's negligence, he must first establish that a nurse-patient relationship was in existence between himself and the nurse.

Which *one* of the following offers of proof by the patient would most effectively establish this fact?

☐   proof that he was over 21 years of age and could legally enter into a contractual relationship

☐   proof that the nurse was employed as a full-time staff nurse at the hospital

☐   proof that the nurse provided nursing care to him while he was a patient at the hospital

1-56 ☑ *If you checked the wrong*
      ☐ *answer, turn to p. 48, Note A.*
      ☐

1-57 *proof that the nurse provided*
      nursing care to him while he
      was a patient at the hospital

1-58   Consider the following situation:

- Operating room (OR) Nurse N, while on a coffee break, strikes up a conversation in the hallway with Patient P while the latter is waiting to undergo a diagnostic test for stomach pain. Based on P's description of his symptoms, N tells P that he definitely needs surgery and suggests that he do so promptly. P decides to take the advice and shortly thereafter undergoes surgery. Even though N is not a member of the surgical team, when P's surgery turns out poorly, P sues N along with the operating surgeon. Before the trial, N's attorney moves to have N dismissed as a defendant.

What is the court most likely to say about the inclusion of N as a defendant in this case?

☐   N should be dismissed as a defendant because N was under no obligation to treat P and, hence, there was no nurse-patient relationship between N and P.

☐   N should be dismissed as a defendant because N was not in actual attendance during the surgical procedure.

☐   N is a proper defendant because, even though P was not N's patient, N's advice had a direct bearing on P's decision to undergo surgery, which led to the poor result.

1-58   *N should be dismissed as a defendant because N was under no obligation to treat P and, hence, there was no nurse-patient relationship between N and P.*

1-59 In contrast to general-duty hospital nurses who normally are expected to provide nursing care to all assigned hospital patients, private-duty nurses are considered free agents and may decide for themselves whether they wish to accept employment by any particular person. Their refusal to accept an offer of private employment will not subject them to any legal liability because no nurse-patient relationship has come into being.

Consider the following situation.

■ The family of a hospitalized patient hires a private-duty nurse through a local nurses' registry. When the nurse arrives at the patient's room, she recognizes him as the same disagreeable, uncooperative patient she had attended during a prior illness. The nurse tells the family member present that she will not accept the assignment and will arrange for the registry to send another nurse immediately. She then leaves, and on her way out arranges with the regular nursing staff to provide necessary nursing care until her replacement arrives.

Indicate whether each of the following statements is true or false:

True	False	
☐	☐	The nurse had a legal right to refuse the assignment.
☐	☐	The moment the nurses' registry made the assignment, a nurse-patient relationship came into being.
☐	☐	The nurse's reasons for not wishing to accept the assignment are unimportant in determining whether a nurse-patient relationship came into being.
☐	☐	The nurse had no legal right to refuse the assignment.

1-60 If, while leaving the hospital, the private-duty nurse discussed in the previous frame had gone to the assistance of another patient and committed an act of malpractice while so doing, would the law consider that a nurse-patient relationship had come into being?

                        Yes   *No*
                         ☐   ☐

1-61 Would the fact that the private-duty nurse was not employed either by the hospital or the patient have any bearing on the establishment of a nurse-patient relationship?

                        Yes   *No*
                         ☐   ☐

1-62 The nurse-patient relationship is not an exclusive legal status, so it is possible for several nurses to have a nurse-patient relationship with a particular patient at the same time.

Consider the following situation:

■ A private-duty nurse engaged to care for an elderly hospitalized patient leaves the patient's bedside for 10 minutes to make some personal telephone calls. During the nurse's absence the patient suffers an acute coronary episode, and a nurse from the pediatric unit, on the way to lunch, rushes to the patient's aid. Because of limited experience with geriatric patients, the pediatric nurse makes a serious error of professional judgment in assisting the patient, causing him further harm.

Assuming these facts, which of the following statements is correct?

☐ Since the patient already had a specially assigned private-duty nurse, it was legally impossible for a new nurse-patient relationship to come into being with the pediatric nurse.

☐ Although the private-duty nurse had a valid nurse-patient relationship with the patient, as soon as the pediatric nurse went to the patient's assistance this relationship was temporarily suspended.

☐ Upon going to the patient's assistance, the pediatric nurse established a new nurse-patient relationship with him.

1-60 *Yes*   **1-61** *No*   **1-62** ☐
                                                       ☐
                                                       ☑

1-63 In the previous example, who do you think would be held liable for the harm that resulted to the patient?

☐ the private-duty nurse only

☐ the pediatric nurse only

☐ both nurses

NOTE: Frames 1-59 through 1-63, relating to private-duty nurses, were included simply to illustrate how a nurse-patient relationship can be created between a patient and a nurse not on the hospital's regular nursing staff. Although the private-duty nurse (PDN) is a vanishing breed, several aspects of private-duty nursing merit brief discussion at this point.

The PDN is an independent contractor who normally bills and is paid directly by the patient, the patient's family, or a third party insurer. Many hospitals maintain referral lists of PDNs, and most PDNs get patient referrals either from those sources or from nurse registries. As an independent contractor, the PDN is solely liable for any harm caused by his or her negligent conduct, and thus assumes much greater exposure to the risks of malpractice liability than do hospital staff nurses. This is especially true where the PDN's services are provided in the patient's home, since home care often involves providing not only the traditional skilled nursing services but knowledge of how to use complex technical equipment for treating specialized medical conditions.

Many if not most PDNs who provide home health care prefer to work through and be affiliated with home health care agencies—organizations established and licensed expressly to provide home health services in accordance with government regulations under Medicare and Medicaid. Liability for the PDN's negligent conduct when employed in this manner is lessened to the extent that it may be shared with the referring agency, but this is not always the case, as we shall discuss more fully in Part 2. Because of the greater risks involved in their independent contractor status, it is essential that PDNs obtain adequate professional liability (malpractice) insurance coverage.

It should be noted that a hospital also may engage the services of a PDN to provide care to patients in the hospital, in which case the hospital, as well as the PDN, can be held liable for the PDN's negligent conduct, a subject that is also discussed more fully in Part 2.

1-63 ☐   *If you checked either the first or*
         ☐   *2d box, turn to p. 49, Note B.*
         ☑

THE DUTY TO GIVE EMERGENCY CARE

1-64 You have just seen how an emergency situation may be the basis for the establishment of a nurse-patient relationship. We will now discuss the nurse's legal obligations to give emergency care.

As the last example illustrated, an emergency that occurs in the normal hospital setting may call for immediate action on the part of a nurse to provide care to a patient even though the patient may not be specifically assigned to the nurse. This is so because a general-duty nurse employed by a hospital assumes a duty of care to all patients for whose benefit that nurse's professional services are engaged. The same may be said for nurses who are employed by school systems, industrial plants, public health departments, and the like.

A general-duty nurse employed by a hospital would be legally responsible for providing emergency care

☐ only to those patients to which the nurse is specifically assigned

☐ to any patient in the hospital in need of such care

☐ both to patients in the hospital and to members of the general public in need of such care

---

1-65

■ A secondary school in Toronto, Canada, plays host to a visiting group of school children from the United States. Several of the American visitors are injured in a minor bus accident on the school property, and the Canadian school nurse deliberates whether she is legally obligated to give them treatment.

Which of the following statements correctly states her responsibility?

☐ A Canadian nurse is under no legal obligation to treat nonresidents of Canada.

☐ Since the injured children are not enrolled in the school where she is employed, the nurse has no legal obligation to give them emergency care.

☐ The duties of the school nurse include the legal responsibility to furnish emergency care to all persons in need of such care while on the school property where she is employed, and this would include the injured children in question.

1-64 *to any patient in the hospital in need of such care*   **1-65** ☐ ☐ ☑

> **NOTE:**   The same rule would apply if the injured children were Canadians visiting an American school. The choice of a Toronto school was made simply to show that the general legal principles concerning establishment of the nurse-patient relationship and the duty to give emergency care are the same both in Canada and the United States.

THE HOSPITAL EMERGENCY DEPARTMENT

In recent years, a variety of court decisions, statutes, and government regulations have made it mandatory for hospitals with emergency rooms to admit and treat patients in need of immediate or medically indicated emergency care. For growing numbers of persons, the hospital emergency department (ED) has become their entry point into the health care system, thus making the ED both a trauma center and a frequent substitute for a personal provider. As a consequence, ED personnel—and nurses in particular—must be familiar with ambulatory and emergency care and must be able to demonstrate superior skill and judgment in assessing patients' needs.

ED nursing is fast gaining recognition as a nursing specialty, and most ED nurses continually update their skills to better help them deal with the wide variety of medical emergencies they face in the ED. After taking appropriate advanced courses, such as Advanced Cardiac Life Support, many ED nurses become certified in emergency nursing (CEN) and in so doing become responsible for meeting the higher standards applicable to nurses in this specialty. Since ED care calls for such a high level of assessment and treatment skills, it is possible that nurses in the future may have to qualify as clinical specialists in emergency care before being assigned to the ED. Certainly, the ED is no place for the inexperienced nurse, since the very nature of the ED environment—often requiring life-or-death decisions without hesitation—creates greatly expanded nursing responsibilities, resulting in proportionately greater exposure to malpractice claims.

What are the standards of care applicable to nurses who provide care in the ED? First and foremost, ED nurses must be capable of acting swiftly, often basing their actions as much on instinct as on pure technical knowledge. The first thing the nurse must do is evaluate the patient's condition, often with little opportunity to obtain a complete history, and make an initial decision regarding the urgency of treatment and the need to summon a physician. This process is called *triage* ("sorting out"), and because patients' lives often are at stake, the margin for error is exceedingly slim. Nurses customarily perform triage in accordance with guidelines developed by the American Hospital Association, appropriately adapted to each hospital's needs and made a part of its own protocols and standing orders.

Most courts have ruled that the applicable standard of care in providing ED care is a nursing standard (i.e., what would a reasonably prudent ED nurse do under the particular treatment circumstances?). In the landmark case of *Fein v. Permanente Medical Group*, 175 Cal. Rptr. 177 (Cal. App. 1981), the trial court in California held the nurse-practitioner working in the ED to the standard of care expected of a physician. On appeal, however, the California Supreme Court said that the decision went too far and held that the nurse-practitioner's conduct should be measured against the standard of care of other nurse-specialists practicing under the same or similar conditions (*Fein v. Permanente Medical Group*, 695 P. 2d 665 [Cal. 1985]). This decision has been widely viewed as an important step for the autonomy of nursing.

The types of acts or omissions that have been major sources of malpractice claims against ED nurses and their hospital employees include failure to make a proper assessment and interpretation of the patient's condition; failure to promptly communicate significant changes in the patient's condition; failure to recognize the possible dangers of a physician's order, failure to adequately protect against falls and other sources of patient injury; medication/treatment/procedure errors; equipment-related problems; and failure to prevent patients from leaving the ED without medical consent. These acts and omissions have all resulted in costly claims against hospitals and nurses. Part 3 discusses at greater length other types of negligent conduct in the hospital setting.

We resume our discussion of the nurse's duty to provide emergency care in the nonhospital setting.

1-66   The nurse's legal responsibility to provide emergency care to persons within a normal employment setting is quite different from the nurse's legal responsibility under other circumstances. In a noncontractual and nontherapeutic setting nurses have no *legal* obligation to render emergency care to someone in need, even though they may have a *moral* and *ethical* obligation to render such care.* Thus, a nurse ordinarily cannot be held legally liable for refusing to offer emergency care to the victim of highway accident or other similar occurrence, no matter how life threatening the circumstances.

In hospitals, schools, or industrial plants where they are employed, the obligation of nurses to provide emergency nursing care to persons noted to be in physical or mental distress is
☐   greater than   ☐   the same as   ☐   less than   their obligation to provide such care to persons in distress outside such environment.

---

*This general rule of the common law has a few statutory exceptions, discussed more fully on p. 52.

1-67   A nurse's legal obligation to go to the aid of someone in need of emergency care normally extends

☐   to all persons in need of such care (i.e., the general public)

☐   only to those persons encompassed within the terms of the contract of employment

☐   to no one

1-66   *greater than*   **1-67**   *only to those persons encompassed within the terms of the contract of employment*

1-68 The reason a nurse ordinarily is not required to aid someone who is the victim of a high-way accident or other similar emergency is that

☐ the nurse has no way of being assured of payment for the services

☐ the nurse has no opportunity to ascertain the patient's medical history

☐ the nurse stands in no special relationship to such person and therefore owes him or her no special duty of care

---

1-69

■ A general-duty nurse coming home from work at the local hospital stops briefly to watch a holiday parade. Just as the nurse approaches the parade grounds a grandstand collapses, causing injury to many persons. A local physician watching the parade immediately begins giving emergency aid to the injured. Noticing the nurse (still in uniform), the physician beckons for assistance with the injured. However, because of a strong personal dislike of the physician, the nurse ignores the request and refuses to render any help to the injured.

Under the given facts:

Yes	No	
☐	☐	Has the nurse violated any legal duty to render care to the injured persons?
☐	☐	Will the injured persons, or their legal representatives, have a legal basis for suing the nurse for her conduct?
☐	☐	Do you think the nurse exercised good judgment in refusing to offer help for the stated reason?

1-68   *the nurse in no special
relationship to such person . . .*

1-69   Yes   No
☐   ☑
☐   ☑
☐   ☐   ← *You decide. See p.
49, Note C.*

EXPLANATORY NOTES

Note A (from Frame 1-56)

It was pointed out previously that a nurse-patient relationship can come into being in a number of ways, and the precise manner in which this relationship develops is not really important. Moreover, whether a nurse-patient relationship exists does not depend on the nurse's employment status. As stated earlier, the *manner* in which a nurse is employed, *by whom* the nurse is employed, or *whether* the nurse is technically employed at all has no bearing on the creation of a nurse-patient relationship. The only thing that counts (in the legal sense) is the nurse's *actual providing of nursing care.*

The occupational health nurse in this example may have had no contractual duty to give care to the injured employee for the neighboring firm, and indeed could have declined to give any help whatsoever. (We will discuss this point in detail very shortly.) However, the fact is the nurse *did* undertake to give care to the injured person, and that in itself is sufficient to create a nurse-patient relationship.

If the nurse is held liable at all in the given situation, it would be for malpractice, not ordinary negligence, because professional nursing services were rendered. We're discussing the nurse-patient relationship at this point; note, however, that giving emergency care brings into play special rules that may relieve the nurse of legal liability, depending on the surrounding circumstances. The role and applicability of the so-called emergency rule and of state Good Samaritan laws to nurses will be discussed shortly.

Proceed to Frame 1-57.

EXPLANATORY NOTES

Note B (from Frame 1-63)

Both nurses would be held liable, but each for a different reason. The pediatric nurse's "error of professional judgment" is just another way of saying "malpractice," and the nurse will be held legally responsible for such an error of judgment. However, limited experience with geriatric patients and the emergency circumstances that prompted the nurse's assistance in the first place would be important factors in assessing the *extent* of liability—that is, how much money damages, if any, the nurse will be required to pay.

The private-duty nurse, on the other hand, clearly would be held liable, along with the pediatric nurse, for the harm that resulted to the patient since it was her neglect of the patient that necessitated the emergency care by the pediatric nurse. The private-duty nurse cannot escape liability for neglect by claiming interference with her sole responsibility for the patient when the pediatric nurse went to the patient's assistance. As you have been informed, it is perfectly possible for more than one nurse-patient relationship to exist with respect to the same patient at any one time and, as this example clearly illustrates, it is the act of *giving* professional nursing care—not what prompted such care—that brings the nurse-patient relationship into existence, with all its legal consequences.

Proceed to Frame 1-64.

Note C (from Frame 1-69)

Most members of the nursing profession would say that the nurse exercised very poor judgment in this case. There is no doubt that the nurse had a legal right to refuse to volunteer services, but morally and ethically there was a clear-cut obligation to assist at the scene of the accident. What is a profession, after all, if not a public trust? And nursing is a profession whose express purpose is to serve the health needs of suffering humanity. Nurses who are unable to subordinate their personal feelings at a time when their professional services are so urgently needed not only bring criticism upon themselves but dishonor the fundamental ethical concepts upon which the nursing profession was founded.

Proceed to Frame 1-70.

1-70 Even though a nurse is under no *legal* obligation to provide emergency care to persons not within the nurse's normal work responsibilities, once he or she volunteers to offer such assistance, a nurse-patient relationship is automatically established with respect to that emergency. At that point, the nurse has the legal obligation to act as other reasonably prudent nurses would act under the same emergency circumstances.

If a nurse were to volunteer emergency care to someone to whom the nurse owed no special duty of care, which of the following would be true?

☐ The nurse would be expected to act no differently than any other citizen in giving such care.

☐ The nurse would be legally required to exercise no greater care than other nurses would exercise under similar circumstances.

☐ The nurse would be legally required to exercise the highest degree of care to assure the victim's well-being.

1-71

■ Two nurses licensed to practice in New Jersey are on a summer vacation in the Southwest, and while motoring through Arizona they come upon the scene of a serious railroad accident causing injury to many persons. Their discussion concerning whether or not to stop and give emergency care to the victims is as follows:

Nurse A: "I really think we should help out. I know we're not legally obligated to do so, but I believe we have a moral obligation to render help under these circumstances."

Nurse B: "Well, we may have no legal obligation to offer our help, but you know as well as I do that once we start caring for these people, we run the risk of being sued for malpractice if we don't act with 'reasonable care.'"

Which nurse (if either) is legally correct?

Nurse A   *Nurse B*   *Both nurses*   *Neither nurse*
☐   ☐   ☐   ☐

1-70 *The nurse would be legally required to exercise no greater care than other nurses would exercise under similar circumstances.*

We will discuss this concept in more detail shortly.

1-71 *Both nurses*

GOOD SAMARITAN STATUTES

Beginning in the late 1950s, as fears of medical malpractice suits began to permeate the medical profession, much attention was focused on the growing reluctance of physicians to give emergency assistance to victims of highway accidents and other similar medical emergencies. While fears of being sued by injured accident victims or their families undoubtedly were exaggerated—the risk of being sued for negligence occurring in daily practice has always been infinitely greater—surveys of doctors at the time clearly showed that they would not stop to treat injured persons at the scene of an accident because of the threat of litigation.

Thus came into being the rash of so-called Good Samaritan laws, passed by state and provincial legislatures in the hope that persons with the necessary knowledge and training would no longer be discouraged from going to the aid of accident victims out of fear of being sued. These statutes offer protection to "good samaritans" by granting either absolute or qualified immunity from suit to some or all classes of persons who render emergency medical assistance.

The first Good Samaritan statute was enacted by California in 1959. Since that time, Good Samaritan laws have been enacted by every state, the District of Columbia, and the Virgin Islands. In addition, five of the ten Canadian provinces and one Canadian territory have enacted Good Samaritan laws. Originally, these laws expressly limited the liability of physicians only, but later encompassed other health care professionals through legislative amendments. Nurses are frequently mentioned in the statutes, but some grant immunity only to registered nurses, while others include licensed practical or vocational nurses. Many of the laws extend immunity to "any person," a term certainly broad enough to include doctors and nurses, as well as persons without medical training.

There has never been uniformity in state Good Samaritan laws. Some of them grant absolute immunity against liability to physicians and nurses who render emergency assistance; most extend immunity from liability only for ordinary, not gross, negligence. A few statutes not only provide immunity from liability, but protect the doctor or nurse from even being sued. By far, the majority of the Good Samaritan laws confine immunity to care given to injured persons "at the scene" of an accident and in need of immediate medical attention or in imminent danger of loss of life or impairment of health. This is not always the case. The Texas statute, for example, specifies that the "scene" may include a hospital, and California's law has also been construed to include certain emergencies in the hospital if the responding physician had no legal duty to render aid to the patient in question.

Because of the wide differences between jurisdictions in the scope, applicability, and coverage of these Good Samaritan laws, it is virtually impossible for a physician or nurse to know with reasonable certainty whether he or she really enjoys any legal advantage when rendering emergency care in a state that has such a law. For example, Nevada and Pennsylvania extend protection only to "registered nurses," thus affording no immunity to LPNs or vocational nurses who happen to be passing through those states. Because of problems like this, a number of legal commentators have concluded that the Good Samaritan laws as a whole are relatively useless and will never achieve their intended goals until there is greater uniformity among them.

Neither before nor since the enactment of the Good Samaritan laws have there been any reported cases against nurses who have been held liable for negligence in treating victims at the scene of an accident or other emergency. Most of the reported Good Samaritan cases against doctors have focused on the rendering of emergency care in the hospital setting. (These cases are cited in the Selected References at the end of Part 1.) In any event, all members of the nursing profession should recognize their ethical and moral obligation to render emergency medical assistance to persons in genuine need of such assistance, without regard to any possible legal protection afforded by state or provincial Good Samaritan laws. The responsible trained nurse has nothing to fear when acting competently and within the standard of care, taking into consideration the exigent circumstances. The giving of *reasonable care* should be all the protection needed. Still, the prudent nurse should not hesitate to procure and maintain adequate malpractice insurance coverage just in case someone files suit in a Good Samaritan situation.

COMPULSORY ASSISTANCE AND DUTY-TO-RESCUE STATUTES

In recent years, there has been some call for Good Samaritan legislation of the compulsory-assistance type. Vermont, Minnesota, and most Canadian provinces have enacted compulsory-assistance statutes—laws requiring *all* persons to render aid to persons who are "exposed to grave physical harm," or containing similar language. The Vermont statute grants civil immunity to one who provides reasonable assistance "unless his acts constitute gross negligence or unless he will receive or expects to receive remuneration." The immunity given, therefore, is not absolute, and the question still remains as to when liability might attach to the careless acts of a well-intentioned samaritan. The Vermont statute, which is not limited to roadside accidents, provides for criminal penalties for failure to render assistance as required under the law. By contrast, the Quebec statute, which specifies that "every person must come to the aid of anyone whose life is in peril," provides no penalties for violation of its mandate (Quebec Statutes 1975, Chapter 6, section 2). The Minnesota statute makes the failure to render "reasonable assistance at the scene of an emergency" a petty misdemeanor.

Both Wisconsin and Wyoming, in addition to their Good Samaritan laws, have enacted duty-to-rescue laws that apply either to special circumstances (e.g., in Wisconsin, the duty to rescue crime victims) or special persons (e.g., in Wyoming, the duty to rescue applies only to doctors). Incidentally, most European countries have long had compulsory-assistance statutes, and studies made of their impact indicate that they have had a measurably positive effect on public attitudes toward giving assistance.

POINTS TO REMEMBER

1. The legal consequences of an act amounting to nursing malpractice cannot occur until a nurse-patient relationship exists between the parties.

2. The nurse-patient relationship is a legal status that arises whenever a nurse renders nursing care to another person.

3. How a nurse's services are engaged, by whom they are engaged, or whether they are technically engaged at all is of no significance insofar as the nurse-patient relationship is concerned. The act of providing nursing care is what creates the relationship.

4. Once a nurse-patient relationship comes into being, the law automatically imposes certain legal responsibilities upon the nurse with respect to the patient, and these are greater than the general legal responsibilities (i.e., the duty of care) the nurse owes to members of the general public.

5. Nurses are under no *legal* obligation to provide emergency care to those to whom they owe no special duty of care, although they may have an *ethical* responsibility to provide such care. Special statutes in Vermont, Minnesota, and the Canadian provinces are exceptions to this widely recognized common law rule. A nurse (or other person) in these areas has an affirmative obligation to render medical or other assistance to persons exposed to "grave physical harm."

6. In most jurisdictions Good Samaritan laws have been passed to encourage physicians and nurses to give emergency medical assistance to the victims of highway accidents, but because of the wide differences between the various state laws, nurses are not assured of any greater protection from malpractice suits then they already enjoy.

7. Nurses will not be held liable for malpractice in the giving of emergency medical care provided they do what other reasonable and prudent nurses would do under the same emergency circumstances.

> **NOTE:**　In the material that follows we will examine the legal principles at the heart of the nurse's liability for malpractice. You will learn about the nurse's legal duty of care, about legal standards of care, and how the law determines whether a nurse's conduct conforms to the particular standard of care applicable in a given situation.

THE NURSE'S LEGAL STANDARD OF CARE

1-72　You will recall that the law imposes an absolute duty on *every* person to act in a reasonable and prudent manner to avoid causing injury to others. When individuals do not act with reasonable care and cause harm to others, we say they are negligent, and they will be held legally liable to the injured persons if the latter bring lawsuits seeking damages.

This fundamental standard of conduct applies with equal force to the acts of nurses and other health care professionals insofar as their *nonprofessional* activities are concerned. The standard is much higher, however, when it comes to the providing of *professional* services. Thus, because the nurse is regarded as a person possessing special skills and learning related to the art of nursing, the laws says that the reasonableness of the individual nurse's conduct must be measured against that of other reasonably prudent members of the nursing profession under the same or similar circumstances.

The duty to exercise reasonable care to avoid injury to others is an obligation the law imposes on　　☐　laypersons only　　☐　professional persons only　　☐　all persons
☐　no one

1-73　In any given situation, the nature and degree of the reasonable care expected of someone may vary, depending on

☐　the individual's sense of social responsibility

☐　the individual's understanding of the law

☐　the individual's status as a professional

1-72　*all persons*	**1-73**	*the individual's status as a professional*
		For a definition of the term "professional," see p. 75, Note A.

1-74 The higher standard of reasonable care expected of a professional person does not apply to all that person's actions but only to those that directly relate to his or her professional functions and responsibilities.

Consider the following example:

■ A registered nurse and a plumber drive their automobiles to the local shopping center in order to do their shopping. While they are there, their vehicles collide. There is reliable evidence that both drivers were equally negligent.

In a court case arising out of this incident, the nurse would not be held to any higher standard of care for negligent conduct than the plumber because

☐ the nurse was not on the way to work at the time of the accident

☐ the nurse's conduct was not related to any professional nursing duties

☐ all persons are presumed to be equally competent in driving automobiles

---

1-75 In the previous example, the negligent conduct occurred while the nurse was off duty. However, the negligence having occurred while the nurse was not officially on duty has no bearing on the applicable standard of care. The critical factor is whether the nurse's conduct involves the providing of professional nursing services to the person who suffers the harm.

If a passenger in the plumber's automobile in the previous example was injured when the vehicles collided, and the nurse administered emergency first aid, the nurse
☐ would   ☐ would not   be held to a higher standard of care than the plumber in so doing because

☐ a nurse has a legal responsibility to give first aid to injured persons

☐ the nurse would be carrying out a professional nursing function

☐ a layperson is not expected to know how to administer first aid

---

1-74 *the nurse's conduct was not related to any professional nursing duties*

1-75 *would*
☐ *If you checked the first box,*
☑ *reread Frames 1-66 through*
☐ *1-71.*

1-76   In each of the following fact situations, indicate whether the standard of care applicable to the nurse's conduct would be ordinary negligence or professional negligence (malpractice):

ordinary negligence	*professional negligence*	
☐	☐	Just before going off duty, a recovery room nurse is directed by the supervisor to raise the siderails on the bed of a patient still recovering from anesthesia. The nurse forgets and leaves without doing so. The patient later falls out of bed, fracturing his nose.
☐	☐	A mother brings her small child to the ED for suturing of a bad cut. While watching, the mother feels faint and the ED nurse tells her to sit down, pointing to a wooden stool nearby. The stool breaks under the mother's weight, resulting in injury to the mother.
☐	☐	In a hurry, a nurse on a coffee break accidentally collides with a gurney carrying a patient to the operating room for emergency surgery. The impact causes blood plasma being fed intravenously to shake loose and spill on the floor. The delay in getting replacement plasma hastens the patient's death.

1-76   *ordinary negligence   professional negligence*

ordinary negligence	*professional negligence*
☐	☑
☑	☐
☑	☐

If you are still uncertain about this distinction, reread Frames 1-41 through 1-46.

1-77 For the most part, statutes that define and prescribe the areas of control of professional and practical nursing are drawn in broad, general terms and do not lay down legal guidelines for *specific* conduct. Statements of functions issued by the Joint Commission on Accreditation of Healthcare Organizations and by nursing organizations likewise tend to lay down fairly general guidelines, although sometimes they can be quite specific.

By and large, however, it is the courts that have filled in most of the gaps by applying general legal principles to specific fact situations. The law of nursing malpractice has thus been developed principally by the courts as a part of the evolving common law.

The most common source of the nurse's legal duty of care to patients is

- ☐ judicial pronouncements in court cases
- ☐ state and provincial nurse practice acts
- ☐ statements of functions by professional nursing organizations

---

1-78 The courts have generally expressed the nurse's legal duty of care in the following manner:

In the performance of professional nursing duties, a nurse is required to exercise the degree of care and skill that a reasonably prudent nurse with similar training and experience practicing in the same community would exercise under the same or similar circumstances.

A nurse's failure to exercise the required degree of care and skill is considered professional negligence (malpractice) and the nurse will be held legally liable to the person who is harmed by the negligent conduct if the latter should bring a malpractice suit.

Which of the following situations would give rise to a charge of malpractice on the part of a nurse?

- ☐ failure of the nurse to allay the patient's fears
- ☐ failure of the nurse to exercise reasonable care in treating the patient
- ☐ failure of the nurse to establish a good therapeutic relationship with the patient

---

1-77 *judicial pronouncements in court cases*

1-78 *failure of the nurse to exercise reasonable care in treating the patient*

1-79

- An individual sues a general-duty hospital nurse for an act of alleged malpractice that occurred while the individual was a patient at the hospital.

If the patient is to win the suit, which of the following offers of proof by the patient would *best* establish the nurse's liability?

☐   proof that the nurse failed to carry out a standard nursing procedure prescribed by the hospital

☐   proof that the nurse failed to do what other nurses with similar skills and training would have done in the given situation

☐   proof that the nurse failed to follow a physician's standing order for the type of medical problem presented

---

1-80   In determining whether a nurse acted with reasonable care in any given situation, the nurse's qualifications, experience, and training are major factors to be considered. The degree of care expected is a relative one; the conduct required of the nurse is only that required of other nurses with similar background and training under the particular circumstances presented.

- A malpractice suit is filed against a licensed practical nurse for harm resulting from an alleged failure to properly execute the order of a registered nurse in carrying out a therapeutic procedure.

In determining the nurse's legal liability for malpractice, the court would take into consideration the following:

☐   the nurse's specific conduct, but not his or her background or training

☐   the nurse's professional background and training, as well as the specific conduct

☐   the nurse's professional background and training exclusively

---

1-79   ☐   *If you checked either the 1st or*
        ☑   *3d box, see p. 75, Note B.*
        ☐

1-80   *the nurse's professional background and training, as well as the specific conduct*

1-81 An RN with 1 year of hospital experience normally would be expected to exercise a degree of care in carrying out professional nursing duties that

☐ equals

☐ is higher than

☐ is less than

than of an LPN with 5 years of experience in the same hospital.

1-82 The single most crucial factor in determining whether a particular nurse acted with reasonable care in a given situation is

☐ how many years the nurse has had his or her license

☐ how the nurse's conduct compared with that of other nurses of similar background and experience

☐ how experienced the nurse is in a particular nursing specialty

---

1-83 *True*   *False*

☐   ☐   In determining an industrial nurse's liability for malpractice, a court probably would measure the nurse's conduct against that of a hospital surgical nurse.

☐   ☐   A nurse's previous experience in handling a certain treatment situation would be a pertinent factor in assessing his or her negligence in any similar treatment situation thereafter.

☐   ☐   A general-duty nurse employed by a nursing home would be held to the same standard of care as a general-duty nurse employed by a hospital when carrying out normal nursing functions.

1-81 *is higher than*   **1-82** *how the nurse's conduct compared with that of other nurses of similar background and experience*   **1-83** *False*
True
True

> **NOTE:**   In the discussion on the standard of care expected of nurses, no mention has been made of any distinction between nursing care rendered in one state versus another. This is because the modern trend of the courts is to accept a national standard of nursing care. See, for example, *Shilkret* v. *Annapolis Emergency Hospital Association*, 349 A. 2d 245 (Md. 1975) and *Hall* v. *Hibun*, 466 So. 2d. 856 (Miss. 1985).
>
> In addition, within the past two decades, most states and provinces have recognized the expanded role of professional nurses by including in their nurse practice acts special provisions authorizing nurses with the requisite training to undertake many highly technical procedures previously considered beyond the scope of registered nursing practice. These changes reflect growing public trust in professional nursing and clear recognition that nurses with specialized training can undertake many independent nursing functions that once were deemed to be solely within the province of the physician.
>
> While this increase in nursing specialization clearly has its rewarding aspects from a career standpoint, it has brought with it a decided increase in the nurse's legal accountability. Thus, as we shall see, the performance of the nurse-specialist is measured by a yardstick that is far more demanding than that of the nonspecialist.

STANDARD OF CARE OF THE NURSE-SPECIALIST

1-84   When nurses have acquired the necessary education and training to engage in specialized fields of nursing such as pediatrics, nurse-midwifery, anesthesiology, critical care, school health, psychiatric/mental health, emergency care, or surgical nursing, they are held to a higher standard of care than general-duty nurses in carrying out their duties, *but only while performing services in their specialty*. The standard of care expected of the nurse-specialist (referred to as the nurse-clinician in Canada) is the degree of care and skill customarily exercised by other nurses who practice that specialty. Here, again, we see that the greater the nurse's educational background and training, the higher the standard of care generally expected by the law.

■ Nurse N is a certified registered nurse-anesthetist (CRNA) in a large hospital.

Under what circumstances would Nurse N be held to a higher standard of care than a general-duty nurse in the same hospital?

☐   when counting sponges used during an operation

☐   when monitoring circulatory and respiratory sufficiency during an operation

☐   when administering a preoperative sedative

1-84   *when monitoring circulatory and respiratory sufficiency during an operation*

1-85 Nurse N's conduct in the operating room would be measured against that expected of a reasonably prudent

☐ nurse-anesthetist   ☐ scrub nurse   ☐ anesthesiologist

1-86 Nurse N is a pediatric nurse-specialist with 5 years of experience in that specialty. One day, a staff physician summons Nurse N, who is in the vicinity of the coronary intensive care unit, to assist in defibrillating a patient who has just gone into ventricular fibrillation.

In so assisting the physician, what legal standard of care would be applicable to Nurse N's conduct?

☐ the standard of care applicable to nurse-specialists in coronary care

☐ the standard of care applicable to general-duty nurses with similar experience in defibrillating patients

☐ the standard of care applicable to other nurse-specialists in pediatric nursing

---

1-87

- Nurse N, a duly certified nurse-practitioner under the state nurse practice act, is employed by a health maintenance organization (HMO). P, a 30-year-old man complaining of recent episodes of chest pain, is examined by Nurse N, who diagnoses muscle spasm and prescribes diazepam (Valium). The pain persists and P returns the following day, at which time he is seen by an emergency department physician who orders a chest x-ray and prescribes stronger medication for the "muscle spasms." P returns the following day because the pain now is constant, and a different physician orders an ECG. This reveals an acute myocardial infarction, and P is admitted immediately to the hospital for treatment. He later sues the HMO, Nurse N, and the first doctor for failure to diagnose his true condition promptly.

Nurse N was not legally authorized to examine and diagnose P, especially since staff physicians were readily available.

	True	*False*
	☐	☐

1-85 *nurse-anesthetist*	**1-86** *The standard of care applicable to general-duty nurses with similar experience . . .*	**1-87** *False*

1-88   Nurse N's conduct in this case would be measured against that of

□   other nurses employed by HMOs

□   other nurse-practitioners in the same locality

□   doctors specializing in cardiology

1-89   A finding by the jury that the first physician was negligent would automatically relieve Nurse N of any liability for negligence

True   *False*

□   □

NOTE: The fact situation just outlined was taken from the 1985 California Supreme Court case of *Fein* v. *Permanente Medical Group*, 211 Cal. Rptr. 368, 695 P. 2d 665. This case, which reversed the lower court's decision, clearly confirmed the legal principle that a nurse-practitioner's conduct will be measured against that of other nurse-practitioners acting under similar circumstances. In the trial court, the applicable standard of care was proved not by testimony from another nurse-practitioner, but by the head of cardiology at a nearby major medical center. As the law evolves in this area, it is to be expected that nurse-practitioners, and not physicians, will be the principal experts on the governing standards of care. Within the hospital setting, there is little doubt that the category of nursing specialist most vulnerable to malpractice suits is the nurse-anesthetist. The liability of the Certified Registered Nurse Anesthetist (CRNA) has been established in a multitude of situations involving either the selection, administration, or management of anesthesia. Other OR nursing personnel, as well as Critical Care Unit (CCU) and Intensive Care Unit (ICU) personnel, have also been held liable in malpractice suits, although to a somewhat lesser extent. Future cases undoubtedly will be asserted with increasing frequency against other categories of advanced nursing practice specialists, including certified nurse midwives, neonatal intensive care nurses, psychiatric/mental health nurses, geriatric care nurses and others. (A more detailed description of these various categories is set forth in Part 5.)

1-88   *other nurse-practitioners in the same locality*   **1-89**   *False*

1-90

■ N is a Critical Care Registered Nurse (CCRN) assigned to care for a patient in the ICU who had just undergone a gastroplasty for treatment of obesity. X-rays indicate large amounts of air in the patient's abdomen and signs of infection, but because of a critical staffing shortage, N leaves the patient unattended for a lengthy period to care for other ICU patients. During this period, the patient experiences respiratory arrest, with resulting brain damage. A suit is brought against the hospital and Nurse N for the resulting harm.

Based on the foregoing fact situation, indicate whether the following statements are true or false.

True	*False*	
☐	☐	Nurse N could be held personally liable in this suit for failing to meet the standard of care expected of a critical care nursing specialist.
☐	☐	Nurse N could not be held liable because the patient's injuries were not the result of any direct action on N's part.
☐	☐	The standard of nursing care applicable in this case would be higher than that expected of general-duty RNs assigned to care for postoperative patients.
☐	☐	The hospital, but not Nurse N, could be held liable in this case because it is the hospital's legal responsibility to provide safe care to all hospitalized patients, whether or not there is a staffing shortage.

1-90   *True*
         False
         True
         False

NOTE: The previous material deliberately focused only on the standard of care applicable to nurses who are clinical specialists. The more comprehensive issue of the authority of clinical nurse specialists and nurse-practitioners to diagnose, prescribe medications, and undertake other specialized medical/nursing procedures encompasses the area generally referred to as "scope of nursing practice," which is discussed separately in Part 5. We resume our discussion at this point with the standards of care applicable to other categories of nurses.

STANDARD OF CARE OF THE NURSING STUDENT

1-91   There is an important exception to the general rule regarding the standard of care to be applied to a nurse's conduct: When a nursing student performs duties customarily performed only by an RN, the courts have held the nursing student to the higher standard of care of the RN. This rule applies even though the duties may have been specifically assigned to the nursing student by the clinical instructor.

The reason for this exception is that a patient has a right to assume that all professional services furnished in the hospital, including nursing services, will be provided by persons with the requisite degree of professional training and skill.

Consider the following situation:

■ A nursing student is assigned by his clinical instructor to perform a complex nursing procedure normally performed only by registered nurses. The student's ineptness causes injury to the patient, who later sues him, claiming that the student's conduct did not meet the standard of care of other reasonably prudent *RNs*. In defense of his conduct the nursing student points out at the trial that:

A.   Nursing students ordinarily are not given assignments of the type in question and, accordingly, he should not be held liable.

B.   He should not be held liable because he was only following the orders of his clinical instructor.

C.   Since he is only a student, his conduct should be judged by the standard of care applicable to other nursing students under similar circumstances.

Which, if any, of these defenses would protect the student from liability?

A	B	C	None of these
☐	☐	☐	☐

1-91   *None of these*

1-92 The nursing student in the previous example could have avoided being held liable to the patient by proving that

☐   he performed the procedure in question at the specific direction of his clinical instructor

☐   he exercised the degree of care expected of reasonably prudent registered nurses in the same or similar circumstances

☐   he exercised the degree of care expected of other reasonably prudent nursing students in the same or similar circumstances

---

1-93 Where injury to a patient is caused by a nursing student in the course of clinical training, there is little doubt that the law's principal concern is with

☐   compensating the injured patient

☐   improving the quality of patient care

☐   punishing the student's negligent conduct

1-94

■ N is a nursing student who has been assigned to the medical ward of a local hospital to obtain clinical experience.

If N's conduct causes harm to a patient assigned to her care, she would most likely be held liable for

☐   ordinary negligence

☐   nursing malpractice

☐   neither of the above

☐   both of the above

1-92 ☐
      ☑
      ☐

1-93 *compensating the injured patient*

1-94 *nursing malpratice*

NOTE: Our focus here is on the standard of care applicable to nursing students, but the reader may be wondering about the *legal authority* of nursing students to provide hands-on nursing care to patients in the first place. The authority to do so is granted by the state practice acts, which generally exempt nursing students from their provisions and allow them to practice nursing without a license—and not be prosecuted—while learning to become nurses. Licensing laws and their role and effect are discussed in detail in Part 5.

1-95   Knowing one's own limitations of training and experience is a good rule for *every* nurse, but it is particularly important for nursing students to be aware of their limitations and to bring these to the attention of the clinical instructor whenever they are assigned tasks that call for skills they do not possess.

Acting with reasonable care may well require nursing students to decline to carry out tasks that they know they are not qualified to perform, *even at the risk of appearing insubordinate.*

Consider the following situation:

■ The charge nurse in a large hospital is suddenly diverted from her normal supervisory and administrative duties and is required to assist in a technical nursing procedure at a patient's bedside. She is somewhat irritated by this diversion, and when she notices a nursing student in the hallway, she directs the latter to take over for her. The student has never performed the nursing function in question but is too frightened to inform the charge nurse of this fact. His inexperience in carrying out the procedure results in harm to the patient, who later sues the nurse for malpractice.

Based on the foregoing fact situation, indicate whether the following statements are true or false.

True   **False**

☐   ☐   The student could not avoid personal liability for the harm done once he undertook to perform the procedure as ordered.

☐   ☐   The student could avoid personal liability for the harm done by pointing out that his fear of being regarded as insubordinate kept him from refusing the assignment.

☐   ☐   The student could avoid personal liability for the harm done by proving he was clearly untrained in the procedure in question.

1-95   True
        False
        False

1-96 In the described situation, what course of action should the nursing student have taken in order to avoid liability?

☐ He should have ignored the charge nurse's order, since he knew he could not give the required care competently.

☐ He should have protested his inexperience to the patient or a member of the patient's family.

☐ He should have informed the charge nurse of his inability to carry out the procedure and his consequent refusal to do so.

1-97 Assume that the charge nurse in the previous example had directed an RN to take over for her instead of the nursing student. In what way (if any) would the situation differ?

☐ An RN presumably would be more competent than a nursing student to carry out a technical nursing function.

☐ The situation would not differ in any respect from that involving the nursing student.

☐ An RN could not refuse to perform a procedure when directed to do so by a charge nurse.

1-98 The law's insistence that a nurse not undertake to perform a function he or she is not qualified or competent to perform is for the purpose of

☐ bringing about better and safer patient care

☐ protecting nurses and hospitals from liability suits

☐ assuring compliance with the nurse's professional liability policy

---

1-96 *He should have informed the charge nurse of his inability . . .*

1-97 *An RN presumably would be more competent than a nursing student to carry out a technical nursing function.*

1-98 *bringing about better and safer patient care*

NOTE: As we have shown, the mere fact that a nursing student is given a nursing assignment by the clinical instructor or by a unit or charge nurse does not absolve the student from personal liability for any harm caused. The nursing student who is directed to carry out an assignment that he or she is not qualified to perform, and that he or she justifiably believes is likely to harm the patient, should immediately bring the matter to the attention of the clinical instructor or other responsible hospital staff member. In the final analysis, both patient and nursing student will benefit from the student's clear understanding of his or her legal responsibilities and forthright conduct in these difficult situations.

One final point: The fact that the nursing student may be held liable does not necessarily relieve the clinical instructor or charge nurse from liability for supervisory negligence when the supervisor assigns a task to a student that is clearly beyond his or her capabilities. This subject is covered in greater detail later in this course.

POINTS TO REMEMBER

1. Professional and lay persons alike are required to act with reasonable care, but the reasonableness of a professional person's conduct is measured not against the conduct of laypersons but against the conduct of other reasonably prudent members of the same profession.

2. The higher standard of care imposed on a professional person applies only to conduct that is related to that person's professional duties.

3. In the performance of professional duties, a nurse is required to exercise the degree of care and skill that a reasonably prudent nurse with similar training and experience would exercise under the same general circumstances.

4. When it is necessary to determine in a court case whether a nurse acted with care in a given situation, the nurse's educational background and professional training are always taken into consideration.

5. The nurse who is a specialist is held to the higher standard of care that applies to other nurse-specialists who practice that specialty, but only while the nurse is performing services in that specialty.

6. Legally, every patient has the right to expect competent nursing care, even if provided by students as part of their clinical training. Thus, a nursing student will be held to the standard of care of the RN when performing duties in a hospital that are customarily performed only by registered nurses.

7. When a nursing student does not possess the skills needed to carry out an assigned nursing function, acting with reasonable care requires that the student refuse to perform the function, even at the risk of appearing insubordinate. The patient's safety is always the paramount concern.

OTHER FACTORS AFFECTING NEGLIGENT CONDUCT

1-99   It is sometimes said that professional negligence does not exist in a vacuum, which simply means that in determining what is negligent conduct, the "surrounding circumstances" must always be taken into account. The types of surrounding circumstances normally considered in a nursing malpractice suit are (1) the nature and complexity of the nursing function involved, (2) the foreseeability of harm if care is not exercised, (3) the nurse's known or presumed professional qualifications to perform that function, and (4) the urgency of the overall situation.

Which of the following statements *best* illustrates the point of the preceding paragraph?

☐   Negligent conduct usually involves a variety of surrounding circumstances.

☐   All the surrounding circumstances must be considered in determining whether particular conduct is negligent.

☐   There are four major types of surrounding circumstances involved in every malpractice case.

1-100 Select from the following list *two* factors that would be legally significant surrounding circumstances in a malpractice suit against a general-duty nurse:

☐   the alleged malpractice involved nursing care customarily given by a nurse-specialist

☐   the alleged malpractice occurred while carrying out a difficult and novel nursing procedure

☐   the nurse had been sued for malpractice on at least one prior occasion

☐   the nurse was generally antagonistic to the patients and was not well-liked

---

1-99	*All the surrounding circumstances must be considered . . .*	**1-100**	☑
			☑
			☐
			☐

1-101 In view of the law's consideration of the surrounding circumstances in determining liability in a malpractice suit, how likely is it that two nurses sued for the same type of allegedly negligent conduct would fare *differently* in the outcome of their lawsuits?

☐ not likely

☐ quite possible

☐ impossible

1-102 As noted, one legally significant surrounding circumstance in determining liability is the foreseeability of harm to the patient if proper care is not exercised. Under the doctrine of foreseeability, every person is held legally liable for all the reasonably foreseeable consequences of that person's negligent conduct, provided those consequences are naturally and proximately* related to such conduct. Thus, an important asepct of determining whether a nurse has been negligent is the extent to which he or she is able to foresee that his or her action (or inaction) will cause harm to the patient.

The doctrine of foreseeability of harm applies

☐ only to health care providers

☐ to everyone

☐ only to nurses

---

*Proximately means closely related in time.

1-103 If most reasonably prudent nurses would anticipate harmful consequences to a patient from specific nursing conduct, whether acts or omissions, then proof of such conduct by a nurse in a malpractice case would be a clear basis for holding the nurse liable for any injuries suffered.

True	*False*
☐	☐

1-101   *quite possible*   **1-102**   *to everyone*   **1-103**   *True*

1-104

■ Doctor D orders Nurse N to give an elderly female patient a particular medication, but the order fails to specify the route of administration.

What is the correct legal position of Nurse N in these circumstances?

☐ N can assume the doctor wished him to exercise his own judgment regarding the route of administration.

☐ N can assume the medication will not be harmful to the patient without regard to the route of administration.

☐ N can assume that some harm is likely to result if the route of administration is not specified.

1-105

■ Pediatric Nurse N knows that a 6-year-old boy has experienced convulsions previously when his temperature rose above 102 degrees. Late one evening, Nurse N records a temperature of 102.5 degrees, but concludes this is a momentary spike. Shortly thereafter, the child has a violent seizure, goes into a coma, and dies 2 days later. The parents sue Nurse N for the child's wrongful death.

Which of the following most accurately characterizes Nurse N's legal position?

☐ N could not reasonably have foreseen that her inaction might lead to the child's death.

☐ N could be held liable for all the consequences of her inaction, including liability for his death.

☐ N could be held liable, but only for the normal consequences of an episodic seizure.

1-104 ☐
            ☐
            ☑

1-105 *N could be held liable for all the consequences of her inaction. . .*

1-106 When a nurse's liability in a given situation is being determined, circumstances relating to the nurse's *personal* state of mind or physical condition are generally considered irrelevant. Since nurses are charged with responsibility for their patients' welfare, they are expected to maintain themselves in a physical and mental condition that will enable them to meet their normal professional responsibilities at all times.

- While on duty at the hospital, Nurse N receives a call from her husband who tells her he has been arrested for drunken driving. They argue vehemently and the conversation leaves Nurse N very distraught. Shortly thereafter, she forgets to disconnect a heat lamp, which causes severe burns to a patient.

Indicate which, if any, of the following would afford Nurse N a good defense in the patient's later lawsuit against her.

☐   N has no valid defense against the lawsuit.

☐   N can defend by showing that the heat lamp was set up by someone else before she came on duty.

☐   N can defend by showing that her failure to disconnect the lamp was due to her severe emotional state.

1-107 Under *ordinary* circumstances a nurse's claim of fatigue and inability to act with the customary degree of care and judgment would not be a relevant defense in a malpractice suit. Which of the following circumstances (if any) *might* be relevant in a malpractice action brought against a nurse?

☐   The nurse had been on duty continuously for 36 hours to help meet an acute shortage of nurses during a mass casualty situation at the hospital.

☐   The nurse had been up late the evening before as the result of getting stuck in a traffic jam on the way back from a holiday weekend.

☐   The nurse was exhausted from studying until 2 AM for a special nursing examination scheduled 2 days later.

| 1-106 | *N has no valid defense against the lawsuit.* | 1-107 | ☑ ☐ ☐ | *If you checked either the 2d or 3d box, see p. 76, Note C.* |

THE PROBLEM OF THE IMPAIRED NURSE

While on the subject of the nurse's physical condition and ability to perform normal nursing duties, it is appropriate to discuss the growing problem of substance abuse and alcoholism by nurses. It is reliably reported that the incidence of chemical dependency by nurses is 50% higher than in the general population, with an estimated 7% of the 1.9 million nurses in the United States presently addicted to drugs or alcohol. There is little doubt that the primary cause is the high stress level associated with nursing practice today, attributable to increased work loads, double shifts, floating to unfamiliar units, and other similar causes of fatigue and loneliness. In addition, nurses face the usual assortment of stressors placed on them by family and financial obligations, which all too often prompt them to turn to the escape mechanisms of drugs and alcohol.

Past attitudes towards this problem focused on disciplinary action—bringing the accused nurse before the state nursing board, initiating an investigation, and revoking the nurse's license if found guilty of the charges brought. Colleagues seldom reported nurses suspected of alcoholism or drug abuse, knowing that the latter would almost certainly lose their licenses. In the process, however, the best interests of addicted nurses as well as the safety of their patients were essentially ignored. As these problems have become more widely discussed and understood, the nursing profession has increasingly begun to deal with substance abusers as persons with treatable disorders rather than as pariahs who should be run out of the profession. In fact, some nurse practice acts now specify these more modern treatment approaches to rehabilitation of nurses who have become chemically dependent, in lieu of summary license revocation.

Sooner or later, every nurse will encounter a colleague with a drug abuse or alcoholism problem and will react to that individual in a variety of ways (e.g., resentment for having to assume the problem nurse's workload, concern about the latter's potential for causing harm to patients, anxiety over whether to report the colleague to nursing management combined with feelings of guilt for being seen as disloyal to a fellow nurse and a whistle-blower). Notwithstanding these feelings, the preferred response of the profession today is to focus on the end result—complete rehabilitation of the nurse with a substance abuse problem—with intervention being the key. Intervention is a three-stage process: (1) recognizing the signs and symptoms of substance abuse, (2) documenting and reporting those signs and symptoms, and (3) confronting the substance abuser with the facts and explaining the available options.

Most, if not all, hospitals now have formal policies for dealing with substance abuse by employees, often based on the three-stage intervention process previously noted. It behooves all staff nurses to understand and adhere to the policies in their respective hospitals and to become familiar with the signs of substance abuse in colleagues. Some of the more prominent ones include increased errors in treatment, particularly dosage calculations; slurred speech, unsteady gait, flushed face or red eyes, rapid mood swings from depression to elation; poor personal hygiene; patients' complaints of nonreceipt of their prescribed pain-killing narcotics; discrepancies in narcotics supplies at the end of the nurse's shift; excessive reports of broken vials or spilled narcotics by the nurse; and so forth. If such signs are noted, the ethically responsible nurse will document them and report them to nursing management promptly. In the final analysis, this is not only the morally correct way of dealing with the problem of substance abuse by a colleague, but the action most likely to lead to the latter's rehabilitation as well as enhancing the safety of his or her patients.

EXPLANATORY NOTES

Note A (from Frame 1-73)

A word about terminology: The term "professional" is used in its primary dictionary sense, namely, "of, relating to, or characteristic of a profession." The intention is to distinguish professional activities (i.e., those that require special skills and learning) from those of a nonprofessional nature, which are performed by laypersons. Within this general context, the term professional is intended to apply to the acts of LPNs as well as registered professional nurses, at both the student and graduate level.

Proceed to Frame 1-74.

Note B (from Frame 1-79)

The nurse's failure to comply with a standard hospital procedure or a physician's standing order would certainly appear to be evidence of a failure to exercise reasonable care, but this is not *necessarily* the case. Under some circumstances a nurse's rigid adherence to a particular standard procedure or a physician's standing order might actually be considered *unreasonable*, or even dangerous.

We must never forget that nurses are supposed to be aware of the total nursing needs of their patients, and if they carry out orders that they know are wrong and are likely to be harmful to their patients, they will be held legally liable for so doing. In the eyes of the law, the patient's welfare is paramount over any standard procedure or method of conduct.

Without knowing the particular circumstances, therefore, we cannot characterize the conduct as unreasonable or negligent merely because the nurse failed to follow the hospital's prescribed procedure or the physician's standing order.

Proceed to Frame 1-80.

EXPLANATORY NOTES

Note C (from Frame 1-107)

Both the second and third choices describe circumstances that are purely *personal* to the nurse, even though the third choice appears to have some relevance to the nurse's professional activities. Nevertheless, a nurse who is too fatigued to carry out the normal patient care responsibilities because of a decision to stay up late to study for an examination has acted neither with reasonable care nor in the patients' best interests.

The test of reasonableness in this situation is what other reasonably prudent nurses would have done under the circumstances. Here the answer becomes clear: The prudent nurse either would have *avoided* becoming fatigued by getting the proper amount of sleep or (alternatively) would have informed the nursing supervisor of his or her fatigued condition and consequent inability to work on the assigned shift.

In contrast with the latter two situations, the first one describes unusual emergency circumstances that were *not of the nurse's own making*, and these would be sufficient to alter the usual rule regarding the irrelevance of the nurse's personal physical condition.

Proceed to Frame 1-108.

1-108 A nurse who is suddenly confronted with an emergency situation within his or her normal work environment presenting imminent (perhaps life-threatening) danger to a patient is not legally required to use the same degree of prudence and judgment that he or she would use under normal circumstances. In such an emergency a nurse's legal duty is merely to exercise the degree of care and skill that an ordinarily prudent nurse of similar training and experience would exercise under similar circumstances.

■ Five hospital nurses are sued in separate malpractice actions involving different types of alleged negligent conduct. At the trials of these malpractice suits, all the nurses *admit* they deviated from the standard of care applicable but each raises a particular circumstance in defense.

Which of the five nurses (if any) has raised an issue that might alter the standard of care the law normally requires?

☐ Nurse A, who claims that the patient in question was someone she had not previously attended

☐ Nurse B, who claims that he was off duty at the time the nursing care in question was given

☐ Nurse C, who claims that she was directed by the head nurse to assist in an emergency procedure in which she had no prior experience

☐ Nurse D, who claims that vitally-needed resuscitation equipment, which he ordered, was not brought to the patient's room because of a sudden strike of paramedical personnel at the hospital

☐ Nurse E, who claims that she gave the patient an injection with an unsterile needle because his condition was rapidly deteriorating and time did not permit her to obtain a sterile needle

☐ None of the nurses has raised an issue that would alter the standard of care normally required

---

1-109 In emergency circumstances, a nurse is not legally required to exercise reasonable care in treating a patient.

True	*False*
☐	☐

1-108 ☐ *At this point you may wish to*   **1-109**   *False*
          ☐ *review the material in Frames*
          ☑ *1-64 through 1-71 dealing with*
          ☑ *the nurse's responsibility to give*
          ☑ *emergency care to someone.*
          ☐

1-110 The fact that a nurse or nursing student is legally considered a minor under the pertinent state law will not in and of itself exempt him or her from liability for negligence in carrying out nursing duties. This fact emphasizes the need for all nurses to be fully aware of their legal responsibilities in caring for patients. Except for care rendered in emergency circumstances, age and relative inexperience will not shield them from liability for negligent conduct if they are sued.

Which *two* of the following would be considered *legally significant* in assessing a nurse's liability for an act of malpractice?

☐   the fact that the nurse graduated with honors from a highly-rated nursing school

☐   actual experience as a nurse

☐   the particular conduct complained of

☐   prior status as an LPN

☐   the fact that the nurse is legally a minor

1-111 When a nursing student is treating hospitalized patients as a part of nursing training, the student's exposure to liability (i.e., risk of being sued for malpractice) is   ☐   greater than   ☐   the same as   ☐   less than   a hospital staff RN's exposure to liability.

1-112 The fact that a nurse who is sued for malpractice is a minor

☐   is of no legal significance in determining the outcome of the case

☐   will usually resolve the case in the nurse's favor

☐   is a clear indication that the nurse probably was negligent

---

1-110	*actual experience as a nurse*	**1-111**	*the same as*	**1-112**	*is of no legal significance in determining the outcome of the case*
	the particular conduct complained of		*The importance of this conclusion cannot be overemphasized. If in doubt, reread Frames 1-91 through 1-98.*		

VIOLATION OF STATUTES

1-113 Earlier it was pointed out that statutes *generally* do not lay down legal guidelines for specific types of nursing functions, but this is not *always* the case. Sometimes the applicable standard of care is expressly set forth in a statute intended to prohibit a particular type of nursing activity or function, and in this situation, deviation from the standard of care is shown merely by proof of the statutory violation.

- A provincial statute states that nurses shall not perform nursing duties during any period in which they are suffering contagious or communicable diseases. Nurse N applies for work at a small hospital in the province, knowing that she has TB at the time. After three patients at the hospital contract TB, it is discovered that Nurse N was the infecting carrier.

What would be necessary to hold Nurse N liable for the resulting harm to the three patients?

- ☐ proof of her negligence in treating one or more of the patients

- ☐ proof of her knowing violation of the provincial statute

- ☐ proof of her violation of the standard of care normally applicable when a nurse has a contagious disease

---

1-114 The nurse practice act of State X expressly prohibits a nurse from prescribing medication for a patient except under the specific order of a licensed physician. Nurse N, certified as an OB/GYN nurse-practitioner by the Nurses' Association of the American College of Obstetrics and Gynecology, and employed in a family planning clinic in State X, prescribes birth control pills to a patient, acting entirely on her own.

The fact that Nurse N is appropriately certified as an OB/GYN nurse-practitioner   ☐ will   ☐ will not   protect her against a claim that she violated the nurse practice act of State X.

1-115 The language of the nurse practice act in the previous frame is an example of
    ☐ a statutory impediment   ☐ a standard of care   ☐ a suggested guideline

---

1-113	*proof of her knowing violation of the provincial statute*	1-114	*will not*	1-115	*a standard of care*

1-116

■ The nurse practice act of State Y provides that only a licensed professional nurse may administer inoculations. Nurse N, who is licensed as a practical nurse in State Y, is employed by Doctor D as her office assistant. One day, concerned about the large number of patients waiting to see the doctor, N takes it upon herself to administer a polio booster shot to a 2-year-old child. The needle breaks in the child's buttock, and cannot be removed without surgery. The parents sue both Doctor D and Nurse N for the resulting damages.

In a lawsuit of this type, proof of N's violation of the state's nurse practice act would be

☐ sufficient legally to hold N liable for the child's injuries

☐ taken into consideration, but would not be legally significant on the issue of N's liability

☐ of little legal significance on the issue of N's liability

1-117 Apart from N's violation of the statute in the previous frame, the standard of care by which her conduct would be measured in this case would be

☐ that of a licensed practical nurse

☐ that of a licensed professional nurse

☐ that of a reasonably prudent office nurse

NOTE: A nurse's proven violation of a statute will not automatically hold him or her liable—there must be a clear cause-and-effect relationship between the violation and the resultant harm or injury. This is called the rule of proximate causation and is an essential element in every malpractice case. In effect, the injured party (the plaintiff) must prove a direct and clear chain of events leading from the nurse's wrongful act to the resultant harm. No intervening act of another must have been capable of producing the harm or injury to the patient. This rule is discussed more fully in Part 6.

1-116 *sufficient legally to hold N liable for the child's injuries*

1-117 *that of a licensed professional nurse*

An LPN who acts as a professional nurse will be held to that standard.

1-118 When the major issue in a malpractice case is the nurse's failure to conform to a standard of care set forth in a statute, in what manner is negligence (if any) proved?

☐ by the testimony of other nurses as to what they would have done under the circumstances

☐ by the testimony of experts in the field of nursing as to what should have been done under the circumstances

☐ by proof of the nurse's violation of the statute that prescribed the standard of care

OTHER APPLICABLE STANDARDS OF CARE

In addition to the general standards applicable to nursing practice laid down in state and provincial statutes, over the years some very specific standards have been promulgated by the Joint Commission on Accreditation of Healthcare Organizations, by national, provincial, and state nursing associations, and by various nursing specialty groups. In actual practice, however, the most significant regulation of the nurse's professional conduct comes from the state or provincial nurse practice act and the rules and regulations issued thereunder by the respective boards of nursing.

The state and provincial boards of nursing are customarily delegated broad authority, including the authority (1) to prescribe regulations setting forth educational requirements and admission standards for licensure of nurses and, in some states and Canadian provinces, nurse-practitioners; (2) to delineate the tasks nurses and nurse-practitioners are permitted to carry out either independently or in collaboration with physicians; and (3) to establish criteria and administrative mechanisms for disciplining nurses who violate the rules, including authority to impose appropriate penalties.

Professional nursing is continually expanding its statutory basis for practice, with increasing numbers of states and Canadian provinces amending their nurse practice and medical practice acts so as to make more explicit those nursing functions that are deemed independent and do not require specific physicians' orders. The overlapping nature of many medical and nursing functions—such as those relating to diagnosing and the establishment of treatment plans or regimens—has made it difficult at times to determine who is primarily responsible and should be held legally liable when a diagnosis proves to be wrong or a particular treatment regimen results in injury to the patient. These scope of practice issues are discussed at greater length in Part 5.

1-118 *by proof of the nurse's violation of the statute that prescribed the standard of care*

POINTS TO REMEMBER

1. Whether an act constitutes negligent nursing conduct depends not only on the act itself but on all the surrounding circumstances.

2. Four surrounding circumstances deemed to be of prime concern are (1) the nature of the nursing function involved, (2) the nurse's qualifications to perform that function, (3) the foreseeability of harm if care is not exercised, and (4) the urgency of the overall situation.

3. Under ordinary circumstances, a nurse's personal state of mind or physical condition is not considered relevant as a defense to a malpractice claim.

4. In an emergency, a nurse is not held to the same standard of care expected under normal circumstances.

5. Being a minor does not, in and of itself, exempt a nurse from liability for acts of malpractice.

6. When a statute lays down a specific standard of nursing conduct, liability normally will result upon clear proof of violation of the statute and harm flowing therefrom.

Summary of Basic Elements
Comprising the Nurse's Liability for Malpractice

Element	Explanation	Example
1. A nurse-patient relationship must be in existence before liability of the nurse can accrue.	This legal status is created whenever professional nursing care is actually provided.	A staff RN in a community general hospital is assigned to provide care to all medical ward patients.
2. Nurse has the duty to meet the applicable standard of care, whether based on statute (federal or state), administrative agency regulations, or common law court decisions.	The basic standard of care is what the reasonably prudent nurse would have done under the same or similar circumstances.	The nurse's duty is to give the patient the proper drug, in the proper dosage, on time , and through the proper route of administration.
3. Proof of conduct that fails to meet the applicable standard of care is essential.	Acts or omissions that legally amount to negligent conduct, by statute or common law.	The nurse administers the wrong drug to the patient, through neglect or inattention.
4. Surrounding circumstances may alter (reduce or increase) the nurse's liability.	• Foreseeability of harm • Possible emergency circumstances • Complexity of the function being performed (Q—Is this a task for a nurse specialist?) • The nurse's qualifications to perform the act in question	• Contraindicated medication is very likely to harm the patient • No emergency circumstances • Giving medications is a routine nursing task • An RN is clearly competent to perform the act in question
5. The negligent act in question must be the proximate cause of injury or death to the patient.	The nurse's conduct must be the material or substantial cause of the patient's injury. There must be no other likely or intervening cause.	The patient suffers an anaphylactic reaction to the improperly-administered drug, goes into cardiac arrest, and dies.
6. Damages (economic loss) must be incurred by the patient or the patient's family.	Compensatory damages will be awarded for measurable economic loss and pain and suffering; emotional loss suffered by the patient's family is sometimes allowed (depending on the state).	The patient's death causes immediate as well as anticipated future financial loss, loss of consortium, and emotional grief to the patient's family.

SELECTED REFERENCES—PART ONE

Common Law and Statutory Law Distinguished

McCormack v. *Oklahoma Publishing Co.*, 613 P. 2d 737 (Okla. 1980)
Hogan v. *State*, 441 P. 2d 620 (Nev. 1968)
In re Davis' Estate, 35 A. 2d 880 (N.J. 1944)

Tort Law Defined

74 *Am Jur 2d*, TORTS, §1
Abel R, "A Critique of Torts," *UCLA L Rev* 37:785, 1990.
Freeman v. *Busch Jewelry Co.*, 98 F. Supp. 963 (Ga. 1951)

Tort Law and Contract Law Distinguished

Prosser W, *Handbook of the Law of Torts*, ed 4, West Publishing, St. Paul, 1971, §92, pp. 613-622.
74 *Am Jur 2d*, TORTS, §23
Glisson v. *Loxley*, 366 S.E. 2d 68 (Va. 1988)
Mitchell v. *Spataro*, 452 N.Y.S. 2d 646 (N.Y. 1982)
Hinkes v. *City of Newark*, 295 A. 2d 399 (N.J. 1972)
Bankers Fidelity Life Ins. Co. v. *Harrison*, 123 S.E. 2d 438 (Ga. 1961)

Criminal Law and the Nurse

Kelly ME, "Criminal Law Overview," in *Legal Issues In Nursing* (Northrop CE and Kelly ME, eds.), C.V. Mosby, St. Louis, 1987, Ch. 24.
LaFave WR and Scott AW, *Substantive Criminal Law*, West Publishing, St. Paul, 1972.
Fiesta J, "Criminal Liability for the Nurse," *Nurs Management* 23(4):16, 1992.
Fiesta J, "Criminal Liability for the Nurse—Part II," *Nurs Management* 23(5):16, 1992.
Dawson JS and Schimeca JA, "Hospital Crimes: Expecting the Unexpected," *Healthspan* 7:10, 1990.
Wiley S, "Liability for Death: Nine Nurses' Ordeals," *Nursing '81* 9:34, 1982.
People of the State of New York v. *Simon*, 549 N.Y.S. 2d 701 (N.Y. 1990)
Rachals v. *State of Georgia*, 361 S.E. 2d 671 (Ga. 1987)
State of North Carolina v. *Raines*, 344 S.E. 2d 138 (N.C. 1987)
Jones v. *State of Texas*, 716 S.W. 2d 142 (Texas 1986)

Concept of Legal Liability

University of Florida Institute of Agricultural Services v. *Karch*, 393 So. 2d 621 (Fla. 1981)
Marrico v. *Misericordia Hospital*, 398 N.Y.S. 2d 660 (N.Y. 1977)
Stuyvesant Insurance Co. v. *Bournazian*, 342 So. 2d 471 (Fla. 1977)
Continental Insurance Co. v. *Echols*, 243 S.E. 2d 88 (Ga. 1951)

Negligence Defined

Prosser W, *Handbook of the Law of Torts*, ed 4, West Publishing, St. Paul, 1971, §35-36, pp. 149-163.
57 *Am Jur 2d* NEGLIGENCE, §6
Note: "Contributory Negligence in Medical Malpractice," *Univ of Dayton L Rev* 17:151, 1991.
Wielgus v. *Lopez*, 525 N.E. 2d 1272 (Ind. 1988)
Trapanni v. *State Farm Fire & Casualty Company*, 424 So. 2d 449 (La. 1982)
Palsgraf v. *Long Island R. Co.*, 162 N.E. 99 (N.Y. 1928)

Malpractice Defined

Kansas Malpractice Victims Coalition v. *Bell*, 757 P. 2d 251 (Kan. 1988)
Boudreaux v. *Panger*, 481 So. 2d 1382 (La. 1986)

Matthews v. *Walker*, 296 N.E. 2d 569 (Ohio 1973)
Kosberg v. *Washington Hospital Center, Inc.*, 394 F. 2d 947 (D.C. 1968)
Louie v. *Chinese Hospital Association*, 57 Cal. Rptr. 906 (Cal. 1967)
Valentin v. *La Société Française*, 172 P. 2d 359 (Cal. 1956)

Negligence and Malpractice Distinguished

Chafin v. *Wesley Homes, Inc.*, 367 S.E. 2d 236 (Ga. 1988)
Corgan v. *Muehling*, 522 N.E. 2d 153 (Ill. 1988)
Candler General Hosptial, Inc. v. *McNorrill*, 354 S.E. 2d 872 (Ga. 1987)
Cubito v. *Kreisberg*, 419 N.Y.S. 2d 78 (N.Y. 1979)
Duling v. *Bluefield Sanitorium*, 142 S.E. 2d 754 (W. Va. 1965)

Creation of the Nurse-Patient Relationship

Murphy C, "Models of the Nurse-Patient Relationship," in *Ethical Problems in the Nurse-Patient Relationship* (Murphy C and Hunter H, eds.), Allyn and Bacon, New York, 1982, pp. 8-25
Clough v. *Lively*, 367 S.E. 2d 295 (Ga. 1988)
Burrows v. *Hawaiian Trust Company*, 417 P. 2d 816 (Haw. 1966)
Noland v. *Brown*, 129 S.E. 2d 477 (N.C. 1963)
Harvey v. *Silber*, 2 N.W. 2d 483 (Mich. 1942)

Standard of Care Applicable to Nurses Generally

Standards of Clinical Nursing Practice, American Nurses Association, 1990.
Cushing M, *Nursing Jurisprudence*, Appleton-Lange, Norwalk, Conn., 1988, pp. 32-34.
Annotation, 51 ALR 2d 970, "Nurse's Liability for Her Own Negligence or Malpractice."
Fiesta J, "Legal Aspects—Standards of Care: Part I," *Nurs Management* 24(7):30, 1993.
Fiesta J, "Legal Aspects—Standards of Care: Part II," *Nurs Management* 24(8):16, 1993.
Bullough B, "The Current Phase in the Development of Nurse Practice Acts," *St. Louis U L J* 28:365, 1984.
Guariello D, "The Legal Boobytraps in Nursing Standards," *RN* 47(6):19, 1984.
Eccard WT, "A Revolution in White—New Approaches in Treating Nurses as Professionals," *Vanderbilt L Rev* 30:839, 1977.
McMillan v. *Durant*, 439 S.E. 2d 829 (S.C. 1993)
Alef v. *Alta Bates Hospital*, 6 Cal. Rptr. 2d 900 (Cal. 1992)
Gibson v. *Bossier City General Hospital*, 594 So. 2d 1332 (La. 1991)
Northern Trust Co. v. *Upjohn Co.*, 572 N.E. 2d 1030 (Ill. 1991)
Cangelosi v. *Our Lady of Lake Medical Center*, 564 So. 2d 654 (La. 1989)
Ellinghausen v. *Flushing Hospital & Medical Center*, 531 N.Y.S. 2d 824 (N.Y. 1988)
Ewing v. *Aubert*, 532 So. 2d 876 (La. App. 1988), *writ den.*, 551 So. 2d 1333 (La. 1989)
Koeninger v. *Eckrich*, 422 N.W. 2d 600 (S.D. 1988)
Hodges v. *Effingham County Hospital Authority*, 355 S.E. 2d 104 (Ga. 1987)
Hall v. *Hibun*, 466 S.E. 2d 856 (Miss. 1985)
Reynolds v. *Swigert*, 697 P. 2d 504 (N.M. 1985)
Shilkret v. *Annapolis Emergency Hospital Association*, 349 A. 2d 245 (Md. 1985)
Fraijo v. *Hartlane Hospital*, 99 Cal. App. 3d 331 (Cal. 1979)

Standard of Care of Nurse-Specialists

Prosser W, *Handbook of the Law of Torts*, ed 4, West Publishing, St. Paul, 1971, §32, pp. 161-166.
61 *Am Jur 2d*, PHYSICIANS & SURGEONS §26
Restatement (Second) TORTS §299A, Comment d
Shore NL, "Advanced Nursing Practice and Prescriptive Authority: A Victory for New Jersey Nurses," *Seton Hall Legisl J* 17:576, 1993.

Salatka MA, "Professional Liability in Critical Care Nursing," *Ohio N U L Rev* 19:85, 1992.

Note: "Nursing and the Future of Health Care: The Independent Practice Imperative," *Golden Gate U L Rev*, 20:593, 1990.

Fralic MF, "Nursing's Precious Resource: The Clinical Nurse Specialist," *J Nurs Admin* 18(2):5, 1988.

Comment, "Critical Care Nurses: A Case for Legal Recognition of the Growing Responsibilities and Accountability in the Nursing Profession," *J Contemp L* 11:239, 1984.

Regan W, "Nurse Specialists: Authority and Accountability," *Regan Rep Nurs L* 24(5):1, 1983.

Cushing M, "When Medical Standards Apply to Nurse Practitioners," *Am J Nurs* 82:1274, 1982.

Mitchell v. *Amarillo Hospital District*, 855 S.W. 2d 857 (Texas 1993)

Gibson v. *Bossier City General Hospital*, 594 So. 2d 1332 (La. 1991)

Cangelosi v. *Our Lady of Lake Medical Center*, 564 So. 2d 654 (La. 1989)

Planned Parenthood of Northwest Indiana v. *Vines*, 543 N.E. 2d 654 (Ind. 1989)

Northern Trust Co. v. *Louis A. Weiss Memorial Hospital*, 493 N.E. 2d 6 (Ill. 1986)

Fein v. *Permanente Medical Group*, 211 Cal. Rptr. 368, 695 P. 2d 665 (Cal. 1985)

Parks v. *Perry*, 314 S.E. 2d 287 (N.C. 1984)

Czubinsky v. *Doctors Hospital*, 188 Cal. Rptr. 684 (Cal. 1983)

Guillory v. *Employers Mutual*, 441 So. 2d 505 (La. 1983)

Tice v. *Hall*, 303 S.E. 2d 832 (N.C. 1983)

Standard of Care of Nursing Students

Northrop CE, "Nursing Students," in *Legal Issues in Nursing* (Northrop CE and Kelly ME, eds.), C.V. Mosby, St. Louis, 1987, Ch. 19.

Creighton H, *Law Every Nurse Should Know*, ed 4, WB Saunders, Philadelphia, 1981, pp. 137-141

Tschikota S, "The Clinical Decision-Making Processes of Student Nurses," *J Nurs Educ* 32(9):389, 1993.

Northrop CE, "Student Nurses and Legal Accountability," *IMPRINT* 32:16, 1985.

Raicevich v. *Plum Creek Medical P.C.*, 819 F. Supp. 2d 929 (Col. 1993)

Hampton v. *Greenfield*, 576 So. 2d 630 (La. 1991)

Central Anesthesia Associates v. *Worthy*, 333 S.E. 2d 829 (Ga. 1985)

Habuda v. *Trustees of Rex Hospital*, 164 S.E. 2d 17 (N.C. 1968)

Honeywell v. *Rogers*, 251 F. Supp. 841 (Pa. 1966)

Payne v. *Garvey*, 142 S.E. 2d 158 (N.C. 1965)

Standard of Care in an Emergency

Buschiazzo L, *The Handbook of Emergency Nursing Management*, Aspen Publishers, Inc., Rockville, Md., 1987.

Louisell D and Williams H, *Medical Malpractice*, Matthew Bender & Co., New York, 1983, §9.05

Mancini M and Gale A, *Emergency Care and the Law*, Aspen Systems, Rockville, Md., 1981.

Prosser W, *Handbook of the Law of Torts*, ed 4, West Publishing, St. Paul, 1971, §33, pp. 169-170

Fiesta J, "Emergency Department Liability: General Legal Issues for Nurses," *Nurs Management* 21(11):18, 1990.

Marhoefer v. *Nacozy*, 2 Cal. Rptr. 2d 466 (Cal. 1991)

Brown v. *North Broward Hospital District*, 521 So. 2d 143 (Fla. 1988)

Floyd v. *Willacy County Hospital District*, 706 S.W. 2d 731 (Texas 1986)

Anthony v. *Hospital Service District No. 1*, 477 So. 2d 1180 (La. 1985)

Hammond v. *Grissom*, 470 So. 2d 1049 (Miss. 1985)

People v. *Flushing Hospital & Medical Center*, 471 N.Y.S. 2d 745 (N.Y. 1984)

Bartimus v. *Paxton Community Hospital*, 458 N.E. 2d 1072 (Ill. 1983)

Lunsford v. *Board of Nurse Examiners*, 648 S.W. 2d 391 (Texas 1983)

Murphy v. *Rowland*, 609 S.W. 2d 292 (Texas 1981)

Ulma v. *Yonkers General Hospital*, 384 N.Y.S. 2d 201 (N.Y. 1981)

Good Samaritan Laws and Their Effect

57 *Am Jur 2d*, NEGLIGENCE, §§5-46

Annotation, 68 ALR 4th 294, "Construction and Application of Good Samaritan Statutes."

Griffith GLH, "The Standard of Care Expected of a First Aid Volunteer," *Mod L Rev* 53:255, 1990.

Northrop CE, "How Good Samaritan Laws Do and Don't Protect You," *Nursing '90* 20(2):50, 1990.

Murphy EK, "Good Samaritan Laws—Who They Protect and How," *AORN J* 50:640, 1989.

Rozovsky LE and Rozovsky FA, "The Nurse as 'Good Samaritan,'" *Canadian O R Nurs J* 7(3):20, 1989.

Tuttle R, "Hospital Emergency Rooms—Application of Good Samaritan Laws," *Med Tr Tech Q* 31:141, 1984.

Brandt EA, "Good Samaritan Laws—The Legal Placebo: A Current Analysis," *Akron L Rev* 17:303, 1983.

Johnson v. *Matviuw*, 531 N.E. 2d 970 (Ill. 1988)

Kearns v. *Superior Court (Von Rader)*, 204 Cal. App. 3d 1325 (Cal. 1988)

McCain v. *Batson*, 760 P. 2d 725 (Mont. 1988)

Clayton v. *Kelly*, 357 S.E. 2d 865 (Ga. 1987)

Burciaga v. *St. John's Hospital*, 187 Cal. App. 3d 710 (Cal. 1986)

Gregg v. *Neurological Associates*, 263 S.E. 2d 496 (Ga. 1979)

Hamburger v. *Henry Ford Hospital*, 248 N.W. 2d 155 (Mich. 1979)

McKenna v. *Cedars of Lebanon Hospital*, 93 Cal. App. 3d 282 (Cal. 1979)

Wallace v. *Hall*, 244 S.E. 2d 129 (Ga. 1978)

Compulsory Assistance/Rescue Statutes

Restatement (Second) TORTS, §314, comment c

Annotations: 64 ALR 4th 1200, "Liability for Injury or Death Allegedly Caused by Activities of Hospital Rescue Team."; 33 ALR 3d 301, "Duty of One Other Than Carrier or Employer to Render Assistance to One For Whose Initial Injury He Is Not Liable."; 64 ALR 2d 1179, "Duty and Liability of One Who Voluntarily Undertakes to Care for Injured Person."

Minnesota Statutes, §604.05

Vermont Statutes Annotated, Title 12, §519

Wisconsin Statutes, §895.48

Wyoming Statutes, §1-1-120

Quebec Statutes, 1975, Ch. 6, sec. 2

Note, "Creation of a Duty Absent a Special Relationship—Legal Duty Based on a Moral Obligation," *Whittier L Rev* 6:605, 1984.

Soldano v. *O'Daniels*, 141 Cal. App. 3d 443, 190 Cal. Rptr. 310 (Cal. 1983)

Determining Negligence—Effect of Surrounding Circumstances

Louisell D and Williams H, *Medical Malpractice*, Matthew Bender & Company, New York, 1983, §9.05.

57 *Am Jur 2d*, NEGLIGENCE, §1

Restatement (Second) TORTS, §11

Casucci v. *Kenmore Mercy Hospital*, 534 N.Y.S. 2d 606 (N.Y. 1988)

Kirk v. *Michael Reese Hospital*, 513 N.E. 2d 397 (Ill. 1987)

Chapman v. *Carlson*, 240 So. 2d 263 (Miss. 1970)

Long v. *Sledge*, 209 So. 2d 814 (Miss. 1968)

Lince v. *Monson*, 108 N.W. 2d 845 (Mich. 1961)

Impaired Nurses

Annotation, 55 ALR 3d 1141, "Revocation of Nurse's License to Practice Profession."

"Impairment: To Report or Not to Report—Is There a Choice?" *J Nurs* 22:7, 1992.

Alexander D and O'Quinn-Larson J, "When Nurses are Addicted to Drugs: Confronting an Impaired Co-Worker," *Nursing '90* 20(8):55, 1990.

Baywood T, "Substance Abuse and Obligations to Colleagues," *Nurs Management* 21(8):40, 1990.

Fiesta J, "The Impaired Nurse—Who Is Liable?" *Nurs Management* 21(10):20, 1990.
Fry ST, "Whistle-Blowing by Nurses: A Matter of Ethics," *Nurs Outlook* 37(1):56, 1990.
Selbach KH, "Chemical Dependency in Nursing," *AORN J* 52(3):531, 1990.
Green P, "The Chemically Dependent Nurse," *Nurs Clin N Am* 24(1):81, 1989.
Kotyk V, "Manitoba's Response: Nurses at Risk," *Canadian Nurse* 84(4):18, 1988.
Burns v. *Board of Nursing*, 495 N.W. 2d 698 (Iowa 1993)
Navarro v. *George*, 615 A. 2d 890 (Pa. 1992)
Alabama Board of Nursing v. *Herrick*, 454 So. 2d 1041 (Ala. 1984)
Arthur v. *District of Columbia Nurses' Examining Board*, 459 A. 2d 141 (D.C. 1984)
Leib v. *Board of Examiners for Nursing*, 411 A. 2d 42 (Conn. 1979)

Standard of Care—Violation of Statutes

Prosser W, *Handbook of the Law of Torts*, ed 4, West Publishing, St. Paul, 1971, §36, p. 190
Restatement (Second) TORTS, §285
Mitchell v. *Amarillo Hospital District*, 855 S.W. 2d 857 (Texas 1993)
Central Anesthesia Associates v. *Worthy*, 325 S.E. 2d 819 (Ga. 1985)
Rafferty v. *Commonwealth, State Board of Nursing*, 499 A. 2d 289 (Pa. 1984)
McCarl v. *State Board*, 396 A. 2d 866 (Pa. 1978)

PART TWO

SPECIAL RULES
OF LIABILITY

Part 2

INTRODUCTORY NOTE

Is the nurse who has committed an act of malpractice held liable even though the nurse is employed by a physician or a hospital? Is it possible that the physician or hospital can be held liable and the nurse escape liability? To what extent is the nurse's employment status a factor in liability for malpractice? Are the school nurse and industrial nurse *more* likely or *less* likely to be sued for malpractice than their general-duty colleagues? These are some of the problems treated in Part 2 of this course, in which we will examine in greater depth the nature and extent of the nurse's liability.

The various legal doctrines explained in this part will give you insight into the ways in which the law fixes liability for acts of malpractice and will show how you may be subjected to a greater exposure to liability based on such factors as your state of employment or the unique legal status of your employer. The fundamental doctrines covered in Part 2 are the rule of personal liability, the liability of the nurse for the acts of others, the doctrine of *respondeat superior*, the doctrines of charitable immunity and governmental immunity, and the special liability of occupational health nurses.

RULE OF PERSONAL LIABILITY

2-1   If there is one rule that all nurses should know and clearly understand, it is the fundamental rule of law that *every person is liable for his or her own tortious conduct.* (Remember: A tort is a private legal wrong.) This is called the rule of personal liability.

While the rule of personal liability is simple enough, it is often misunderstood. Stating the rule in a different way may help clarify its meaning: The law does not permit a wrongdoer (in the tort-liability sense) to avoid legal liability for his or her own wrongdoing even though someone else also may be sued and held legally liable for the wrongful conduct in question under another rule of law.

The rule of personal liability is a rule that

☐   protects nurses against lawsuits for malpractice

☐   holds everyone personally liable for his or her own tortious conduct

☐   makes some persons liable for the tortious conduct of others

---

2-2   The rule of personal liability applies to the conduct of

☐   nurses only

☐   doctors and nurses only

☐   professional persons only

☐   everyone

2-3

■ Doctor D writes an order: "Walk the patient 3x daily, even if she protests." Nurse N tells Doctor D that carrying out his order *literally* could result in harm to the patient. Doctor D assures N that he will take full responsibility for any harmful consequences. N complies with the order and the patient is harmed. She later sues Nurse N.

Doctor D's verbal assurance to Nurse N is legally sufficient to protect N from liability to the patient for the harm suffered.

     True   **False**

      ☐   ☐

2-1 *holds everyone personally liable for his or her own tortious conduct*   **2-2** *everyone*   **2-3** *False*

If you checked the wrong answer, turn to p. 100, Note A.

2-4

■ While employed as a general-duty nurse in a hospital, Nurse N negligently injures a patient.

Assuming that under the applicable law the hospital can be held liable for the negligent acts of its employees, which of the following conclusions (if any) would apply?

☐ If the injured person sues and collects damages from the hospital, Nurse N cannot be held personally liable.

☐ Nurse N cannot be held liable under any circumstances since N's hospital employer automatically assumes liability for its nurses' negligent conduct.

☐ Both Nurse N and N's hospital employer can be held liable for N's negligent conduct.

☐ None of the above

2-5   The law will absolve nurses from personal liability for their negligent conduct

☐ provided they are employed by hospitals that are insured against the negligent conduct of employees

☐ if they can show they were carrying out the specific orders of a physician

☐ in both of the above instances

☐ in neither of the above instances

2-4   *Both Nurse N and N's hospital employer can be held liable for N's negligent conduct.*

2-5   *in neither of the above instances*

2-6   The rule of personal liability becomes particularly pertinent when applied to the acts of nurses who are supervised by other nurses. In every instance the fundamental rule is the same: *The nurse who is negligent is always personally liable even though someone else also may be sued and held liable.*

- Nurse N (an RN) directs Nurse P (a practical nurse) to perform a nursing function that N knows the latter is not qualified to carry out. P follows N's orders without question, however, and harm results to the patient, who then sues both N and P.

Yes   No

☐   ☐   If P is found to be negligent, can N also be held liable in the given circumstances?

☐   ☐   If N is found to be negligent, would P thereby be relieved of liability?

SUPERVISOR'S LIABILITY FOR THE ACTS OF SUBORDINATES

2-7   While all professional persons are held liable for their own negligent conduct (malpractice), there are certain circumstances under which a person who supervises others may be held liable for the negligent acts of those he or she supervises. Thus, a nursing supervisor is expected to know whether the one to whom he or she has assigned specific nursing duties is competent to perform them with or without supervision. The supervisor's inability to properly evaluate the patient's nursing needs and the nurse's capabilities will be sufficient to hold the supervisor liable for any harm that results to the patient.

True   False

☐   ☐   A nursing supervisor may not safely assume that an RN is competent to carry out every assigned nursing function.

☐   ☐   The complexity of a patient's nursing needs might make it legally improper for a supervisor to assign a particular nurse to the patient even if the nurse is an RN.

☐   ☐   Provided a nurse is properly licensed, it is not a supervisor's responsibility to assess the nurse's competence to perform particular nursing functions.

2-6   *Yes*   **2-7**   *True   False*
           No   ☐   ☑
           At this point you may   ☑   ☐
           wish to review Frames 1- ☐   ☑
           91 through 1-98.

2-8

■ Nursing supervisor S gives Nurse N a routine nursing assignment that, as an RN, N should be able to perform without difficulty. Nevertheless, N's negligence causes the patient to be seriously burned.

Under these facts, which of the following would be true?

☐ S can be held liable because he or she made the nursing assignment in question.

☐ S can be held liable for failing to ascertain Nurse N's competence to perform the assignment.

☐ Nurse N alone can be held liable for her negligence in carrying out an assignment clearly within her capabilities.

2-9

■ OR supervisor S directs a nursing student to assist at a major abdominal surgery even though S knows the student has assisted during minor surgical procedures on only two occasions. As a result of the student's negligence, a laparotomy sponge is left in the patient, with serious consequences.

On what basis could the nursing student be held liable in the event of a malpractice suit?

☐ for failure to discuss his or her limitations with S prior to assisting at the surgery

☐ for lack of care in counting the sponges

☐ for both of the above

☐ for neither of the above

2-10 On what basis could the OR supervisor be held liable?

☐ for the assignment of the nursing student despite the knowledge of the latter's limited qualifications to assist at major surgery

☐ for failure to supervise the nursing student more closely during the operation

☐ for both of the above

☐ for neither of the above

2-8 ☐
☐
☑

2-9 *for both of the above*

2-10 *for both of the above*

ASSIGNMENT PROBLEMS FACED BY SUPERVISORY NURSES

Supervisory nurses have responsibilities that necessarily put them at greater risk of personal liability, so a little further discussion of their legal position is in order. To begin, the basic rule is clear: Every nurse, whether subordinate or supervisor, is expected to provide the same degree of care that a reasonably prudent nurse with the same level of expertise and training would give under comparable circumstances. Since it is a supervisor's job to supervise, he or she is held to the standard of care of other reasonably prudent supervisors in the same or similar circumstances. What does the law expect of such persons?

Whether the title is head nurse, charge nurse, operating room supervisor, cardiac care unit supervisor, recovery room supervisor, emergency room supervisor, or simply the unit manager, nurses in charge are directly responsible for the quality of care rendered by everyone working under their overall area of responsibility. The list may include nurses, licensed practical nurses, nursing students, medical and surgical technicians, special duty nurses, nurses' aides, orderlies, and other persons who have direct patient care functions.

Supervisory nurses can be held liable for errors or misjudgments in a number of other areas, apart from making nursing assignments to nurses that are beyond their known competence. For example, supervisory nurses can be held liable for errors or misjudgments in the hiring or firing of nurses, inadequate staff orientation, inadequate evaluation of the competence of staff nurses, failing to adequately document staff problems, or failing to take appropriate remedial measures when significant problems arise in the nursing unit.

A major part of the supervisor's responsibility is the making of careful nursing assignments, sometimes in the face of drastic staffing shortages. Even though the standards of the Joint Commission on Accreditation of Healthcare Organizations (JCAHO) require hospitals to maintain a sufficient number of duly licensed registered nurses on duty "at all times" to plan, supervise, and evaluate nursing care, as well as to give patients the professional nursing care they require, supervisors often are forced to "float" nurses from their normally assigned units to others that may call for nursing skills they simply do not possess. The legal risks of so doing are apparent (for supervisor and float nurse alike), but this does not always solve the *practical* problems supervisory nurses have to face when dealing with staffing crises not of their own making.

Supervisors who believe their units are inadequately staffed must make their views known to hospital administration promptly and emphatically, *preferably in writing*. They should carefully document incidents in which patients have been endangered through lack of proper staffing, pointing out how substandard assignments expose patients to physical harm and the hospital as well as themselves to consequent malpractice suits. The failure to take vigorous action of this type will inevitably lead to the emotional trauma of litigation and an unnecessary challenge to a supervisor's professional competence.

POINTS TO REMEMBER

1. It is a fundamental rule of law that every person is legally responsible for his or her own tortious conduct. This is called the rule of personal liability.

2. Under the rule of personal liability a wrongdoer cannot avoid legal liability for his or her own wrongful conduct, even though someone else may share that liability under some other rule of law.

3. Physicians cannot alter the rule of personal liability by their agreement to assume responsibility for the negligent acts of their nurses. In the final analysis, nurses will always be held liable for their own negligent conduct.

4. Supervisors ordinarily will not be held liable for the negligent acts of those whom they supervise, since all professional persons are held liable for their own negligent conduct.

5. A supervisor *may* be held liable for the acts of someone he or she supervises if the supervisor is either negligent in making an assignment clearly beyond the latter's capabilities or does not provide adequate supervision of a nurse or nursing student who, because of inexperience, requires close supervision in carrying out a specific function.

6. A nursing supervisor who believes that crisis staffing with float nurses will jeopardize patient safety and precipitate litigation should document his or her position and promptly inform the hospital administration.

THE DOCTRINE OF *RESPONDEAT SUPERIOR*

2-11　The preceding frames explained the rule of personal liability. Now we turn to a related legal doctrine that has a significant effect on the nurse's legal liability: the doctrine of *respondeat superior.* This doctrine is a form of vicarious (substituted) liability in which the law imputes the liability of one person or entity for the negligent acts of someone else because of a special relationship between the parties. More specifically, under the doctrine of *respondeat superior*, an employer—such as a hospital, private physician, or industrial concern—is held liable for employees' negligent acts that occur within the scope of employment (i.e., while performing their normal duties or otherwise serving the employer's interests). Since most nurses are employed by others, this doctrine assumes a position of great importance and accordingly should be clearly understood.

What is the legal effect of the doctrine of *respondeat superior*?

☐　It establishes the legal relationship of employer-employee.

☐　It absolves an employee of personal liability for his or her negligent acts.

☐　It creates liability on the part of an employer for the negligent acts of his or her employees.

2-12　In what way does the doctrine of *respondeat superior* affect the nurse's personal liability for a negligent act?

☐　It shifts the nurse's liability for negligence to the employer and thereby relieves the nurse of all personal liability.

☐　It subjects the nurse's employer to liability for the nurse's negligence but does not relieve the nurse of personal liability for the conduct in question.

☐　It has no effect on the nurse's liability for negligence in that he or she is always held solely responsible.

2-11　*It creates liability on the part of an employer for the negligent acts of his or her employees.*

2-12　*It subjects the nurse's employer to liability for the nurse's negligence . . .*

2-13 The doctrine of *respondeat superior* applies (1) only when there is an employer-employee relationship and (2) only with respect to negligent acts committed within the scope of the employment. The theory behind the doctrine is that one who is an employer should be held legally responsible for the conduct of those persons (employees) whose actions he or she has the right to direct or control.

■ Supervisory Nurse S and general-duty Nurse N are employed by Hospital H. In the course of treating a patient, S negligently directs N to give the patient the wrong medication, and in the process of administering the drug, N negligently injures the patient.

Who can be held liable to the patient for the resulting harm?

☐ only Nurse S

☐ only Nurse N

☐ only Hospital H

☐ both nurses, but not the hospital

☐ all three parties

2-14 Why would Nurse S *not* be held liable under *respondeat superior* for Nurse N's negligence?

☐ S was not N's employer

☐ both nurses were negligent

☐ *respondeat superior* does not apply in a case where two employees are equally negligent

2-13   *all three parties*   **2-14**   *S was not N's employer*
                                                 The liability of nursing supervisors is discussed on p. 100, Note B.

EXPLANATORY NOTES

Note A (from Frame 2-3)

Although many nurses undoubtedly share your view, this is not correct. As persons with professional training, nurses must always do what their education, training, and experience indicate is best for their patients, and if they knowingly perform acts that do not meet the required standards of care, they will be held personally liable. In other words, they cannot avoid legal responsibility for the consequences of their own negligent conduct, regardless of any assurances given to them by well-intentioned (but legally mistaken) physicians.

In the given example, the physician also will be held liable to the injured patient. The fact remains, however, that *the rule of personal liability cannot be bypassed merely on the verbal assurances of a physician*, and the nurse should always exercise his or her own professional judgment notwithstanding such assurances.

Proceed to Frame 2-4.

Note B (from Frame 2-14)

It is important to note that a nurse with supervisory responsibility is not held liable merely because a nurse to whom he or she has assigned nursing duties negligently injures a patient. The supervisor is liable only for his or her own negligence in carrying out the supervisory duties. Note also that the supervisor's liability is based on his or her own conduct, while the hospital's liability under *respondeat superior* arises by virtue of its employer status. The nurse with supervisory responsibilities is not the employer of the nursing personnel who work under his or her direction.

As a general rule, a nursing supervisor can assume that a subordinate nurse's registration, license, or other form of certification qualifies the individual to carry out the usual responsibilities assigned to persons with such evidence of nursing skills. Nevertheless, the supervisor can be held liable for making an assignment to a nurse who he or she has reason to believe may carry out the task negligently.

Proceed to Frame 2-15.

EXPLANATORY NOTES

Note C (from Frame 2-16)

It is remotely possible (but not likely) that the nurse, as an employee of the hospital in question, would be expected to give emergency care to highway-accident victims within his or her own city, but this theoretical obligation would certainly not extend to highway-accident victims in an adjoining state. (See, however, the exceptions noted on page 52.)

You must not forget that the *respondeat superior* doctrine applies only to an employee's acts of negligence that occur in the course of his or her employment, and the giving of emergency care to highway-accident victims is not normally a part of a nurse's employment duties. As pointed out in Part 1, while there is no *legal* obligation that nurses render such care outside their normal employment settings, the ethics of the profession encourage such humanitarian assistance.

Proceed to Frame 2-17.

2-15 Bear in mind that *respondeat superior* holds the employer liable only for negligent conduct that occurs within the scope of the employment relationship.

- Nurse N is employed by a hospital in a large city. While on a summer vacation in an adjoining state, N has occasion to give emergency care to a victim of a highway accident. N's negligence causes further injury and the victim later sues for malpractice.

Why would the doctrine of *respondeat superior* not apply in this case?

☐   the care that was given took place in a state in which the nurse was not licensed

☐   the negligent conduct did not occur within the scope of the nurse's employment

☐   the negligent conduct arose out of emergency care

2-16 If the nurse had not been on vacation, would the doctrine of *respondeat superior* apply to N's conduct in giving the emergency care?

       Yes   *No*
       ☐   ☐

2-17 Under *respondeat superior*, an employer who is sued for the alleged negligence of a nurse-employee could be held liable for a patient's injury even if the nurse-employee is found not to be negligent.

       True   *False*
       ☐   ☐

2-15   *the negligent conduct did not occur within the scope of the nurse's employment*

2-16   *No*

If you checked Yes, see p. 101, Note C.

2-17   *False*

2-18 Since most nurses are not self-employed but work for others, the doctrine of *respondeat superior* significantly affects their legal liability for acts of negligence. In the absence of both an employment relationship and negligent conduct, however, the doctrine will not apply.

Consider the following situation:

■ Nurse N is employed by Doctor D, and Nurse F, a friend of Nurse N, is employed by Doctor Z. Both doctors have their offices in the same building. One day as the nurses are leaving for lunch together, they notice an elderly lady in obvious respiratory distress in the lobby of the building. Nurse N recognizes the lady as a patient of Doctor D and immediately runs back to summon Doctor D to the lobby. Meanwhile, Nurse F goes to the victim's aid, but injures her in the attempt.

The patient later dies and her estate sues both Doctor D and Doctor Z, claiming negligence on the part of Nurse F.

Assuming Nurse F was in fact negligent, against whom would the doctrine of *respondeat superior* apply in this case?

☐ against Doctor D only

☐ against Doctor Z only

☐ against both doctors

☐ against neither doctor

2-19 Indicate which of the following legal doctrines, if any, are directly relevant in the given fact situation:

☐ emergency care rule

☐ establishment of a nurse-patient relationship

☐ rule of personal liability

☐ none of the above

2-18	☐	*If you did not select the correct*	**2-19**	☑
	☐	*answer, turn to p. 105, Note A.*		☑
	☐			☑
	☑			☐

2-20   The doctrine of *respondeat superior* is primarily concerned with the following three elements:

☐   nurse   patient   liability

☐   employer   employee   negligent conduct

☐   hospital   employee   safety rules

2-21   The rule of *respondeat superior* ordinarily does not apply when the nurse offers his or her services as a private-duty nurse, since the relationship thus established is not one of employer-employee. The private-duty nurse is considered an independent contractor who is held legally responsible for his or her own conduct. This does not apply, however, when the private-duty nurse works under the direction, supervision, and control of a hospital, nursing home, home health agency, or private physician.

The doctrine of *respondeat superior* does not apply to the negligent conduct of a nurse when he or she is employed (select two)

☐   by someone who is uninsured against malpractice claims

☐   by a particular person as a private-duty nurse at home

☐   by an employer who legally cannot be sued for the negligence of his or her employees

☐   in a state where he or she is not licensed to practice

2-22   Assume negligent conduct in the course of his or her duties on the part of each of the following nurses. With respect to which of them would the doctrine of *respondeat superior* apply?

Would apply	Would not apply	
☐	☐	An RN employed by a hospital
☐	☐	A private-duty nurse employed by a hospitalized patient
☐	☐	A practical nurse employed by a convalescent individual at home
☐	☐	A private-duty nurse employed by a hospital
☐	☐	A practical nurse employed by a physician

2-20		2-21		2-22	Would apply	Would not apply	*If you checked two or*
	☐		☐		☑	☐	*more wrong boxes,*
	☑		☑		☐	☑	*turn to p. 105, Note B.*
	☐		☑		☐	☑	
			☐		☑	☐	
					☑	☐	

EXPLANATORY NOTES

Note A (from Frame 2-18)

This was a fairly complex problem, but a little careful analysis should help clarify the matter. Doctor D could not be held liable because *respondeat superior* applies only to the act of an employee, and the negligent act in this case was committed by Doctor Z's nurse.

Theoretically, Doctor Z could be held liable since the negligent nurse was Z's employee; however, this would not sufficient to hold Doctor Z liable under *respondeat superior* because you will recall that Nurse F was on lunch hour and was not acting within the scope of her employment by Doctor Z at the time of the incident.

The correct response, therefore, is that *neither* doctor could be held liable. Just by way of review, *respondeat superior* holds an *employer* liable for the negligent act of an *employee* that arises out of and in the course of the *employment.* All three elements must be present or the employer cannot be held liable. In the given example, neither doctor would be held liable because Doctor D's nurse committed no negligent act, and Doctor Z's nurse (who *did* commit a negligent act) was not acting within the scope of her employment at the time.

Proceed to Frame 2-19.

Note B (from Frame 2-22)

Respondeat superior generally applies to the acts of a nurse employed by a hospital, home health care agency, or private physician. Thus, you should have had little difficulty in deciding that the rule applies to the first and last nurses listed—the registered nurse employed by the hospital and the practical nurse employed by the physician. Private duty nurses are *usually* (but not always) employed by private persons, and when they *are* so employed, they are solely responsible for their own conduct. The second and third examples illustrated this type of employment status—the private-duty nurse employed by the hospitalized patient and the practical nurse employed by the convalescent individual at home.

The fourth example was perhaps more troublesome, since the private-duty nurse was employed by a hospital rather than by a private person. Nevertheless, the legal responsibility in such a situation is the same as if the nurse were a full-time staff nurse at the hospital. Remember: The doctrine of *respondeat superior* is strictly tied to the nurse's *employment status at the time of the alleged malpractice,* not the employment status he or she usually enjoys.

Proceed to Frame 2-23.

2-23   Even though the doctrine of *respondeat superior* provides the injured patient with another party to sue, it does *not* relieve negligent nurses of their own liability. Thus, if the employer is otherwise blameless for the negligent conduct of a nurse-employee but is held liable under *respondeat superior* to pay damages to the injured patient, the employer has the legal right to recover in a separate action against the nurse-employee the amount the employer has thus been required to pay.

   ■ Nurse N, employed by a large midwestern hospital, commits an act of malpractice in the course of nursing duties that results in serious injury to Patient P.

   Under these facts, which of the following statements would be true?

   ☐   P can sue either Nurse N or the hospital for N's negligent conduct, but not both.

   ☐   If P is successful in a suit against N's employer and the latter pays the judgment rendered in the case, N can be held liable to the hospital for the judgment paid.

   ☐   If P is successful in a suit against Nurse N and N pays the judgment, N is legally entitled to recover from the hospital the amount thus paid.

NOTE: It bears repeating that while the doctrine of *respondeat superior* gives the patient someone else to sue, it does not relieve the negligent nurse of his or her ultimate liability to the patient. Moreover, an employer who is required to pay a judgment because of the negligence of a nurse-employee is less likely to seek reimbursement from the nurse than to terminate his or her employment. Thus, while *respondeat superior* affords the nurse a certain degree of protection against being sued personally, it is *not* (and should not be thought of as) a shield against liability for acts of malpractice.

2-24   Who benefits the *most* from the doctrine of *respondeat superior*: the nurse, the nurse's employer, or the injured person?

   ☐   the nurse, because it enable him or her to escape liability for negligent conduct

   ☐   the injured person, who is given an additional party (one generally in a better financial position to make payment) to sue for damages

   ☐   the employer, who can always recover any damages paid from the negligent nurse-employee

---

2-23	☐	2-24	*the injured person, who*
	☑		*is given an additional*
	☐		*party . . .*

POINTS TO REMEMBER

1. The doctrine of *respondeat superior* holds an employer legally liable for the negligent acts of his or her employees that arise out of and in the course of the employment. The legal basis of *respondeat superior* is an employer-employee relationship, with the employer being held responsible for the acts of those whom he or she has a right to supervise or control.

2. Even though *respondeat superior* may apply in a particular case, the negligent employee is always liable for his or her own negligent conduct and may be sued alone or jointly with the employer.

3. Ordinarily (but not always) the doctrine of *respondeat superior* applies to the acts of nurses when they are employed by a hospital, nursing home, or a private physician.

4. Ordinarily (but not always) the doctrine of *respondeat superior* does not apply when nurses offer their services as private-duty nurses. However, when private-duty nurses come under the direct supervision and control of a physician, nursing home, or hospital, the doctrine *will* be applicable to their conduct.

5. Employers who are required (under *respondeat superior*) to pay money damages to injured persons because of the negligence of their employees have the legal right to recover from such negligent employees the amounts thus paid.

2-25 In what way is the doctrine of *respondeat superior* related to the rule of personal liability?

☐ It completely nullifies the rule of personal liability.

☐ While it creates an additional liability, it does not hold negligent employees free from liability for their own conduct.

☐ It forces the injured person to sue someone who is blameless for the negligent acts of his or her employee.

HOSPITAL LIABILITY UNDER *RESPONDEAT SUPERIOR*

2-26 With a few exceptions, which we will discuss shortly, a hospital generally is held liable under *respondeat superior* for the negligent acts of *all* its employees—including, of course, its nurses. Many of the lawsuits brought against hospitals involve claims arising out of alleged nursing malpractice, and when liability is proved, such claims generally are paid by the hospital's liability insurance carrier.

A hospital's liability under *respondeat superior* applies to

☐ the acts of its physicians and nurses only

☐ the acts of its professional employees only

☐ the acts of its nonprofessional employees only

☐ the acts of all the hospital's employees

2-27 The underlying reason for holding a hospital liable under *respondeat superior* is that

☐ the hospital's insurance carrier is in a better financial position to pay malpractice claims than are negligent hospital employees

☐ the hospital has the legal right and authority to exercise direction and control over its employees' actions

☐ in the absence of such liability, hospitals would be unable to hire doctors, nurses, and other employees involved in patient care

2-25 *While it creates an additional liability, it does not hold negligent employees free from liability for their own conduct.*

2-26 *the acts of all the hospital's employees*

2-27 ☐ ☑ ☐

NOTE: Thus far in this discussion of *respondeat superior* we have concerned ourselves solely with acts of negligence committed by a nurse when performing nursing functions in a professional capacity, but the doctrine applies with equal force to negligent conduct of a nonprofessional nature. For example, if a nurse employed by a nursing home was directed to take a patient's blood sample to an outside laboratory by automobile and while en route injured a pedestrian, the nurse's negligence in driving the automobile (clearly not a professional nursing act) would nevertheless make the nursing home-employer liable to the pedestrian under the doctrine of *respondeat superior*.

2-28 Before one could determine whether the doctrine of *respondeat superior* would apply to the conduct of a nurse in a given situation, one would have to know

☐   who employed the nurse and paid for his or her services

☐   whether the negligent act arose out of the nurse's professional (i.e., nursing) or non-professional activities

☐   who had the legal right to direct and control the nurse's activities at the time the negligent act was committed

2-29 If a hospital were to engage the services of a private-duty nurse for general-duty nursing over a weekend, would the hospital be liable under *respondeat superior* for the nurse's negligent acts?

	Yes	*No*
	☐	☐

2-30 From the legal standpoint, *any* negligent act or omission on the part of an employed nurse, whether in a professional capacity or not, will give rise to liability on the part of the nurse's employer as long as the act or omission occurred within the scope of the employment, i.e., while on duty during working hours.

	True	*False*
	☐	☐

2-28 *who had the legal right to direct and control the nurse's activities at the time the negligent act was committed*   **2-29** *Yes*   **2-30** *True*

> **NOTE:**   We come now to a special application of the doctrine of *respondeat superior* that has particular relevance for nurses engaged in OR activities. This special application of the rule arises from the fact that an employee (the nurse) may serve two employers (the doctor and the hospital) simultaneously . . . even if only for brief periods.

THE "BORROWED SERVANT" DOCTRINE

2-31   Ordinarily, a staff physician is not liable for the failure of a hospital nurse to carry out reasonable orders in treating a patient. The mere fact that a physician gives instructions—whether verbally, on the chart, or in some other manner—does not create an employer-employee relationship between the physician and the nurse. In many if not most instances, the physician does not know *which* nurse will actually be assigned to execute the instructions. The nurse is still under the direction and control of the hospital, and the hospital *only* will be held liable for any negligence on the nurse's part in carrying out those instructions.

Indicate whether the following statements are true or false.

True	*False*	
☐	☐	A hospital is liable under *respondeat superior* for the acts of all nurses in its employ, but not when they are carrying out the orders of attending physicians.
☐	☐	General-duty nurses, but not their hospital-employers, will be held liable if they deviate from the orders of an attending physician and the patient suffers injury.
☐	☐	The attending physician, but not the hospital, will be held liable for the negligence of a hospital nurse when executing the physician's medically sound order.
☐	☐	Generally, a hospital-employed nurse is considered to be under the direction and control of the hospital, regardless of whose orders the nurse is carrying out.

	2-31	*True*	*False*
		☐	☑
		☐	☑
		☐	☑
		☑	☐

2-32

■ Doctor D, an attending physician at a local hospital, performs a thoracotomy and gives written orders for the postoperative care of the patient. One order calls for giving the patient intramuscular injections of an antibiotic at stated intervals. In administering the injection, Nurse N strikes the patient's sciatic nerve, resulting in nerve damage and a "foot drop" condition. The patient sues Nurse N, Doctor D, and the hospital.

Assuming Nurse N's negligence in giving the injection, which party is most likely to be held liable to the patient under the rule of *respondeat superior*?

☐   Nurse N

☐   the hospital

☐   Doctor D

☐   both Doctor D and the hospital

2-33 In certain circumstances, the courts have imposed legal liability on an attending physician or surgeon for a hospital nurse's negligence, while absolving the hospital of its normal liability as the nurse's employer. This exception to the rule of *respondeat superior* usually arises when a hospital nurse, although not in the regular employ of an operating surgeon, technically becomes the surgeon's temporary employee ("borrowed servant") while working under the direct supervision and control of the surgeon during an operation. This special application of *respondeat superior* rule is thus aptly called the "borrowed servant" doctrine.

The "borrowed servant" doctrine applies to an OR nurse's conduct

☐   whenever a hospital assigns him or her to OR duty

☐   whenever the OR nurse's activities require special skills and he or she is subject to the direct control of the surgeon

☐   whenever the nurse is technically "borrowed" from another unit of the hospital

---

2-32 ☐   *If you did not choose the correct*   **2-33**   *whenever the OR nurse's*
         ☑   *answer, turn to p. 135, Note A.*   *activities require special*
         ☐   *skills and he or she is*
         ☐   *subject . . .*

2-34   The key to the borrowed servant doctrine is the matter of control. Before the physician or surgeon can be held liable, it must be shown that he or she had the right to control the assisting nurse in details relating to the *specific act* that produced the injury for which liability is sought to be imposed. Unless such control can be shown, either the hospital (or possibly some other physician present) will be held liable for the nurse's negligent conduct under *respondeat superior*.

In the following fact situations, who (apart from the nurse) would be held liable for the nurse's conduct

Hospital	Doctor	
☐	☐	A scrub nurse negligently prepares the operating room for surgery.
☐	☐	An OR nurse improperly counts the sponges used during an operation.
☐	☐	A nurse anesthetist administers anesthesia at an improper rate, as prescribed by the surgeon.
☐	☐	An OR nurse improperly positions an electrosurgical machine, causing burns to the patient.

2-35   During abdominal surgery, an anesthesiologist directs a nurse in the OR to intubate a patient. The nurse does so improperly, causing injury to the patient's mouth and teeth.

Indicate whether the following statements are true or false.

True	False	
☐	☐	The anesthesiologist, but not the surgeon, could be held liable for the nurse's negligence under the borrowed servant theory.
☐	☐	The surgeon, but not the anesthesiologist, could be held liable for the nurse's negligence under the borrowed servant theory.
☐	☐	The hospital, but neither the surgeon nor the anesthesiologist, could be held liable for the nurse's negligence under *respondeat superior*.
☐	☐	The nurse, but no one else, could be held liable for the harm caused by the nurse's negligence.

2-34	Hospital	Doctor		2-35	True	False
	☑	☐			☑	☐
	☑	☐			☐	☑
	☐	☑			☐	☑
	☑	☐			☐	☑

2-36   While the borrowed servant rule most often applies to OR situations, it is equally applicable in theory to other situations in the hospital context. The critical factor in each case is whether the physician in fact becomes the nurse's temporary employer by exercising direct control over the nurse's acts.

A physician can avoid liability under the borrowed servant rule by proving

☐   the nurse was assigned by the hospital without the physician's approval

☐   the nurse was carrying out a routine nursing function

☐   the nurse was not in the operating room at the time of the incident

---

2-37   In a non–operating-room situation, it is rare for an attending physician to be held liable for a hospital nurse's negligence in carrying out treatment prescribed by the physician.

True	*False*
☐	☐

NOTE: It should be emphasized that the borrowed servant doctrine is an exception to the usual rule of *respondeat superior*. Physicians who are not employed by the hospital but are on staff and treat patients at the hospital are normally considered independent contractors and the hospital is not liable for their negligent conduct. By the same token, these physicians are not normally responsible for a nurse's negligence. The borrowed servant rule comes into play only when the physician exercises *direct control over the details of the specific nursing procedure* that caused harm to the patient.

2-36   *the nurse was carrying out a routine nursing function*   **2-37**   *True*

THE "CAPTAIN OF THE SHIP" DOCTRINE

An offshoot of the borrowed servant doctrine is the "captain of the ship" doctrine, which imposes liability on the surgeon in charge of an operation for the negligence of any of his or her nonphysician assistants during the time an operation is in progress, even though they remain employees of the hospital. This rather harsh legal doctrine has not gained widespread acceptance, and even in those few jurisdictions where it is followed its use is restricted to acts of negligence that occur in the operating room, in the presence of the surgeon, and under his or her immediate direction.

Even in the operating room, many courts make a distinction between nursing acts that are medical in nature and those considered to be essentially routine administrative or clerical tasks. In this sense, the captain of the ship doctrine has been held totally inapplicable to preoperative preparations and postoperative care. Thus, it does not apply to the negligent acts of nurses during preliminary cleaning and preparation of the operating room, sterilization of the instruments to be used, making ready the sterile drapes, placing the patient on the operating table, or any of the myriad acts carried out by nurses in the recovery room after surgery has been completed.

The majority of jurisdictions that do not adhere to the captain of the ship doctrine take the position that a surgeon's mere presence in the operating room is not enough to make the surgeon liable for the negligence of nurses who have been assigned by the hospital to assist during surgery. This is especially true where the nurse is a trained and certified anesthetist or other OR specialist. Clearly, there is a trend away from the captain of the ship doctrine and toward the recognition of the independent professional nature of nursing, both in and out of the operating room.

The borrowed servant and captain of the ship doctrines are simply special applications of the *respondeat superior* doctrine. They are of far greater importance to the hospital and physician than to the nurse because they fix liability on those parties for acts they did not directly supervise or carry out. The legal phrase characterizing this form of substituted liability is *vicarious liability*.

THE DOCTRINE OF HOSPITAL CORPORATE LIABILITY

Up to this point, we have been discussing the hospital's liability for the negligent acts of its employees under the doctrine of *respondeat superior*. There is another basis for liability of the hospital, however—known as the doctrine of hospital corporate liability—that holds that the hospital has a direct and independent responsibility to provide due care to every hospitalized patient. This legal doctrine was first enunciated in the landmark case of *Darling* v. *Charleston Community Hospital*, 211 N.E. 2d 53 (Ill. 1965), in which the court found that the hospital failed to comply with various standards designed to ensure patient safety, including the JCAHO standards, the rules and regulations of the state health department, and the hospital's own bylaws and regulations.

Under the doctrine of hospital corporate liability as it has evolved over the years, a hospital can be held liable to its patient for negligence in maintaining its facilities, negligence in providing and maintaining medical equipment, negligence in hiring, supervising, and retaining nurses and other employees, and failing to have in place basic procedures to protect patients. It can also be held liable for the negligent acts of a private staff physician if the hospital knew of the physician's incompetence or could have detected it through reasonable screening or supervision. The doctrine also has been applied to impose obligations on hospitals to maintain responsibility for essential functions, such as emergency rooms. Thus, in *Jackson v. Power*, 743 P. 2d 1376 (Alaska 1987), the court held that the hospital-defendant in a malpractice suit had "a nondelegable duty to provide non-negligent physician care in its emergency room," and could not shift that responsibility to its independent contractor ER physicians.

At least one state, Florida, has by statute incorporated "institutional liability" or "corporate negligence" in its regulation of hospitals. West's Florida Statutes Annotated § 768.60.

Cases involving hospital corporate liability have arisen out of the failure of hospitals to provide proper and safe instrumentalities for the treatment of conditions they undertake to treat, especially in emergency situations, such as failure to provide an adequate 24-hour anesthesia service, failure to have an on-call system capable of producing specialists in emergency situations, failure to send a patient to a trauma center, and failure to have on hand essential ER equipment for making prompt and accurate diagnoses.

An increasingly significant basis for holding hospitals liable is their failure to have sufficient numbers of nurses on duty to provide the fundamental quality of care that is required. Because of the shortage of nurses, many hospital units are routinely (or at least intermittently) understaffed and the nurses on duty are consequently overworked, often being floated to units calling for nursing skills they may not have. It goes without saying that in this sort of environment patient safety is more likely to be compromised, harmful errors are more likely to occur, and malpractice lawsuits are more likely to follow.

Yet another basis for holding hospitals liable as corporate entities was the enactment by Congress in 1986 of the federal Emergency Medical Treatment and Active Labor Act (EMTALA) 42 U.S.C. § 1395dd(d)(2)(A), often called the "Anti-dumping Act." This legislation was aimed at reducing the practice of some hospitals of dumping patients—that is, transferring them to other hospitals or simply refusing to treat them because of the patient's inability to pay.

Despite the growing importance of the hospital corporate liability doctrine as a quality control mechanism, from the standpoint of the hospital-based nurse, *respondeat superior* continues to play the most significant role in determining who ultimately is held liable for the nurse's negligent acts or omissions. The doctrine has several notable exceptions, however, which we will now examine.

THE DOCTRINE OF CHARITABLE IMMUNITY

2-38 The first important exception to the *respondeat superior* doctrine can have far-reaching financial consequences for nurses who practice in a few American states. In these states the doctrine of *charitable immunity* applies, which holds that a charitable (i.e., nonprofit) hospital cannot be held liable in tort by a person who has been injured due to the negligence of a hospital employee. The practical effect of this rule is to force the injured person to sue the negligent hospital employee personally.

In a state that recognizes the charitable immunity doctrine, which of the following classes of nurses would be affected the most?

☐ school nurses

☐ occupational health nurses

☐ nonprofit hospital nurses

☐ public health nurses

☐ all categories of nurses

2-39 In a state that adheres to the charitable immunity doctrine, would a proprietary (profit-making) hospital be liable for the negligent acts of its nurses under *respondeat superior*?

Yes *No*
☐ ☐

2-40 What is the significant legal consequence when the charitable immunity rule applies to hospital care in a particular jurisdiction?

☐ An injured patient cannot prevail in a suit against a charitable hospital whose negligent employee caused the injury.

☐ A negligent charitable hospital employee is protected against being held personally liable to the injured patient.

☐ The law in that jurisdiction permits the injured patient to hold both the hospital and its negligent employee liable.

2-38 *nonprofit hospital nurses*	**2-39** *Yes* *If you checked the wrong answer, turn to p. 135, Note B.*	**2-40** *An injured patient cannot prevail in a suit against a charitable hospital . . .*

NOTE: At one time, a large number of jurisdictions adhered to the charitable immunity rule. The rationale for the rule was the duty of a public charity (such as a nonprofit hospital) as a trustee to apply all of its funds to its charitable purpose, and that to permit the invasion of these funds to satisfy tort claims would destroy the sources of charitable support on which the enterprise depends. This rationale faded significantly with the growth and prevalence of hospitalization insurance and Medicare and Medicaid benefits, while the availability of hospital liability insurance further reduced the impact of tort claims on the hospital's finances. The average so-called "nonprofit" hospital today is a large, well-run corporation so businesslike in its monetary requirements for admission and its methods for collection of accounts that it could hardly be called a "charity." Consequently, a vast majority of states have abolished the charitable immunity rule either directly by statute or indirectly by judicial decision.

Approximately 35 states have rejected the rule in its entirety, while several others have retained the rule in varying degrees and in the following ways: (1) by limiting the amount of damages recoverable against a charitable hospital (20,000 dollars in Massachusetts; 10,000 dollars in New Jersey; 100,000 dollars in Maryland), (2) by limiting the amount recoverable only to the extent of existing hospital liability insurance (as in Maine, Rhode Island, and Tennessee), or (3) by limiting damage recovery to paying patients (as in Georgia, Alabama, and Utah).

In Arkansas, charitable immunity has been retained for the hospital itself but a statute permits a direct action against the hospital's liability insurer. In Colorado, case law provides that a judgment against a charitable hospital may not be satisfied out of the trust funds of the institution, but recovery may be available out of liability insurance proceeds. In Georgia, charitable immunity has been retained for care rendered to true charity patients but does not apply to patients who pay full compensation for their medical services.

Nurses who practice in charitable (nonprofit) hospitals in states that still recognize the charitable immunity rule—either in its entirety or partially—are thereby exposed to a greater risk of being sued and held *personally* liable for their acts of negligence in treating hospitalized patients. Thus, it is essential that nurses who practice in these states purchase malpractice insurance to protect themselves against suits brought by patients who cannot recover damages from the hospital.

In Canada the doctrine of charitable immunity has not been adopted. Accordingly, a hospital in Canada can be held liable for the negligence of its employees under the usual rule of *respondeat superior*.

THE DOCTRINE OF GOVERNMENTAL IMMUNITY

2-41 Another exception to the *respondeat superior* doctrine comes into play when the nurse's employer is a state or provincial government. The common-law rule of *governmental immunity* provides that state and provincial governments cannot be held liable for the negligent acts of their employees while carrying out governmental activities. However, some states and provinces have changed this rule by statute, and in these particular jurisdictions the doctrine of *respondeat superior* continues to apply to the acts of nurses employed by the state or provincial government. Consider the following situation:

■ Public Nurse N is employed by State X in one of its mental health clinics. While performing encephalography on a patient, N negligently injures his scalp.

Under these facts can the patient sue State X for his injury?

Yes	*No*	*Can't be sure*
☐	☐	☐

2-42 If State X has *not* passed any special legislation with respect to liability for acts of its employees, against whom can suit be brought by the patient for his injury?

☐ only Nurse N

☐ only State X

☐ both Nurse N and State X

☐ none of the above

2-43 If State X *has* enacted a statute waiving (relinquishing) its governmental immunity, against whom can suit be brought by the patient for his injury?

☐ only Nurse N

☐ only State X

☐ both Nurse N and State X

☐ none of the above

2-41 *Can't be sure*

No information has been given about the state's position on immunity; hence, we really don't know enough to make a proper choice.

2-42 *only Nurse N*

2-43 *both Nurse N and State X*

GOVERNMENTAL IMMUNITY FROM TORT SUITS

The doctrine of governmental immunity from suit—occasionally referred to as "sovereign immunity"—descended from early British law. In England it was a cardinal rule that, since the sovereign (the king) was considered the "giver" of law, he was held to be beyond the law and no judgment could be rendered against him. The doctrine of sovereign or governmental immunity became entrenched in U.S. jurisprudence, much like the doctrine of charitable immunity. Unlike charitable immunity, however, the states have been much slower to reject the doctrine of governmental immunity as applied to government-operated hospitals, even though the trend is clearly in that direction.

In those states that still adhere to the doctrine of governmental immunity, the courts have held to their basic legal position that a state, in its discharge of purely governmental functions, should not (and therefore cannot) be held liable in tort. Some have cited the direct economic consequences to the state if it were forced to pay for the tortious conduct of its agents and employees. On the other hand, many states, either by legislation or judicial decision, have substantially rejected immunity, either completely or by allowing damage claims up to a specified dollar amount, or the amount of the state's existing liability insurance coverage.

The following states still adhere to the doctrine of governmental immunity, either completely or within specified limitations: Alabama, Colorado, Delaware, Maine, Maryland, Michigan, Missouri, North Dakota, South Dakota, Texas, Virginia, Wisconsin, and Wyoming. It bears repeating that nurses who practice in state-operated hospitals or other medical facilities in these states are more likely to be sued personally, a fact that makes the purchase of malpractice insurance a virtual necessity.

LIABILITY OF THE SCHOOL NURSE

2-44   In the United States the rules relating to governmental immunity affect not only nurses employed directly by state governments but also nurses employed by school districts. These rules apply because education is a state function in the United States, and a school district is therefore legally considered a subdivision of the state government. Accordingly, a nurse employed by a school district will be subject to the same legal liabilities for his or her tortious conduct as are other government employees in that jurisdiction.

The school nurse employed in a state that is immune from tort liability is exposed to a ☐ greater   ☐ lesser   risk of personal liability than a school nurse in a state that has waived its immunity to tort liability.

2-45

   ■ Nurse N is a school nurse in State X, which has waived its immunity to tort liability.

If Nurse N commits a negligent act while in the employ of a school district in State X, which of the following would apply?

   ☐   The rule of *respondeat superior* would apply to N's conduct, making the school district liable.

   ☐   The rule of *respondeat superior* would not apply to N's conduct, making the nurse the only party against whom suit could be brought.

2-46   If state X in the previous example had not waived its immunity to tort liability, which of the following would apply?

   ☐   Nurse N could expect to be sued and held liable personally for the negligent conduct.

   ☐   The state would most likely bring suit against Nurse N to recover the damages paid out because of the negligence.

   ☐   The person injured as a result of Nurse N's negligence would have no legal basis for suing Nurse N or State X.

2-44 *greater*	**2-45** *The rule of* respondeat superior *would apply to N's conduct, making the school district liable.*	**2-46** *Nurse N could expect to be sued and held liable personally . . .*

2-47   The school nurse is held to the same standard of care applicable to other professional nurses with comparable backgrounds and training and working in similar circumstances, unless that standard is modified by statute.

- School Nurse N administers an anticonvulsant drug to a 7-year-old child during school hours, pursuant to parental consent and a physician's order. Hurried, Nurse N negligently administers too large a dose, however, causing the child to suffer a severe reaction and consequent injury requiring hospitalization.

    In a lawsuit brought by the child's parents, Nurse N's conduct would be measured against

    ☐   that of reasonably prudent general-duty hospital nurses

    ☐   that of reasonably prudent special-duty nurses

    ☐   that of reasonably prudent school nurses

    ☐   all of the above

2-48   In the previous example, assume that the state law specifically provides that a school nurse who administers medications to a child pursuant to parental consent and a physician's written order cannot be held liable for ordinary negligence in so doing, and that gross or willful negligence is the only basis for holding a nurse liable.

This statute would

☐   have no effect on the outcome of this case

☐   absolve the nurse of liability in this case

☐   establish the standard of care governing this case

NOTE: In point of fact, nearly a dozen states now have laws regulating the administration of medications by school nurses and other school personnel. The Connecticut statute is one that provides immunity to nurses for ordinary negligence, as in the example just given.

2-47   *that of reasonably prudent school nurses*

2-48   *establish the standard of care governing this case*

2-49 School nurses usually are not under the direct supervision of physicians, which makes their position legally more perilous than that of nurses who work under the direct supervision of physicians. For this reason, school nurses should be especially alert to their legal responsibilities and exercise the utmost in good judgment in all that they do.

■ Nurse N is the school nurse for a large school in a jurisdiction that has *not* waived its immunity to tort liability. One morning a 16-year-old girl reports to the nurse, complaining of moderately severe abdominal cramps. The nurse decides that the girl is experiencing simple menstrual cramps and applies a hot water bottle to the affected area. Her condition worsens and the child eventually is removed to the hospital, where her condition is diagnosed as acute appendicitis. The child dies in surgery because of the delay in treatment attributable to the nurse's conduct.

In a malpractice suit alleging the foregoing facts, who could be held liable for the child's death?

☐   the nurse alone

☐   the school district alone

☐   both the nurse and the school district

2-50 Because they work in a nonmedical environment, school nurses must exercise considerable independent judgment and must be able to recognize and treat most of the ailments and injuries that school children experience. One of their chief tasks, of course, is knowing how to identify those conditions that require immediate medical attention, and making the necessary arrangements therefor.

What would be the *most significant* professional qualification of a nurse hired by a school district as a school nurse?

☐   the nurse's ability to work closely with school officials in assessing the health status of students

☐   the nurse's ability to exercise independent nursing judgment in critical emergency situations

☐   the nurse's ability to properly counsel students on their medical and dental health problems

2-49 *the nurse alone*   **2-50** *the nurse's ability to exercise independent nursing judgment . . .*

NOTE: Since traumatic injuries are among the most common reasons for students to visit school nurses, the latter must be capable of providing competent emergency care. This responsibility includes, of course, the ability to diagnose injuries and illnesses and to treat them appropriately or refer the injured students to physicians or hospital facilities. Sometimes, nurses are called on to treat sports injuries that occur after school hours—generally outside the scope of the nurse's normal employment. In these situations, the nurse is held to the standard of care of other reasonably prudent nurses in similar emergency circumstances, as discussed in Part 1. Note, however, that the Good Samaritan statutes in a few states have granted specific civil immunity against suit to nurses who render emergency care at school athletic programs or competitive sports events. Ohio and Missouri have such provisions in their Good Samaritan laws.

Finally, unlike the immunity against suit accorded school boards in the United States, in Canada there is no statutory rule of immunity that precludes the bringing of a suit directly against a local school board for the negligence of one of its nurses. Usually, the injured person or that individual's legal representative files suit against both the school board and the nurse in question.

Special Rules and Doctrines
That Relate to the Liability of Nurses

Name of Rule or Doctrine	How the Rule or Doctrine Works
Rule of personal Liability	Every individual is always held personally responsible for his or her own negligent conduct, even though someone else also may be held liable for the particular harm or injury that resulted to another.
Supervisor's Liability for the Acts of Subordinates	A nursing supervisor may be held *personally liable* for the negligent conduct of employees under his or her supervision for, among other things, assigning a nurse to a task beyond the nurse's capabilities.
Respondeat Superior Doctrine	This doctrine holds an employer liable for the negligent acts of employees whose conduct the employer has the right to direct or control. This vicarious (substituted) form of liability applies only to conduct within the scope of the employment.
Borrowed Servant Doctrine	On occasion, though rarely, a hospital nurse may become the temporary "borrowed servant" of a physician in a particular treatment setting (such as the OR) for specific acts carried out under the *direct supervision and control of the physician.*
Captain of the Ship Doctrine	An offshoot of the borrowed servant doctrine that imposes strict liability on the surgeon in charge of an operation for the negligent acts of all nonmedical OR personnel who assist during the operation.
Doctrine of Hospital Corporate Liability	The doctrine that holds a hospital liable for injuries to patients based on its independent, corporate legal responsibility to assure the quality of care of all hospitalized patients.
Doctrine of Charitable Immunity	A doctrine applicable in relatively few states whose laws provide immunity to nonprofit hospitals against liability based on the alleged negligence of hospital employees. In these states, the injured patient is more likely to sue the offending employee alone.
Doctrine of Governmental Immunity	A doctrine applicable in certain jurisdictions that provide immunity to the state against suits based on the alleged negligence of state employees while carrying out their normal governmental activities. Nurses in these states face a greater risk of being sued personally for their acts of negligence.

POINTS TO REMEMBER

1. As a general rule, hospitals are liable under *respondeat superior* for the negligent acts of *all* their employees.

2. The key element in deciding whether *respondeat superior* will apply in a given case is whether another party had the right to direct and control the nurse's activities with respect to the incident in question.

3. The borrowed servant doctrine is a special application of the *respondeat superior* doctrine. It provides that a temporary employer (usually the operating surgeon) is held liable for the negligent acts of nurses in the operating room or elsewhere done under his or her direction and control. Routine nursing functions are not held to be within the purview of the operating surgeon's borrowed servant liability.

4. In a few states, the doctrine of *respondeat superior* does not apply to employees of certain types of hospitals. In these states the doctrine of charitable immunity still applies. Under this doctrine a nonprofit hospital is legally immune from suit for the negligent acts of its employees. The doctrine of charitable immunity does not apply in Canada.

5. In some jurisdictions the common law doctrine of sovereign (governmental) immunity applies, which provides that no claim can be brought against the state or province for the negligent acts of its employees.

6. In U.S. states that adhere to the governmental immunity rule, the local school board (which is considered a branch of the state government) cannot be held liable for the negligence of one of its employees.

7. In Canada a local school board *can* be sued for the negligence of one of its employees, since there is no special rule of immunity applicable to school boards in Canada.

8. Whenever a special exception to the doctrine of *respondeat superior* applies, the nurse is exposed to a greater risk of personal liability for his or her negligent conduct.

> **NOTE:** Since many nurses are employed by the United States and Canadian governments, a brief discussion of their liability is in order. We will not be discussing the liability of nurses who work for state or provincial governments—only those employed by the federal government in both the United States and Canada.

LIABILITY OF FEDERAL GOVERNMENT NURSES

2-51　Before 1946, the United States government could not be sued for the torts of its employees. In that year Congress enacted the Federal Tort Claims Act (FTCA), permitting such suits to be brought by nongovernment individuals who have suffered injury or loss of property due to the negligent acts of federal employees. Acts of medical negligence (malpractice) are included.

In view of the enactment of the Federal Tort Claims Act (FTCA), the United States government is　☐　immune from suit　　☐　subject to suit　　for the negligent acts of its employees.

2-52　Which of the following (if any) is (are) correct?

The FTCA permits

☐　injured federal government employees to sue the government for injuries they incur at work

☐　the federal government to sue one of its negligent employees for injury caused a nongovernment person

☐　someone not employed by the federal government to sue the latter for the negligent conduct of one of its employees

☐　none of the foregoing

2-51　*subject to suit*　　　**2-52**　*someone not employed by the federal government to sue the latter for the negligent conduct of one of its employees*

2-53 By assuming liability for the negligent acts of its employees under the FTCA, the United States government   ☐ is subject to   ☐ is not subject to   the rule of *respondeat superior*.

NOTE: In the years following passage of the FTCA in 1946, the U.S. Congress has enacted a variety of statutes to make clear its intent to immunize certain categories of federal employees against their personal liability for job-related negligence. Medical, dental, and nursing personnel have long been accorded special consideration. Since 1966, nurses employed by the Department of Veteran Affairs have been accorded specific statutory immunity from suit for negligent acts performed in the course of their employment, 38 U.S.C. § 4116, and since 1970, nurses employed by the U.S. Public Health Service have been accorded similar immunity, 42 U.S.C. § 233(a). Although the latter statute doesn't specifically mention nurses, their inclusion within the broad class of covered persons was clearly established in the case of *Flickinger* v. *United States*, 523 F. Supp. 1372 (Pa. 1981), which involved the alleged negligence of a U.S. Public Health Service nurse-practitioner. Medical, nursing, and related personnel of the National Aeronautics and Space Administration and the Department of Defense have also been granted immunity from suit under special federal statutes.

In response to the U.S. Supreme Court's 1988 decision in *Westfall* v. *Erwin*, 484 U.S. 292, which eroded to some degree the FTCA's grant of personal immunity to allegedly-negligent federal employees, Congress enacted The Federal Employees Liability Reform and Tort Compensation Act of 1988 (P.L. 100-694). That legislation closed the loophole created by the Supreme Court in *Westfall* and makes it absolutely clear that the FTCA is to be the *exclusive* remedy against the United States for suits based on the tortious acts of *any* of its employees while acting within the scope of their employment—thus precluding any other action or civil suit against the employee in question or his or her estate.

The Canadian government also has enacted legislation that makes it possible for an injured patient to sue the government for the negligence of its medical employees. By virtue of the Crown Liability Act, the rule of *respondeat superior* applies to the conduct of all nurses employed by the Dominion of Canada.

2-53   *is subject to*

ENHANCED LIABILITY OF THE OCCUPATIONAL HEALTH NURSE

2-54   The occupational health nurse faces a risk of personal liability that in some cases exceeds and in some cases is less than the liability of other classes of nurses. This liability is a result of the unique interplay between the doctrine of *respondeat superior* and state workers' compensation laws.

All state and provincial workers' compensation laws mandate the compensation of employees who are injured while at work in accordance with specific compensation schedules. These same laws make this remedy the injured employee's *sole remedy against the employer*, and thus deny the employee the legal right to sue the employer for damages even if the employer's negligence was the prime cause of the injury.

Indicate which of the following, if any, is a legal consequence of a state or provincial workers' compensation law:

☐   It affords a statutory compensation remedy to an injured employee that makes it unnecessary to sue his or her employer for damages.

☐   It effectively deprives an injured employee of the right to sue the employer for damages incurred in an on-the-job injury.

☐   Both of the above

☐   Neither of the above

2-55   In just a few states, an employee injured on the job can sue any person (other than his or her employer) whose negligence caused the injury, including a co-worker. In most states, however, the immunity from suit granted the employer is also extended to co-workers of the injured employee. Thus, a nurse employed by a company in a state with such a law, and whose negligence causes harm to a fellow employee, would be protected from civil liability for his or her actions in the same manner as the employer.

Based on the foregoing, in a state that accords immunity from suit against the employer and co-workers of an injured employee, a negligent nurse is in a more protected legal position than is a general-duty nurse employed by a hospital.

                           True   *False*
                                ☐   ☐

2-54   *Both of the above*   **2-55**   *True*

2-56 If the nurse (1) is engaged by the employer as an independent contractor, or (2) works for an employer in a state whose workers' compensation law provides immunity from suit only to the employer, the nurse can be held personally liable for his or her negligent conduct that causes injury to an employee.

■ Nurse N is an occupational health nurse employed by a manufacturer in a state that has not granted immunity from suit to co-workers of an employee injured while on the job. Doctor D is the plant physician, and in D's absence Nurse N's activities are guided by special medical directives that cover both routine and emergency situations.

During Doctor D's absence one day, Nurse N negligently evaluates an employee's signs of illness. The employee suffers a permanent disability as the direct result of N's negligence.

Which of the following would most likely be held liable to the disabled employee in this case?

☐ the manufacturing concern

☐ Doctor D

☐ Nurse N

2-57 If Doctor D's standing order to Nurse N was: "In every case do whatever you think is in the patient's best interests," which of the following would be true?

☐ Doctor D automatically would be held liable for all Nurse N's negligent acts under the doctrine of *respondeat superior*.

☐ The lack of specific guidelines for N to carry out nursing functions would expose N to greater liability for negligent conduct.

☐ Nurse N could avoid liability for any negligent conduct by pointing to the broad authority granted by Doctor D.

2-56   *Nurse N*   **2-57**   ☐   *If you selected the wrong*
                                         ☑   *answer, turn to p. 135, Note C.*
                                         ☐

LIABILITY OF THE PRIVATE-DUTY NURSE

2-58 A private-duty nurse contracts to provide care to a specific patient (either in a hospital, a skilled nursing facility, or the patient's home) and legally is considered an independent contractor. Since the private-duty nurse is not in the employ of the hospital or nursing facility, and therefore not subject to their control, any negligent conduct of the nurse will not subject the hospital or nursing facility to liability under the doctrine of *respondeat superior*. However, this independent mode of functioning clearly places the private-duty nurse in a position of considerably greater exposure to personal liability for nursing functions or procedures carried out, particularly since the private-duty nurse usually acts only under the general direction or supervision of a physician in accordance with standing orders.

From the legal liability standpoint, the private-duty nurse who provides nursing care to a patient in the patient's home

- ☐ has less to be concerned about than does his or her hospital nurse counterpart

- ☐ has considerably more to be concerned about than does his or her hospital nurse counterpart

- ☐ has no reason to be either more concerned or less concerned than does his or her hospital nurse counterpart

---

2-59 Private-duty nursing is distinguished from other forms of nursing practice in that

- ☐ the private-duty nurse contracts to give bedside care to only one patient

- ☐ the private-duty nurse is held to a higher standard of care in treating his or her patients than are other nurses

- ☐ the private-duty nurse is totally independent of medical supervision or control while giving nursing care

2-58	*has considerably more to be concerned about . . .*	**2-59**	☑
			☐
			☐

2-60 Even though the private-duty nurse is legally an independent contractor when caring for a private patient in a hospital, the nurse must nevertheless comply with hospital rules and regulations and can be held responsible to the hospital for compromising its corporate legal responsibility to provide safe and effective care for all of its patients.

■ Private-duty Nurse N is engaged to care for Patient P following P's surgery in Hospital H. While so engaged, N violates the hospital's rules regarding sterile technique for preparing syringes and needles for injections and is chastised for so doing by Supervisory Nurse S. Several days later, P experiences severe pain and a gradual worsening of the redness at an injection site. She is diagnosed as having a severe gangrene infection in her arms and legs, necessitating surgery to remove the affected tissue, as well as corrective plastic surgery. P files suit against both Nurse N and Hospital H to recover damages for her injuries.

True	*False*	
☐	☐	Hospital H cannot be held liable for Nurse N's conduct under the doctrine of *respondeat superior* because N was not in Hospital H's employ.
☐	☐	If Nurse N and Hospital H are both held liable for P's injuries, Hospital H would probably be able to recover from Nurse N its share of the damages paid.
☐	☐	Hospital H theoretically could be held liable for Nurse N's conduct under the doctrine of hospital corporate liability.

	2-60	*True*	*False*
		☑	☐
		☑	☐
		☑	☐

SPECIAL PROBLEMS ARISING OUT OF HOME HEALTH CARE

In 1983, Congress decided to change its retrospective payment system for hospital care rendered to Medicare beneficiaries and adopted instead a prospective payment system. Under this new system, reimbursement rates are set *in advance* of treatment by the Health Care Financing Administration, a unit of the U.S. Department of Health and Human Services. Hospitals now receive a flat fee for their services based on the Diagnostic Related Group (DRG) into which a Medicare patient's illness or injury falls, regardless of the actual costs the hospital has incurred.

Implementation of the DRG system resulted in fewer patients being admitted for elective surgery, an increase in ambulatory surgery, patients being discharged from the hospital at earlier stages of recovery, and patients being discharged to home with problems requiring acute and intensive nursing care. Since home care professional and personal care services are covered under Part A of Medicare, and home care supplies, equipment, and intravenous drug therapy services are covered under Part B, the implementation of this new system of reimbursement has created a virtual boom in the home health care industry. Today, a plethora of agencies currently provide home health care nursing services, including visiting nurse associations, health departments, community-based nursing services, hospital-based home health care, nursing registries, hospices, independent professional practices, small and large for-profit agencies and corporations, and so forth. Unfortunately, the ever-increasing competition for revenue among these various entities, as well as with participating Part B pharmacies, infusion therapy companies, and medical equipment suppliers, have sometimes subordinated traditional concerns for quality of patient care to greater concerns for financial gains.

To be eligible to receive Medicare payments for services to covered beneficiaries, a home care agency must meet specified requirements set forth in the Medicare statute and regulations before being granted Medicare certification. Compliance inspections typically are conducted by state-designated Medicare survey agencies—usually the state health department. It should be noted that the states, in administering their state Medicaid program for low-income individuals, have generally followed Medicare's lead in setting service levels, eligibility and provider criteria, and reimbursement methods.

In addition to the regulation of home health care by the federal and state governments, an additional source of home care regulation is the private/voluntary sector of the health care industry. The most significant private organization involved in accrediting home care programs is the Joint Commission on Accreditation of Healthcare Organizations (JCAHO), which published its *Standards for the Accreditation of Home Care* in 1988. Pursuant to regulations adopted in 1993, the Federal Health Care Financing Administration now accepts JCAHO accreditation as meeting all federal requirements.

Two other private organizations also engage in aspects of voluntary home care accreditation. Skilled nursing services delivered in the home are now accredited by the National League for Nursing, and the National Homecaring Council, under the auspices of the Foundation for Home Care, accredits and approves homemaker and home health aide services.

Medicare patients discharged from hospitals most often enter a home health care program through a referral system administered by the treating hospital. The referral process generally begins with consultations between a hospital-employed "discharge planner" and the patient's physician(s), nurses, and therapists. Based on these consultations, the discharge planner makes a recommendation as to the level of home health care a patient needs. The patient's primary physician then writes the order for the discharge planner to place the patient in a home care program. The discharge planner contacts the home health agency, whose representative meets with the attending physician and reviews the treatment plan. Finally, in accord with the physician's plan, the home health provider sets up a schedule, and treatment at home begins.

There is little doubt that home care is less costly and more humane, particularly for the elderly who might otherwise face long-term institutionalization. However, home care brings its own set of problems, especially those attributable to more complex therapies and the use of highly technical equipment. Patients who used to be treated only in the hospital are now being treated at home with IV therapy, parenteral nutrition, enterostomal care, diabetes care, postoperative cardiology care, pulmonary care, and so forth—in many cases calling for oxygen tanks, tubes, indwelling catheters, and a variety of complex monitoring devices. In these circumstances, the danger of injury to the patient through some form of negligence is ever present. The opportunities for equipment failure, in particular, increase enormously where the equipment is not under the day-to-day control of trained technicians as in the hospital setting.

Of the variety of legal problems most likely to arise out of home health care services, the one that stands out is the apparent unwillingness of physicians to provide any meaningful degree of direct supervision of home health care services. This situation is attributable in part to the Medicare program's failure to reimburse physicians for providing such supervision. In addition, many physicians are genuinely ignorant of the role they are expected to play in the planning of home health care and tend to rely on instructions supplied to them by the various home health care providers. This abrogation of professional responsibility by physicians for supervising the patient's care puts home health care providers (including nurses, of course) in an extremely dangerous position from the liability standpoint.

Other legal areas arising out of home health care services include the normal standard-of-care problems associated with the providing of nursing services and fixing legal responsibility for the reliable performance and safety of the high-tech equipment that is often used. One can only speculate as to how many of these problems ultimately will be resolved. However, it is not difficult to predict that when a malpractice suit is filed, everyone associated with the patient's care at home—the hospital, the home care agency, the prescribing/treating physician, the equipment manufacturer, and the home care nurse—will be joined as defendants in the litigation until it can be decided exactly who is responsible for what.

In any event, the legal doctrines discussed earlier, such as the rule of personal liability and the doctrine of *respondeat superior*, will continue to be the basic guidelines for deciding most fact situations. What must still be determined by the courts, however, are the specific standards of care to be applied to home health care. Clearly, there is a fundamental legal obligation on the part of the home-care agency to (1) exercise care in the selection of competent and experienced nursing personnel, (2) carefully train such personnel in the use of specialized equipment and medical technologies, (3) develop operational guidelines and protocols for the provision of home care designed to assure close communication between all the involved parties (especially the handling of potential emergencies), and (4) assure the safety and reliability of all medical equipment used.

Since home health care frequently requires a multidisciplinary approach—involving physicians, nurses, therapists, nutritionists, social workers, and other specialists—and because nursing care consumes most of the direct care time, it is logical for the nurse team member to be the coordinator of care. It is he or she who makes the initial assessment of the family and its home environment, as well as the availability of other resources and personnel in the community. Within this context, clinical nurse-specialists are likely to play an increasing role in home care, particularly since they will be readily able to provide the specialized services needed, such as IV antibiotic therapy, respiratory therapy, and parenteral nutrition. The absence of immediate medical backup may prove to be a problem in some cases, but generally well-trained nurses will be able to function capably in the home environment where they should find their nursing skills utilized to the fullest. Scope-of-practice problems faced by nurse-specialists are covered at length in Part 4.

EXPLANATORY NOTES

Note A (from Frame 2-32)

Certainly, Nurse N would not be held liable in this case under the doctrine of *respondeat superior*, even though N would still be held liable for personal negligence. Do not forget: *respondeat superior* is a substituted liability doctrine.

Since the administration of an intramuscular injection is a common nursing function, Doctor D would not be held liable for the nurse's negligence merely for having ordered the injection.

Under the given facts, only the hospital would be held liable under *respondeat superior*.

Proceed to Frame 2-33.

Note B (from Frame 2-39)

It should be noted that the charitable immunity rule is an exception to the basic doctrine of *respondeat superior*. Accordingly, unless it specifically applies in a given case, the usual rule of *respondeat superior* will continue to apply. The concept of charitable immunity is a dwindling legal doctrine that has all but vanished from U.S. law. When applicable at all, it applies only to so-called charitable (nonprofit) hospitals. For this reason, negligent conduct that occurs in a profit-making hospital would be subject to the doctrine of *respondeat superior*.

Proceed to Frame 2-40.

Note C (from Frame 2-57)

There is little doubt that the lack of clear working guidelines for carrying out nursing functions would expose Nurse N to greater liability for negligent conduct. As a matter of fact, following such an open-ended standing order would not only expose a nurse to greater liability for malpractice but might also be the grounds for a criminal charge of practicing medicine without a license. In the final analysis, the rule of personal liability will always hold nurses personally responsible for their negligent conduct, and all the more so where they have no clear guidelines from the company physician.

The intelligent occupational health nurse must not rely on a "do-whatever-you-think-is-proper" standing order as authority for his or her functions, and he or she should ignore or challenge any such order for the reasons mentioned above. Incidentally, most courts also would hold the company physician liable for negligence in supervision in a case of this type, but our primary concern here is with the nurse's conduct.

Proceed to Frame 2-58.

POINTS TO REMEMBER

1. Under the Federal Tort Claims Act (FTCA), the U.S. government has consented to be sued for the negligent acts of its employees. The doctrine of *respondeat superior* applies, therefore, to the United States government.

2. In all essential respects the principles of malpractice law apply in the same manner to nurses who are in private or government practice.

3. By virtue of special statutory enactments, nurses employed by the U.S. Public Health Service and by the Department of Veterans Affairs have complete immunity from personal liability for acts of negligence in the course of their government nursing duties. However, these statutes do not affect the rights of aggrieved patients from suing the government for the injuries they have sustained.

4. The Canadian government likewise has waived its immunity against suit and can be held liable for the negligent acts of any of its employees so long as the acts are committed in the scope of the employment.

5. Because of the joint effect of the doctrine of *respondeat superior* and workers' compensation laws, occupational health nurses are sometimes exposed to a greater risk of being sued for negligent conduct than are other classes of nurses.

6. Since workers' compensation laws generally prevent an employee from suing an employer for an injury incurred in the course of the employment, in many states the employee whose injury is aggravated by the malpractice of the company nurse can sue only the nurse, and not the employer.

SELECTED REFERENCES—PART TWO

Rule of Personal Liability

Prosser W, *Handbook of the Law of Torts*, ed 4, West Publishing, St. Paul, 1971, §§ 46-51, pp. 291-313.

74 *Am Jur 2d*, TORTS § 10, p. 628

Annotation, 51 ALR 2d 970, "Nurse's Liability for Her Own Negligence or Malpractice."

Morris CW, "The Negligent Nurse—The Physician and the Hospital," *Baylor L Rev* 33:109, 1981.

Sullivan v. *Sumrall by Ritchley*, 618 So. 2d 1274 (Miss. 1993).

Wheeler v. *Yettie Kersting Memorial Hospital*, 866 S.W. 2d 32 (Texas 1993)

Navarro v. *George*, 615 A. 2d 890 (Pa. 1992)

St. Paul Medical Center v. *Cecil*, 842 S.W. 2d 808 (Texas 1992)

Robison v. *Michelaine Faine and Catalano's Nurse Registry*, 525 So. 2d 903 (Fla. 1988)

Theophelis v. *Lansing General Hospital*, 424 N.W. 2d 478 (Mich. 1988)

Trujillo v. *Berry*, 738 P. 2d 1331 (N.M. 1987)

Dessauer v. *Memorial General Hospital*, 628 P. 2d 337 (N.M. 1981)

Hiatt v. *Groce*, 523 P. 2d 320 (Kan. 1974)

Meier v. *Ross General Hospital*, 74 P. 2d 283 (Cal. 1937)

Supervisor's Liability for Acts of Subordinates

Raicevich v. *Plum Creek Medical P.C.*, 819 F. Supp. 2d 929 (Col. 1993)

Salas by Salas v. *Wang*, 846 F. 2d 897 (N.J. 1988)

Bowers v. *Olch*, 260 P. 2d 997 (Cal. 1953)

Valentin v. *La Société Française de Bienfaisance Mutuelle*, 172 P. 2d 359 (Cal. 1946)

Doctrine of *Respondeat Superior*

Prosser W, *Handbook of the Law of Torts*, ed 4, West Publishing, St. Paul, 1971, § 458.

53 *Am Jur 2d*, MASTER AND SERVANT, § 417

Walker N., "Nursing 1980: New Responsibility, New Liability," *Trial* 16:43, 1980.

Hospital Liability under *Respondeat Superior*

Louisell D and Williams H, *Medical Malpractice*, Matthew Bender & Co., New York, 1983, § 16.08.

Vogler v. *Dominguez*, 624 N.E. 2d 56 (Ind. 1993)

Brickner v. *Normandy Osteopathic Hospital, Inc.*, 746 S.W. 2d 108 (Mo. 1988)

Cornell v. *Ohio State University Hospital*, 521 N.E. 2d 857 (Ohio 1988)

Augeri v. *Massoff*, 520 N.Y.S. 2d 787 (N.Y. 1987)

Variety Children's Hospital v. *Perkins*, 382 So. 2d 331 (Fla. 1982)

Su v. *Perkins*, 211 S.E. 2d 421 (Ga. 1974)

Sesselman v. *Muhlenberg Hosital*, 306 A. 2d 474 (N.J. 1973)

Doctrine of Hospital Corporate Liability

Keeton WP et al, *Prosser and Keeton on the Law of Torts*, ed 5, West Publishing, St. Paul, 1993 (reprint of 1983 ed.), § 30.

Fiesta J, "The Evolving Doctrine of Corporate Liability," *Nurs Management* 25(3): 17, 1994.

King DD and Allison JT, "Medical Staff Credentialing: Taking Steps to Avoid Liability," *Def Couns J* 61:107, 1994.

Jackson BS, "Assuring Institutional Control of Private Duty Personnel," *J Nurs Admin* 23:10, 1993.

Nathanson MJ, "Hospital Corporate Negligence: Enforcing the Hospital's Role of Administrator," *Tort & Ins L J* 28:575, 1993.

Schendel NJ, "Patients as Victims—Hospital Liability for Third-Party Crime," *Valparaiso U L Rev* 28:419, 1993.

Weeks SR, "Hospital Liability: The Emerging Trend of Corporate Negligence," *Idaho L Rev* 28:441, 1991-1992.

Huff DLN, "Liability Issues Arising from Hospitals' Use of Temporary Supplemental Staff Nurses," *Loyola U Chi L J* 21:1141, 1990.

Dixon v. Taylor, 431 S.E. 2d 778 (N.C. 1993)

Mundy v. Department of Health & Human Resources, 620 So. 2d 811 (La. 1993)

St. Paul Medical Center v. Cecil, 842 S.W. 2d 808 (Texas 1992)

Doctors Hospital of Augusta, Inc. v. Bonner, 392 S.E. 2d 987 (Ga. 1990)

Douglas v. Freeman, 587 P. 2d 76 (Wash. 1990)

Washington v. Washington Hospital Center, 579 A. 2d 177 (D.C. 1990)

Herrington v. Miller, 883 F. 2d 411 (Texas 1989)

Oehler v. Humana, Inc., 775 P. 2d 1271 (Nev. 1989)

Reynolds v. Mennonite Hospital, 522 N.E. 2d 827 (Ill. 1988)

Sharsmith v. Hill, 764 P. 2d 667 (Wyo. 1988)

Blanton v. Moses H. Cone Memorial Hospital, 354 S.E. 2d 455 (N.C. 1987)

Jackson v. Power, 743 P. 2d 1376 (Alaska 1987)

Darling v. Charleston Memorial Hospital, 211 N.E. 2d 253 (Ill. 1965)

Borrowed Servant Doctrine

Restatement (Second) AGENCY, §§ 226-227

Harris v. Miller, 438 S.E. 2d 731 (N.C. 1994)

Hunnicutt v. Wright, 986 F. 2d 119 (Miss. 1993)

Hoffman v. Wells, 397 S.E. 2d 696 (Ga. 1990)

Mather v. Griffin Hospital, 540 A. 2d 666 (Conn. 1988)

Shepard v. Sisters of Providence in Oregon, 750 P. 2d 500 (Ore. 1988)

City of Somerset v. Hart, 549 S.W. 2d 814 (Ky. 1987)

Fortson v. McNamara, 508 So. 2d 35 (Fla. 1987)

Baird v. Sickler, 433 N.E. 2d 593 (Ohio (1982)

Truhitte v. French Hospital, 180 Cal. Rptr 152 (Cal. 1982)

Captain of the Ship Doctrine

Louisell D and Williams H, *Medical Malpractice*, Matthew Bender & Co., New York, 1983, § 16.07.

Annotation, 29 ALR 3d 1065, "Liability of Hospital for Negligence of Nurse Assisting Operating Surgeon."

Blummenreich GA, "Surgeon's Liability for Negligence of CRNAs: A Recent Case," *Am Assn Nurs Anesth J* 57(2):91, 1989.

Greenlaw J, "Liability for Nursing Negligence in the Operating Room," *Law Med & Health Care* 10(10):222, 1982.

McVey B and Walsh R, "Medical Malpractice—Who is the Captain of the Ship?" *Federat Ins L Couns Q* 27:331, 1977.

Holger v. Irish, 851 P. 2d 1122 (Ore. 1993)

Hunnicutt v. Wright, 986 F. 2d 119 (Miss. 1993)

Leiker ex rel Leiker v. Gafford, 778 P. 2d 823 (Kan. 1989)

Nelson v. Trinity Medical Center, 419 N.W. 2d 886 (N.D. 1988)

Krane v. St. Anthony Hospital Systems, 738 P. 2d 75 (Colo. 1987)

Thomas v. Raleigh General Hospital, 358 S.E. 2d 222 (W.Va. 1987)

Kitto v. Gilbert, 570 P. 2d 544 (Colo. 1977).

Sparger v. Worley Hospital, 547 S.W. 2d 582 (Texas 1977)

Doctrine of Charitable Immunity

Louisell D and Williams H, *Medical Malpractice*, Matthew Bender & Co., New York, 1983, § 17.04.

Bottari A, "The Charitable Immunity Act," *Seton Hall L J* 5:61, 1980.

Restatement (2d) TORTS, § 895E

Child v. *Central Maine Medical Center*, 575 A. 2d 318 (Me. 1990)

Johnson v. *The Mountainside Hospital*, 571 A. 2d 318 (N.J. 1990)

Cutts v. *Fulton DeKalb Hospital Authority*, 385 S.E. 2d 436 (Ga. 1989)

Patterson v. *Fulton DeKalb Hospital Authority*, 384 S.E. 2d 205 (Ga. 1989)

Marsella v. *Monmouth Medical Center*, 540 A. 2d 865 (N.J. 1988)

Perlof v. *Symmes Hospital*, 487 F. Supp. 426 (Mass. 1980)

Lutheran Hospitals & Homes Society of America v. *Yepsen,* 469 P. 2d 409 (Wyo. 1970)

Williams v. *Jefferson Hospital Association*, 442 S.W. 2d 243 (Ark. 1969)

Howard v. *Bishop Byrne Council Home, Inc.*, 238 A. 2d 863 (Md. 1968)

Rhoda v. *Aroostock General Hospital*, 226 A. 2d 530 (Me. 1967)

Hemenway v. *Presbyterian Hospital Association of Colorado*, 419 P. 2d 312 (Colo. 1966)

Doctrine of Governmental or Sovereign Immunity

Hartl WR, "Sovereign Immunity: An Outdated Doctrine Faces Demise in a Changing Judicial Arena," *N D L Rev* 69:401, 1993.

Hickman JD, "It's Time to Call 911 for Government Immunity," *Case W Res L Rev* 43:1067, 1993.

Fields v. *Curators of the University of Missouri*, 848 S.W. 2d 589 (Mo. 1993)

Hunnicutt v. *Wright*, 986 F. 2d 119 (Miss. 1993)

Raicevich v. *Plum Creek Medical P.C.*, 819 F. Supp. 2d 929 (Colo. 1993)

Sullivan v. *Sumrall by Ritchley*, 618 So. 2d 1274 (Miss. 1993)

Hatley v. *Kassen*, 859 S.W. 2d 367 (Texas 1992)

Stacy v. *Truman Medical Center,* 836 S.W. 2d 911 (Mo. 1992)

State v. *Hartsough*, 790 P. 2d 836 (Colo. 1990)

Armendarez v. *Tarrant County Hospital District*, 781 S.W. 2d 301 (Texas 1989)

Stein v. *Southeastern Michigan Family Planning Project, Inc.*, 438 N.W. 2d 76 (Mich. 1989)

Liability of the School Nurse

Newman KD, "Protocols for College Health Nurses: Alive and Well in the 1990s," *J Am Coll Health* 42(3):128, 1993.

Cohn S, "Legal Issues in School Nursing Practice," *Law Med & Health Care* 12:219, 1984.

Gadow L, "Administration of Medications by School Personnel," *J Sch Health* 53:178, 1983.

Kinne M, "Accidents," *J Sch Health* 52(9):564, 1982.

Creighton H, "School Nurses: Legal Aspects of their Work," *Nurs Clin N Am* 9:467, 1974.

Standards for School Nurse Services, National Education Association, Washington, D.C., 1970.

Kersey v. *Harbin*, 531 S.W. 2d 76 (Mo. 1979)

Peck v. *Board of education of the City of Mount Vernon*, 283 N.E. 2d 618 (N.Y. 1972)

Liability for Federal Government Nursing Care

Federal Tort Claims Act, 28 U.S.C. §§ 1346(b), 2671-2680

Federal Employees Liability Reform and Tort Compensation Act of 1988, 28 U.S.C. § 2679(b)(1)

Fiesta J, "Malpractice—and the Federal Employee," *Nurs Management* 25(5):22, 1994.

Bermann GA, "Federal Tort Claims at the Agency Level: The FTCA Administrative Process," *Case W Res L Rev* 35:509, 1984–1985.

Immunity of V.A. medical and nursing personnel, 38 U.S.C. § 4116

Immunity of U.S.P.H.S. medical and nursing personnel, 42 U.S.C. § 233(a)

Immunity of Department of Defense medical and nursing personnel, 10 U.S.C. § 1089

Immunity of N.A.S.A. medical and nursing personnel, 22 U.S.C. § 2458

Johnson v. *Carter*, 983 F. 2d 1316 (Va. 1993)

Davis v. *United States*, 791 F. Supp 793 (Mo. 1992)

Garcia v. *United States*, 697 F. Supp. 1570 (Colo. 1988)

Mendez v. *Belton*, 739 F. 2d 15 (Puerto Rico 1984)
Lojuk v. *Quandt*, 706 F. 2d 1456 (Ill. 1983)
Flickinger v. *United States*, 523 F. Supp. 1372 (Pa. 1981)

Liability of the Occupational Health Nurse

Brown ML, *Occupational Health Nursing: Principles and Practices*, Springer Publishing, New York, 1981.
Bowyer EA, "The Liability of the Occupational Health Nurse," *Law Med Health Care* 11(5):224, 1983.
Cushing M, "An Occupational Nurse's Liability," *Am J Nurs* 79(9):1608, 1979.
Panaro v. *Electrolux Corp.*, 545 A. 2d 1086 (Conn. 1988)
Montgomery v. *Department of Registration & Education*, 496 N.E. 2d 1100 (Ill. 1986)
Samuels v. *American Cyanamid Co.*, 495 N.Y.S. 2d 1006 (N.Y. 1985)
Cooper v. *National Motor Bearing Co.*, 288 P. 2d 581 (Cal. 1955)

Liability of the Private Duty Nurse

Cal. Business and Professions Code, § 2732. 05
Nelson K, "Agency Nurses Pose Growing Liability," *Forum*, Jan. 1989.
Fiesta J, "Agency Nurses—Whose Liability?" *Nurs Management* 21(3):16, 1990.
Avchen v. *Kiddoo*, 246 Cal. Rptr. 152 (Cal. 1988)
Robison v. *Michelaine Faine and Catalano's Nurse Registry*, 525 So. 2d 903 (Fla. 1988)
Shrock v. *Altru Nurses Registry*, 810 F. 2d 658 (Ill. 1987)
Vaughn v. *Baton Rouge General Hospital*, 421 So. 2d 188 (La. 1982)
Meier v. *Ross General Hospital*, 74 P. 2d 283 (Cal. 1937)

Legal Issues in Home Health Nursing

Haddad AM and Kapp MB, *Ethical and Legal Issues in Home Health Care*, Appleton & Lange, Norwalk, Conn., 1991.
Joint Commission on Accreditation of Healthcare Organizations, *Standards for Accreditation of Home Care*, Chicago, JCAHO, 1988.
Sutton S, *Home Health Nursing Manual: Procedures and Documentation*, The Williams & Wilkins Company, Baltimore, 1988.
Kapp MB, "Legal Issues." In Haddad AM, *High Tech Home Care: A Practical Guide*, Aspen Publishers, Rockville, Md., 1987.
Kapp MB, *Preventing Malpractice in Long Term Care: Strategies for Risk Management*, Springer Publishing Co., New York, 1987.
Johnson SH, "Who Sets the Standards for Home Health Care?" *Health Progress*, 69(11):20, 1988.
Van Meter C, "How Times Have Changed in Home Health Care," *RN* 51(4):94, 1988.
Atkinson SC, "Medicare 'Cost Containment' and Home Health Care: Potential Liability for Physicians and Hospitals," *Georgia L Rev* 21:901, 1987.
Jernigan DK, "Managing Risk in the Home Health Setting," *Home Care Econ* 1(2):46, 1987.
Bernzweig E, "Avoiding the Legal Pitfalls in Home Health Care," *RN* 49(8):49, 1986.
Koren MJ, "Home Care—Who Cares?" *New Eng J Med* 314:917, 1986.
Perdew SR, "Litigation in Home Care: What the Future Holds," *Caring* 5(9):84, 1986.
Roach v. *Kelly Health Care*, 742 P. 2d 1190 (Ore. 1987)
Matter of David Gentiel Nursing Service, 483 N.Y.S. 2d 796 (N.Y. 1985)
Homemakers v. *Gonzalez*, 400 So. 2d 965 (Fla. 1981)

SPECIFIC TYPES OF NEGLIGENT CONDUCT

Part 3

INTRODUCTORY NOTE

In Part 1 we discussed the general legal principles that apply to nurses in carrying out their customary duties, and in Part 2 we discussed some of the special rules of liability. Now we shall see examples of how these concepts are applied in specific situations. Many nursing functions and responsibilities have been the subject of court cases, thereby providing authoritative guidelines to proper conduct in future similar cases.

It should be noted that the profession of nursing has undergone dynamic changes within the past decade or so. The nurse has evolved from being the handmaiden of the physician to a recognized professional assistant in carrying out many patient care functions.

Earlier views of the nurse as the physician's aide in carrying out numerous dependent functions have been superseded by changes in nursing curricula and educational standards qualifying the nurse to perform many independent functions without the necessity of medical orders or direct medical supervision. Notwithstanding these changes in activities, the case law does not reveal any undue exposure to liability *solely* because of this expanded nursing role in providing patient care services. Following the general rules outlined earlier in this course, liability is always predicated on failure to exercise the degree of care and skill expected of the nurse—or the nurse-specialist—under similar circumstances.

It would be impossible to cover the entire gamut of factual situations that have been before the courts, but the cases that are included in this part are representative of the more common problems encountered in nursing malpractice suits during recent years.

PATIENT SAFETY ERRORS

3-1   A nurse is required to exercise ordinary or reasonable care to safeguard and protect his or her patient from any known or reasonably foreseeable harm. The courts have held this to be as much the nurse's responsibility as that of the physician. Many of the nurse's routine patient care activities relate to the safety and security of the patient, and the nurse is expected to perform these acts without any special medical order or supervision.

Under what circumstances will a nurse be held legally responsible for seeing that no harm comes to his or her patient?

☐   only when the nurse is engaged to care for the patient as a private-duty nurse

☐   only when the nurse has been specifically directed to protect the patient against harm

☐   whenever the nurse is assigned to caring for the patient

3-2   A nurse's responsibility to safeguard and protect his or her patient from harm is one that

☐   requires a written or verbal order from a physician or nurse-supervisor

☐   the nurse must exercise independently of any special medical order or supervisory directive

☐   the nurse must exercise only when employed by a hospital, nursing home, or other health care institution

---

3-3   The nurse's responsibility to protect his or her patient from harm includes harm that might result from carrying out a physician's specific order.

True   *False*

☐   ☐

3-1   *whenever the nurse is assigned to caring for the patient*

3-2   *the nurse must exercise independently of any special medical order or supervisory directive*

3-3   *True*

3-4

■ P, a 76-year-old woman hospitalized for treatment of congestive heart failure was known to lapse into a semicomatose state from time to time. When lucid, she constantly complained of being cold and asked for hot water bottles around her legs. No specific doctor's orders were given for these complaints, but Nurse N was given general instructions by Supervisory Nurse S to "keep the patient warm."

Nurse N, irritated by P's constant complaints, placed several excessively hot heating pads around P's legs while P was semicomatose, disregarding the patient's immediate objection to the intensity of the heat. Upon checking the patient an hour later, it was noted that she had sustained serious burns on her legs, requiring extensive remedial measures. P later sued Nurse N, Nurse S, her treating physician, and the hospital for the injuries sustained.

What was the *legal* duty owed by Nurse N with respect to the safety of patient P?

☐   the duty to respond immediately to all requests for nursing care made by P

☐   the duty to safeguard and protect P from any known or reasonably foreseeable harm

☐   the duty to carry out whatever treatment the doctor or the supervisor ordered

---

3-5   What was the principal foreseeable danger to guard against in this case?

☐   the danger that P might sustain burns while in a semicomatose state

☐   the danger that P's general condition might worsen

☐   the danger that P might attempt to move the heating pads to another area of her body

---

3-4   ☐   *If you checked the 1st or 3d*   **3-5**   *the danger that P might*
          ☑   *box, turn to p. 160, Note A.*   *sustain burns while in a*
          ☐   *semicomatose state*

3-6   The kind and degree of nursing care necessary to protect a patient from harm will always depend on the particular circumstances of the case. The prime determinant of the type of care necessary is the patient's physical and mental capacity to contribute to his or her own safety and security.

What *legal* significance would be attached to the fact that P was an elderly patient in a weakened condition who occasionally lapsed into a comatose state?

☐   P would be expected to be more aware of the possible harm she might sustain while in a comatose condition.

☐   The foreseeability of harm to P would be greater, and the degree of care to protect against such harm also would be greater.

☐   No particular legal significance would be attached since the degree of care expected of the nursing staff would not differ merely because of these factors.

3-7   Which of the following actions would have afforded *better*, and nevertheless *reasonable*, protection against the type of occurrence that eventually led to P's injuries?

☐   Nurse S could have assigned staff nurses other than Nurse N to check on P's condition every 10 minutes

☐   The hospital could have issued standing orders never to apply heating pads to semi-comatose patients.

☐   Nurse N could have double-checked the temperature of the heating pads after P complained about the intensity of their heat.

	3-6 ☐		3-7 ☐
	☑		☐
	☐		☑

3-8   Supervisory Nurse S gave Nurse N specific instructions to keep Patient P warm. If a jury was to decide that Nurse N was negligent in fulfilling his or her legal responsibilities to P, what likely effect would this have on Nurse S's liability?

☐   No liability would result since the instructions in question were well within the capabilities of a trained nurse.

☐   Nurse S would be held liable for failing to check on P's condition personally.

☐   Nurse S would be held liable for giving only general instructions to Nurse N about keeping Patient P warm.

NOTE: You will recall that a nursing supervisor can be held liable if he or she assigns a task to an individual who is not competent to perform that particular task. A general instruction to "keep the patient warm" is not the type of nursing task that calls for particularized nursing skills, and it is highly unlikely that a nursing supervisor would be held liable for harm resulting from giving such a simple and routine order.

The important thing to note is that a nurse never should rely blindly on someone else's orders and use them as a shield for his or her own negligent conduct. The test is always the same: How would other reasonably prudent nurses have acted in a similar situation?

3-9   Assuming Nurse N's negligence in this case, who else probably would be held liable for N's conduct?

☐   the doctor and the hospital

☐   the hospital

☐   no one else

3-8   *No liability would result since the instructions were well within the capabilities of a trained nurse.*

3-9   *the hospital*

3-10   All nurses should be especially alert to the hazards of smoking by patients who may not
be mentally aware of the dangers involved or physically able to protect themselves from
causing fires and being burned. Under no circumstances should a nurse accommodate a
patient's plea to smoke, regardless how persistent, when the foreseeability of harm to the
patient or others clearly dictates that he or she should not be permitted to smoke.

■ P, a 42-year-old man of below-average intelligence, was hospitalized with paralysis of his arms and
his vocal cords. Nurse N, assigned to care for P, knew him to be a lifelong pipe smoker and frequently lit P's pipe for him and permitted him to smoke. N's only orders from Nurse S, her supervisor, were not to leave him alone when smoking, and N followed these orders faithfully. One day
P's bed caught fire and he suffered burns that resulted in his death. His pipe (which was lit) and
some matches were found on the floor near his bed.

P's estate sues Nurses N and S for malpractice in failing to protect P from harm. At the trial, Nurse
N testifies she was not in the room at the time the fire began and has no way of knowing how P's
pipe might have been lit. Nurse S testifies that he had given Nurse N strict orders not to leave P
alone while he was smoking and that N is a competent and diligent nurse in all respects.

What was the *legal* duty owed by Nurse N with respect to the safety of Patient P?

☐   the duty to light his pipe for him and see that it was out when she left the room

☐   the duty to safeguard and protect him from any known or reasonably foreseeable danger

☐   the duty not to leave him unattended while he was smoking his pipe

---

3-11   What was the principal foreseeable danger to guard against in this case?

☐   the danger that P might fall asleep while smoking

☐   the danger that P might burn himself while attempting to light his pipe

☐   the danger that P might attempt to smoke his pipe while unattended

3-10   ☐
        ☑
        ☐
	3-11 *the danger that P might attempt to smoke his pipe while unattended*

3-12 What *legal* significance would be attached to the fact that P was of below-average intelligence and could neither move his arms nor speak?

☐ P would be expected to know the greater risk presented by his smoking (in view of his condition) and would be expected to assume full responsibility for any consequent harm.

☐ The foreseeability of harm from his smoking would be greater, and the degree of care to protect P against such harm would be proportionately greater.

☐ No particular legal significance would be attached since the degree of care expected of the nursing staff would not differ merely because of these factors.

3-13 Which of the following actions would have afforded *better*, and nevertheless *reasonable*, protection against the type of occurrence that eventually led to P's death?

☐ Nurse S could have assigned staff nurses to check on P's smoking every 10 minutes.

☐ Nurse N could have removed P's pipe and matches from his room and forbidden his smoking while in the hospital.

☐ Nurse N could have posted a sign near the entrance to P's room forbidding all persons to light P's pipe without first consulting her or Nurse S.

3-14 Under the given facts, what is the only *positive* conclusion that can be drawn with respect to the incident in question?

☐ that a passerby probably lit P's pipe for him

☐ that P was not adequately protected against a reasonably foreseeable type of harm

☐ that P probably attempted (unsuccessfully) to light his pipe by himself since no nurse was around to light it for him

---

3-12 ☐	**3-13** ☐	**3-14** *that P was not ade-*
☑	☐	*quately protected against*
☐	☑	*a reasonably foreseeable*
		type of harm

NOTE: While the preceding fact situation may appear far-fetched to some readers, especially since virtually all hospitals today have written protocols against smoking *anywhere within the facility*, hospital fires caused by patients who smoke nevertheless still occur. That is exactly what occurred in the relatively recent case of *Stacy* v. *Truman Medical Center*, 836 S.W. 2d 911 (Mo. 1992), in which a patient with head injuries was permitted by nurses to smoke while unattended even though hospital policy clearly stated that "No smoking shall be permitted in the Truman Medical Center health care facility." Two patients died in the tragic fire that ensued when the patient's cigarette fell onto flammable material in the hospital room.

Another issue is presented in cases like this: can a patient be held responsible for causing, or partly causing, his or her own injury? Two legal doctrines are pertinent to this issue: **contributory negligence** and **assumption of risk**, both of which are legal defenses that can be asserted by nurse-defendants in appropriate cases. Contributory negligence is conduct by the injured person that falls below the standard of care a reasonably prudent person would be expected to exercise for his or her own safety—which conduct contributes to the very injury for which suit has been brought. In most jurisdictions, contributory negligence will bar any recovery against the defendant nurse; in others, this is deemed too harsh a result and these states have adopted what is known as the **comparative negligence** rule, under which damages are apportioned according to the relative degree of negligence between plaintiff and defendant.

Contributory negligence usually is raised in cases in which the patient knowingly and willfully fails to follow a doctor's orders, such as leaving the bed, taking down the side rails, going to the toilet without an attendant, refusing medications, or leaving the hospital against medical advice. On the other hand, when the defense of contributory negligence is asserted the courts always take into consideration the mental state of the patient and all the surrounding circumstances. Thus, the defense of contributory negligence will not be allowed to bar an injured patient's claim for damages where the patient was suffering some impairment of cognition due to drugs, fatigue, pain, Alzheimer's disease or mental incompetency, or was too young to comprehend the dangers involved.

The doctrine of assumption of risk involves a claim that the patient knowingly entered into, or remained in, a position of danger when it was unreasonable to do so, thereby assuming the risk of any foreseeable injury. Both doctrines result in a bar to the plaintiff's recovery of damages, as discussed more fully in Part 6.

The fact that there may be some mitigating circumstances when a malpractice suit is brought does not alter the nurse's fundamental legal obligation to safeguard and protect the patient from any known or reasonably foreseeable harm. Because the patient in the preceding example was allowed to smoke under proper nursing supervision, it is highly unlikely the court would permit the defendant nurses to assert the doctrines of contributory negligence or assumption of risk in this case.

3-15 Not all malpractice claims and suits against nurses are related to errors in carrying out technical nursing procedures. In point of fact, one of the most common causes of such claims and suits is falls from beds, examining tables, or x-ray tables. The prudent nurse always should be alert to the possibility of falling by a patient who is elderly, is under sedation, has suffered a head injury, complains of blacking out, or has not fully recovered from the effects of an anesthetic. Failure to anticipate serious injury to a patient with any of these symptoms is pure and simple negligence.

■ P, an elderly woman who had just undergone an ECG, was removed by Nurse N to an unattended holding room on a stretcher that had no siderails. After being left alone for an hour, P tried unsuccessfully to attract Nurse N's attention. Finally, P got off the stretcher and while trying to reach the bathroom fell and broke her hip.

Was P's fall and broken hip a reasonably foreseeable consequence of leaving her on the stretcher in the manner indicated?

           Yes   *No*
           ☐   ☐

3-16 Assuming that the hospital had no policy on the use of bedrails for patients undergoing ECGs, which of the following conclusions would be most accurate?

☐ In the absence of any hospital policy on the matter, Nurse N could not be held liable for P's injuries.

☐ Even without any hospital policy on the matter, Nurse N had a legal duty to protect P from injury, including a possible fall.

☐ In the absence of any hospital policy on the matter, the hospital could not be held responsible for P's injuries.

3-17 From the standpoint of the degree of care required in this case, what would probably be the single most important fact a jury would consider in a suit brought by P against Nurse N?

☐ the fact that P was left unattended for over an hour

☐ the fact that P was impatient and careless

☐ the fact that the hospital had no policy on siderails

| 3-15 | Yes | 3-16 | Even without any hospital policy on the matter, Nurse N had a legal duty to protect . . . | 3-17 | the fact that P was left unattended for over an hour |

FALLS AND ELDERLY PATIENTS

As pointed out in the preceding example, injuries resulting from falls are a common cause of claims against nurses—based on the nurse's negligence in failing to safeguard his or her patient from reasonably foreseeable harm. Although falls concern all categories of patients, the one category that deserves particular mention is the elderly patient. The nursing student should become sensitive to the mobility problems of older patients.

Hospital or nursing facility policy in most instances will dictate the necessity for bedrails and other forms of restraint to prevent or reduce the likelihood of falls. From a purely litigation-defense standpoint, this posture is understandable, since malpractice insurance statistics consistently rank falls from bed among the most common causes of malpractice claims. There are studies, however, that indicate the routine use of bedrails may actually constitute more of a *hazard* than a *protection* to the average elderly patient. In England, for example, bedrails no longer are routinely used for the elderly, and yet the hospital fall-fracture rate is lower in England than in the United States.

Certainly, there are circumstances when bedrails are clearly indicated for patients of all ages, e.g., when the patient is delirious and thrashing about in bed, when the patient is being transported on a gurney, or when the patient is heavily sedated, unconscious, or intoxicated. Moreover, the elderly present an array of risk factors that go beyond those affecting younger patients, including diminished ability to adjust to unfamiliar surroundings and increased likelihood of becoming disoriented, decreased visual and auditory acuity, increased sensitivity to medication, diminished physical performance (especially locomotion), and so forth.

More often than not, falls are simply the inevitable consequence of leaving the patient unattended when he or she should not be left alone. How long and under what circumstances the patient may be left alone depends on the facts of each case. However, the exercise of reasonable care demands that the nurse be alert to the possibility of a serious fall whenever the patient is elderly, has taken medications that cause orthostatic hypotension, CNS depression, or vestibular toxicity, is recovering from anesthesia, is semiconscious, or is known to suffer dizzy spells. Several recent cases highlight the importance of exercising extra care and attention when dealing with such patients. For example, in *Landes* v. *Women's Christian Association*, 504 N.W. 2d 139 (Iowa 1993), a patient undergoing outpatient arthroscopic surgery and still recovering from the effects of anesthesia fell and was injured when he was taken to the bathroom by the nurse and was left there alone. A somewhat similar situation occurred in *Pierce* v. *Mercy Medical Health Center, Inc.*, 847 P. 2d 822 (Okla. 1992) where shortly after administering Tigan to a patient, the nurse personally escorted her to the shower and left her there unattended, knowing that the drug in question caused drowsiness. The patient fell in the shower and suffered serious injury. *Atkins* v. *Pottstown Medical Center*, 634 A. 2d 258 (Pa. 1993) involved a fall sustained by a patient before surgery; the patient was allowed by a member of the nursing staff to go to the bathroom after preoperative medication was administered.

In *Kadyszeweki* v. *Ellis Hospital Association*, 595 N.Y.S. 2d 841 (N.Y. 1993), a female patient 67 years of age had been administered Demoral, Vistaril, Motrin, and phenobarbital at bedtime and fractured her left hip when she fell in her room after attempting to go to the bathroom at 4:45 AM. At trial, she testified that she tried for approximately a half hour to summon aid and assistance without any response from nursing or other staff before she attempted to walk to the bathroom on her own. Interestingly, the appellate court focused more on the absence of siderails—a violation of the hospital's own rules for medicated patients over 65—than it did about the failure to respond to the patient's call.

In all of these cases, the courts found that the respective nurses failed to exercise ordinary care and attention to protect their patients from harm and were accordingly held to be negligent.

TIPS FOR PROTECTING PATIENTS FROM FALLS

■ Make sure bed siderails are kept up whenever they are indicated or are required by hospital policy

■ Make it a practice to periodically orient the patient to where he or she is and what time it is, especially if the patient is elderly

■ Monitor the patient regularly—or continually, if necessary (i.e., if his or her condition requires it)

■ Offer a bedpan or commode regularly to minimize the need for ambulation

■ Always have someone support and assist the patient whenever he or she gets out of bed

■ Make sure the patient wears proper shoes or slippers when walking

■ Provide adequate lighting and a clutter-free environment in the patient's room

■ Make sure adequate staff is available when the patient is being transferred from one location to another

---

DUTY TO FOLLOW OR QUESTION PHYSICIANS' ORDERS

3-18   Every licensed physician has a right to expect that his or her medical orders will be executed without delay by skilled nurses in the usual and customary manner. The law recognizes this right by requiring the nurse to carry out any procedure directed by a duly licensed physician *unless* the nurse has substantial reason to believe that the doctor's order is clearly erroneous or its execution would not be deemed reasonable and prudent conduct.

■ Doctor D, an obstetrician in private practice, left standing orders that his patients admitted to Hospital H were to be placed on a continuous fetal heart-rate monitor. Obstetrical Patient P arrived at the hospital with severe abdominal pain and tightness in the stomach, but Nurse N did not place a monitor on P, believing that both of the hospital's monitors were in use. In fact, one monitor was not in use and was available. When it was eventually placed on P, it indicated fetal distress, requiring an emergency cesarean section. The infant was born severely brain-damaged. Suit is filed against Hospital H, Nurse N, and Doctor D.

With respect to carrying out Doctor D's order, indicate whether the following statements are true or false.

True   *False*

☐   ☐   Nurse N could be held personally liable for her failure to carry out the order.

☐   ☐   Nurse N could be held liable only if the order came from a house-staff physician.

☐   ☐   Nurse N could avoid liability by showing that the routine use of fetal monitors for obstetric admissions was not standard hospital policy.

3-19   Nurses cannot execute orders blindly. When harm to the patient is a distinct possibility, reasonable care calls for the nurse to question the physician concerning his or her recommended treatment, thereby alerting the physician to the potential harm that may result. If the nurse does not question the physician's order and harm *does* result to the patient, the nurse is clearly negligent and can be held liable to the patient for his or her own negligent conduct.

How can a nurse avoid legal liability for potential harm to a patient resulting from a procedure carried out under a physician's direct order?

☐   by questioning the physician and then proceeding only if the physician agrees to assume full responsibility

☐   by noting his or her objections to the ordered treatment on the patient's chart

☐   by not carrying out the procedure

3-18 ☑ ☐   3-19 ☐   *For information concerning the*
      ☐ ☑   ☐   *correct procedure to follow,*
      ☐ ☑   ☑   *turn to p. 160, Note B.*

3-20 What is the *fundamental* reason why a nurse should *not* follow a physician's order when the nurse has reason to believe some harm will result to the patient?

☐ A reasonably prudent nurse should never carry out an act calculated to be dangerous or harmful to the patient.

☐ A nurse may lose his or her license to practice by blindly following orders that prove harmful to patients.

☐ A nurse is likely to have his or her malpractice insurance canceled if he or she is involved in too many malpractice suits.

3-21

■ A physician writes the following order: "Patient to be walked 5 minutes every day *without fail*." Nurse N, about to get the patient up the following day, is told by her: "I'm terribly sick. My head is swimming, and I feel faint." Nurse N, referring to the doctor's order, insists that the patient walk, but the patient falls and is injured in the process.

Who is *likely* to be held liable for the harm caused?

☐ the doctor only

☐ the nurse and the doctor

☐ the nurse only

3-20 ☑   **3-21** ☐   *If you are uncertain about the*
      ☐   ☐   *correct answer, turn to p. 161,*
      ☐   ☑   *Note C.*

NOTE: While nurses are not expected to follow physicians' orders blindly, they are *not* authorized to unilaterally countermand orders they believe to be erroneous and possibly harmful to the patient. In cases like this, the reasonable and prudent nurse must delay executing the order until the issue is resolved, preferably with the physician directly or, if that is not feasible, by bringing the matter to the immediate attention of the nurse's supervisor. Two recent cases illustrate what can happen when a nurse actually challenges or goes so far as to countermand a doctor's order. In *Frank* v. *South Suburban Hospital Foundation*, 628 N.E. 2d 953 (Ill. 1993), a nursing supervisor who was concerned that her patient might be digtoxic (excessive digoxin in his system) directed an attending nurse *not* to administer further doses of the drug that the physician had ordered until digoxin-level tests *ordered by* Nurse Frank, the supervisor, were completed. When the physician learned that Nurse Frank had interfered with his order to have digoxin administered, she was reported to hospital administration and was immediately suspended and subsequently terminated. This result was unfortunate for a nurse who clearly was doing her best to protect her patient from harm, but the officious manner in which she handled the situation may well have been the real cause of her undoing.

In *Kirk* v. *Mercy Hospital Tri-County*, 851 S.W. 2d 617 (Mo. 1993), a charge nurse made a nursing assessment and diagnosis of her patient as having toxic shock syndrome—a condition that results in almost certain death if untreated. Although her assessment was passed on to the treating physician, the anticipated order from him to combat the life-threatening infection with antibiotics was never received. At that point, proceeding through prescribed hospital channels, the nurse discussed the case with the Chief of the Medical Staff who immediately initiated appropriate treatment, but to no avail—the patient died soon thereafter of massive internal infection. When a member of the patient's family later inquired about her treatment, the charge nurse voiced her displeasure with the treating physician's handling of the case and even offered to obtain the patient's medical records for possible legal action. Once this was made known to management, the nurse was summarily terminated, but she sued the hospital for wrongful discharge. The lower court found for the hospital under the employment-at-will doctrine, but on appeal the Missouri Court of Appeals ruled that a public policy exception to this doctrine—found in the language of the Nurse Practice Act— gave the nurse the right to pursue her wrongful discharge claim. The court held that the duties outlined in the Act reflect the public policy of the state that registered nurses have an obligation to faithfully serve the best interests of their patients. Rulings of this nature should encourage all nurses to act in a forthright manner and take whatever steps are reasonably necessary for the welfare and safety of their patients.

To summarize: when a nurse has reasonable cause to delay executing a physician's order, he or she should bring his or her observations to the attention of those in a position to evaluate—and possibly alter—the questionable order. However, once the order has been properly confirmed, corrected, or modified, as the case may be, the nurse should execute the order without doubt or hesitation about the patient's safety or the nurse's own liability.

3-22   Another problem involves the execution of particular types of physicians' orders. Occasionally, a physician will direct a nurse to carry out a purely medical procedure. Nurse practice acts make it clear that nurses are authorized to carry out many acts that under other circumstances would constitute the unauthorized practice of medicine. This is particularly true in emergency situations.

Under what circumstances can a nurse legally carry out a purely medical procedure?

☐   under no circumstances, since this would constitute the unauthorized practice of medicine

☐   only when ordered to do so by a licensed physician or in an emergency

☐   whenever the patient's condition so requires and no physician is available to order the procedure

---

3-23   Which of the following most accurately states the nurse's legal duty with respect to carrying out a physician's order to perform some medical procedure?

☐   Unless the nurse believes the patient will be harmed, he or she must carry out any procedure ordered by the physician.

☐   The nurse must exercise independent judgment on whether a particular medical procedure will prove effective before carrying it out.

☐   The nurse has the duty to follow the physician's orders without question, at the risk of losing his or her license.

3-22   *only when ordered to do so by a licensed physician or in an emergency*

3-23   *Unless the nurse believes the patient will be harmed, he or she must carry out any procedure ordered by the physician.*

> **NOTE:** In discussing the nurse's duty to follow or question physicians' orders, we have made the implicit assumption that the medical orders in question are *lawful*, even if inappropriate or erroneous. Under no circumstances should nurses carry out physicians' orders directing them to commit acts they know, or should know, to be *unlawful*. If they do, they will subject themselves to criminal liability, whether or not a patient suffers injury, and they cannot avoid such liability by claiming they were merely following the doctor's orders. *United States* v. *Vamos*, 797 F. 2d 1146 (N.Y. 1986), illustrates this point. In that case, a nurse employed by a private physician who specialized in bariatrics (weight control) knowingly assisted him in the distribution of controlled substances outside the scope of medical practice in violation of the pertinent federal drug abuse statute. Despite her defense that she relied on the physician's claim he was dispensing the drugs in question in good faith and in accordance with proper medical practice, the jury found that such reliance was completely unreasonable under all the circumstances. Accordingly, the nurse was found guilty on 19 counts of violating the drug abuse statute and was sent to prison for 6 months.

3-24 In order to meet his or her legal responsibility to the patient, the nurse who is directed to carry out a medical act must understand both *how* to execute the medical procedure in question and the *effect* of the procedure on the patient.

- Nurse N, a first-year nursing student, is directed by a staff physician to administer the anesthetic Novocain to a patient at a bedside operative procedure. Under the particular state nurse practice act the administration of anesthetics is described as a medical function.

Under the described circumstances, would Nurse N be acting illegally by carrying out the physician's order?

Yes | No
☐ | ☐

3-24 *No*

3-25   In order to avoid legal liability in this situation, what would be expected of Nurse N?

☐   Nurse N should get the prior approval of the supervising nurse.

☐   Nurse N should verify the fact that the physician is duly licensed.

☐   Nurse N should know how to administer the anesthetic and be knowledgeable of its effect on the patient.

3-26

■ Nurse N is given an order by a physician to perform a medical procedure that N has reason to believe will result in harm to the patient.

Which of the following accurately states the legal consequences of carrying out or refusing to carry out the procedure?

☐   By carrying out the procedure with due care, Nurse N cannot be held legally liable for any harm to the patient.

☐   By refusing to carry out the procedure, Nurse N may lose his or her license to practice as a nurse.

☐   By carrying out the procedure without question, Nurse N can be held legally liable for any harm that results to the patient.

3-25   *Nurse N should know how to administer the anesthetic . . .*

For amplification of this response, turn to p. 161, Note D.

3-26   *By carrying out the procedure without question, Nurse N can be held legally liable . . .*

EXPLANATORY NOTES

Note A (from Frame 3-4)

Both the first and third items are directly related to the patient's safety, but neither represents a legal duty of care with respect to the patient's safety. The courts always express legal duties in general terms, thereby permitting the pertinent legal rules (or standards) to be applied in a variety of fact situations. The second item expresses a rule in this manner.

Proceed to Frame 3-5.

Note B (from Frame 3-19)

The nurse who is directed to carry out a medical order that he or she is not qualified to perform, or that the nurse believes will result in harm to the patient, should immediately bring the matter to the attention of the nursing supervisor or a responsible hospital official in the event the supervisor is unavailable. If the nurse is a student, he or she should bring the matter to the attention of the nursing instructor or a responsible hospital official in the event the instructor is unavailable. As mentioned in an earlier note, both patient and nurse will benefit from a clear understanding by the nurse of his or her legal responsibilities and forthright conduct in these difficult situations.

Proceed to Frame 3-20.

EXPLANATORY NOTES

Note C (from Frame 3-21)

In retrospect, the doctor's order may have been too inflexible, but since walking a patient is a rather routine medical order, there is no basis for finding the doctor negligent on that basis alone. The nurse, however, is supposed to exercise independent professional judgment in a situation such as this, and the nurse's inflexibility is legally unpardonable. While it is possible that both the doctor and the nurse would be held liable for the harm caused the patient, most courts would fix the blame on the nurse, whose (unsuccessful) defense would be that she was "just following the doctor's orders."

Proceed to Frame 3-22.

Note D (from Frame 3-25)

It is highly unlikely that a first-year nursing student would know, or would be expected to know, how to administer an anesthetic for a bedside surgical procedure. The given example was chosen expressly to illustrate that apart from the *legality* of carrying out a physician's order, there is the separate issue of the nurse's potential *liability* for attempting to carry it out if the nurse (1) does not know how to perform the procedure, and (2) is not aware of the effect of the procedure on the patient.

Proceed to Frame 3-26.

3-27   A nurse's intervention may take the form of requesting the physician to clarify an order or objecting to carrying out the order when the nurse *knows* it to be harmful or erroneous. This responsibility to protect the patient from harm applies to all types of nursing activities, from the most simple to the most complex.

■ Nurse N, a certified registered nurse-anesthetist, is directed by the operating surgeon to administer a general halogenated anesthetic to the patient. Knowing the anesthetic agent in question to be contraindicated because of the patient's past history of hepatitis, Nurse N suggests to the surgeon a more appropriate substitute. The surgeon dismisses the nurse's suggestion and repeats the order to administer the original anesthetic drug.

Why should, or should not, Nurse N follow the surgeon's direct order in this instance?

☐   Nurse N should not follow the order, since it is N's primary responsibility to determine the appropriate anesthetic agent.

☐   Nurse N should not follow the order, since N has a primary legal responsibility to protect the patient from harm.

☐   Nurse N should follow the order, since N gave the surgeon a second opportunity to consider the order and change it as suggested.

3-28   Indicate which of the following classes of nurses is authorized to challenge a physician's order:

☐   private-duty nurses   ☐   occupational health nurses   ☐   nurse-specialists

☐   general-duty nurses   ☐   licensed practical nurses   ☐   all nurses

---

3-27   ☐   *When a dispute of this signifi-*   **3-28**   *all nurses*
        ☑   *cance exists, the surgery should*
        ☐   *be cancelled.*

FOLLOWING THE ORDERS OF PHYSICIANS' ASSISTANTS

What is the nurse's legal duty with respect to following or challenging the order(s) of a legally certified physician's assistant? This brings into focus the entire issue of the relationship between physicians' assistants and the hospitals, nursing homes, and other facilities in which they work. Since the mid-1970s, many state legislatures have enacted statutes defining physicians' assistants and delineating the scope of the services they may provide and the degree of medical supervision they require. There is still a considerable amount of confusion concerning these matters, and nursing organizations have raised many objections about the broad authority granted physicians' assistants under many of these laws.

The Joint Commission on Accreditation of Healthcare Organizations has recognized physicians' assistants as being part of the hospital's medical staff, and the few court cases discussing the point have supported this position. In 1979, the Washington State Nurses' Association challenged a regulation promulgated by the State Board of Medical Examiners (pursuant to statutory authority) for patient care. The Nurses' Association took the position that the State Board of Medical Examiners had exceeded its statutory authority in granting such broad delegated medical authority, and that this would, in effect, require nurses to execute prescriptions issued by physicians' assistants as well as by physicians.

The court ruled in favor of the Board of Medical Examiners, stating in part, "Two provisions in the statutes authorizing physicians' assistants to practice medicine indicate a legislative intent to create an agency relationship. . . . These provisions for control and responsibility indicate that the actions of the assistant are to be considered as actions of the supervising physician" (*Washington States Nurses' Association* v. *Board of Medical Examiners*, 605 P. 2d 1269 [Wash. 1980]).

On the matter of carrying out a physician's assistant's orders, the Iowa Attorney General has ruled that "if the physician's assistant can carry out the intent of the physician under whose supervision he acts and performs his duties . . . only by giving certain orders to a nurse, then he has a legal right to give those orders and the nurse is under a legal obligation to obey them" (Iowa Attorney General Opinion No. 78-12-41, Dec. 30, 1978). the Michigan Attorney General's office ruled similarly (Michigan Attorney General Opinion No. 5220, 1977). By the same token, the nurse has the same legal duty to question and challenge orders transmitted by a physician's assistant as he or she does to question and challenge a physician's order.

Regardless of the foregoing Attorney General opinions, the legal responsibility of the nurse to follow the orders of physicians' assistants is an issue that is still unresolved in a number of states where it is under review. Accordingly, when particular problems arise, nurses should look to their respective state Boards of Nursing for the latest rulings and authoritative guidance on this issue.

3-29 The nurse must be tactful and courteous in questioning a physician's order and must be prepared to justify his or her position. Challenging a physician's apparently harmful order calls for a keen awareness of the physician's professional and psychological position, but the responsible nurse must *never* permit fear of rebuke by the physician to override his or her fundamental concern for the welfare and safety of the patient.

Consider the following case:

- A hospital staff physician writes an order for an unusually large dose of a drug for a patient, and three staff nurses have serious doubts concerning the quantity of the drug ordered. Each broaches the subject to the physician in a different manner.

Which of these nurses has sufficiently alerted the physician to the possible danger involved in carrying out the order?

☐ Nurse A: "Doctor, I simply will *not* give Mrs. P such a massive dose of _____. I'm sure it will harm her. Are you sure you know what you are doing?"

☐ Nurse B: "Doctor, I see you have ordered an injection of 30 ml _____ for Mrs. P. That is a much larger dose than we usually give, and since it might be harmful in that dosage, I thought I'd better check with you. Did you really intend it to be 30 ml?"

☐ Nurse C: "Doctor, will you please explain to me why you have ordered such a large dose of _____ for Mrs. P? All the nurses I've spoken to say that you must have made an error and I'm afraid to risk giving the injection unless you can give me a good explanation."

3-30 Which nurse has brought the matter to the physician's attention in the manner *most likely* to bring about the desired result?

Nurse A	*Nurse B*	*Nurse C*
☐	☐	☐

3-29 ☑
         ☑
         ☑

3-30 *Nurse B*

For information about a related problem, turn to Note A, p. 174.

3-31

- P, a female patient of Doctor D, was noted to be anemic in her thirty-fifth week of pregnancy, and the doctor immediately ordered a blood transfusion in the emergency room (ER) of the local hospital. Doctor D set the amount of blood to be administered at 1000 ml and injected the needle and started administering saline solution prior to the actual transfusion of blood. Doctor D then set the stopcock on the saline solution at the desired rate and left, giving Nurse N instructions only to continue with the procedure.

After the saline solution had been administered, Nurse N connected the container of blood and set the stopcock at the same rate of flow that earlier had been set by Doctor D. The latter returned while the blood was still being transfused and commented that all was in order. When P had received the full 1000 ml of blood, she was permitted to leave the ER but was brought back shortly thereafter, suffering from pulmonary edema. She died, despite all efforts to save her and her child.

P's estate sues Nurse N for alleged malpractice in failing to slow down the rate of flow of the blood being transfused. At the trial all the testifying physicians agree that the attack of pulmonary edema was principally due to the transfusion of such a large quantity of blood into a patient in the last stages of pregnancy and that the *rapid rate of flow* was a contributing factor that probably hastened the patient's death.

The facts as stated indicate that Nurse N   ☐ did have   ☐ did not have   the necessary qualifications to carry out the transfusion.

3-32   Establishment of the rate of flow of blood in this case would be

☐ a matter for Nurse N's independent professional judgment

☐ a matter of medical judgment for the physician

☐ a matter of standard hospital policy

3-31   *did have*   3-32   *a matter of medical judgment for the physician*

3-33 What was Nurse N's legal duty with respect to carrying out the transfusion that was begun by Doctor D?

☐ Nurse N was required to challenge Doctor D's decision to transfuse such a large quantity of blood at such a rapid rate.

☐ Nurse N was required to follow Doctor D's orders unless he or she knew or should have suspected harm would result to the patient.

☐ Nurse N should have slowed the rate of flow of the blood in the exercise of independent professional judgment.

3-34 If Nurse N, *acting on his or her own,* had slowed the rate of flow of the transfusion but P nevertheless died of pulmonary edema, what legal consequence would this have?

☐ Doctor D could sue Nurse N for malpractice.

☐ Nurse N could be charged with practicing medicine without a license.

☐ Nurse N would avoid liability by having acted in the patient's best interests.

3-35 Accepting as true the proposition that the quantity and rapid rate of flow of the blood transfused into the patient was the probable cause of death, who most likely would be held liable for P's death in this case?

☐ Doctor D

☐ Nurse N

☐ the hospital

3-33 ☐
☑
☐

3-34 *Nurse N could be charged with practicing medicine without a license.*

The scope of nursing practice issues is discussed more fully in Part 5.

3-35 *Doctor D*

TIPS FOR DEALING WITH QUESTIONABLE PHYSICIANS' ORDERS

■ Don't execute an order from a doctor if you have any doubt about its accuracy or appropriateness, given the patient's condition.

■ Follow the hospital's existing policy and procedures regarding the clarification of ambiguous orders.

■ Document your efforts to clarify the order—including your efforts to contact the physician who wrote the order or someone else in authority.

■ If, after carrying out an order, the proposed treatment appears to be affecting the patient adversely, discontinue it and report all unfavorable signs and symptoms to the patient's physician at once.

■ Resume treatment only after you've discussed the situation with the doctor and all orders have been clarified.

POINTS TO REMEMBER

1. The nurse is legally required to exercise reasonable care to safeguard his or her patient from any known or reasonably foreseeable harm.

2. The safety and security of the patient is a paramount responsibility of the nurse, although the physician shares this legal responsibility.

3. A nurse is legally authorized and required to carry out any nursing or medical procedure he or she is directed to carry out by a duly licensed physician unless the nurse has substantial reason to believe harm will result to the patient from doing so.

4. Where there is no substantial reason to question a physician's order, failure to carry out such an order will subject the nurse to liability for any consequent harm to the patient.

5. To meet his or her legal responsibility in carrying out a physician's order, the nurse must know *how* to execute the procedure in question, as well as the *effect* of the procedure on the patient.

6. When a nurse has reason to question a physician's order, he or she should do so tactfully, but directly, keeping in mind the fundamental rule that the patient's safety is always of paramount concern.

7. If there are reasonable grounds for believing some harm will come to the patient if he or she carries out a physician's order, the nurse has a legal duty *not* to follow the order. The nurse should bring the matter immediately to the attention of the supervisor (or instructor, in the case of a nursing student). If the supervisor or instructor is not available at the moment, the matter should be brought to the attention of a responsible hospital official.

8. The above legal rules with respect to following or challenging orders given by a physician apply with equal force to orders given to the nurse by a physician's assistant acting on behalf of the physician employer.

DIAGNOSIS, DOCUMENTATION, AND MONITORING ERRORS

3-36 Except in an emergency situation in which a physician is not available, or in which specific authority has been granted to the nurse by statute (such as one relating to nurse practitioners or clinical nurse-specialists), it is unlawful for a nurse to *medically* diagnose a patient's condition for the purpose of instituting positive treatment or therapeutic measures. This is clearly the province and function of the physician. However, the professional nurse is always authorized to make a *nursing diagnosis* in order to evaluate all physical, mental, sociological, and economic factors that may have an influence on the proper course of treatment and the patient's ultimate recovery. In so doing, however, the nurse must exercise reasonable care in ascertaining the essential facts on which his or her diagnosis is based, and failure to do so will result in liability for negligent or improper treatment if harm to the patient results.

Under what circumstances may a nurse make a diagnosis?

☐ whenever the nurse believes he or she has sufficient experience to be able to do so

☐ whenever the nurse is required to evaluate the patient's condition to determine the specific needs for nursing care

☐ under no circumstances, since this is the physician's sole responsibility

3-37 What type of diagnosis is a nurse *prohibited* from making?

☐ one that involves evaluating the patient's state of mind or reaction to a particular course of treatment

☐ one that involves evaluating external influences affecting the patient's condition, such as family relationships or financial problems

☐ one that involves medical judgments concerning the patient's condition for the purpose of instituting specific treatment

NOTE: Most nurses regularly make nursing diagnoses, even though their state nurse practice acts often say nothing specific about their authority to do so. A nursing diagnosis is part of the nursing *assessment* necessary to evaluate the patient's progress, responses to treatment, and nursing care needs. This assessment enables the nurse to develop and carry out the nursing care plan; it is not—and is not supposed to be—a judgment about a patient's medical disorder. The North American Nursing Diagnosis Association (NANDA) is the forerunner in the development of nursing diagnoses to guide nursing practice.

3-36 ☐ / ☑ / ☐   3-37 ☐ / ☐ / ☑

3-38 In an emergency a nurse legally may make a medical diagnosis and undertake whatever medical treatment is reasonable and necessary before a physician can be summoned and arrives.

True   *False*

☐   ☐

3-39 One of the fundamental legal responsibilities of the nurse is the duty to keep accurate records of the patient's physical and mental condition (e.g., temperature, pulse, and other overt physical signs, as well as emotional behavior). This responsibility is one that is shared by practical and registered professional nurses alike, but the RN, because of special training, has the additional responsibility of *interpreting* and *evaluating* the patient's symptoms and reactions to any nursing or medical regimen and reporting them to the physician so he or she may make appropriate adjustments in the prescribed treatment.

Recording and reporting the patient's physical signs and general emotional behavior is the legal responsibility of

☐ all categories of nurses

☐ professional RNs only

☐ licensed practical nurses only

3-40 Why is the RN held to a higher standard of care than the practical nurse with respect to reporting the patient's reactions and symptoms?

☐ the RN is more directly involved in patient care

☐ the RN has been trained to evaluate and interpret reactions and symptoms and to make judgments thereon concerning essential action necessary

☐ practical nurses are not legally required to concern themselves with reactions and symptoms of their patients

---

3-38 *True*

If you checked the wrong answer, turn to p. 175, Note B.

3-39 *all categories of nurses*

3-40 ☐ *The respective roles of*
☑ *the RN and LPN are*
☐ *discussed on p. 176, Note C.*

NOTE: Monitoring the patient's condition and reporting changes therein is one of the nurse's prime responsibilities. Nurses who fail to record their observations run the risk of being unable to convince a jury that such observations actually were made. In *Pirkov-Middaugh* v. *Gillette Children's Hospital*, 479 N.W. 2d 63 (Minn. 1991), a 4-year-old child underwent hip surgery but developed compartment syndrome (muscle swelling beyond the capacity of the fascia) within 48 hours. Due to a breakdown in communication between the surgeon—who was inaccessible by phone over the weekend—and hospital physicians, an emergency fasciotomy to relieve pressure on the vascular and muscular structures was delayed for many hours. By that time, the muscles in the child's right leg had to be surgically removed because the muscle tissue had died. Evidence presented at trial showed that the nurses on duty had failed to monitor the child's condition appropriately after surgery. In addition, they didn't know what equipment was needed to test for compartment syndrome or where it was located. The nurses and the hospital were found negligent for the devastating injuries suffered by the young patient in this case.

An earlier case involving failure to monitor and resulting circulatory compromise was *Collins* v. *Westlake Community Hospital*, 312 N.E. 2d 614 (Ill. 1974). In that case a patient treated for a fractured leg developed ischemia within 3 days, necessitating amputation. The physician had written an order for the nurses to watch the condition of the patient's toes, and although proper nursing care required monitoring the patient's circulation as often as every 15 minutes, the nurse's notes failed to show that the patient's circulation had been monitored *at any time* during the crucial 7-hour period when the patient's condition became critical. The nurses' negligence was upheld by the court.

Good nursing practice dictates that patients who are in casts be monitored frequently to avoid complications of the sort mentioned above. While failure to monitor continues to be a significant cause of nursing malpractice suits, failure to *report* the patient's worsening condition continues to be an equally prominent source of litigation.

3-41

■ Before delivery of Patient P's child, Doctor D made a small incision to relieve the constrictive muscle surrounding the cervix. D left the incision unsutured, but pelvic packs were inserted to control bleeding. Nurse N informed Doctor D while Doctor D was still at the hospital that she believed the patient was bleeding too much, but each time Doctor D insisted her condition was normal.

Doctor D then instructed Nurse N in how to measure the rate of flow of the bleeding and gave orders to call if the postpartum flow was greater than normal. One hour later Nurse N noted excessive bleeding but did not take the patient's blood pressure, temperature, pulse, or respiration, nor did she call Doctor D because, in her opinion, Doctor D would not have come back to the hospital anyhow. A relief nurse who came on duty 30 minutes later could not locate the patient's pulse and immediately called Doctor D, but by the time Doctor D arrived the patient had died from the hemorrhage.

P's estate sues Doctor D and Nurse N for their alleged malpractice in treatment.

What legal duty did Nurse N have with respect to keeping track of P's vital signs?

☐ the duty to record vital signs as soon as the patient's condition began to deteriorate

☐ the duty to record vital signs at regular intervals and to report significant changes to the physician

☐ the duty to use her best professional judgment concerning the desirability of or need for recording vital signs

3-42 Assuming the facts given, Nurse N could *reasonably* conclude that

☐ Doctor D was unwilling to reconsider his assessment of P's postpartum bleeding

☐ Doctor D was unconcerned about P's postpartum bleeding

☐ Doctor D had misdiagnosed the seriousness of P's postpartum bleeding

3-41 *the duty to record vital signs at regular intervals and to report significant changes . . .*

3-42 ☑
☐
☐

3-43   What *significant* error in judgment did Nurse N make in this case?

   ☐   Nurse N made an unwarranted medical diagnosis of P's condition.

   ☐   Nurse N made an unwarranted assumption that Doctor D would not be responsive to any emergency call on her part.

   ☐   Nurse N failed to report Doctor D's handling of the case to her nursing supervisor.

3-44   What would a reasonably prudent nurse have done under the circumstances of this case?

   ☐   He or she would have taken the patient's vital signs regularly and would have called Doctor D as soon as he or she determined the patient's bleeding was excessive.

   ☐   He or she would have waited until the patient's bleeding was serious enough to ensure that Doctor D would respond to an emergency call.

   ☐   He or she would have informed the patient's family of the situation so that they might prevail upon Doctor D to take appropriate remedial action.

3-45   If Doctor D and Nurse N are both sued, and Doctor D is held liable for malpractice in failing to suture the incision immediately after the baby was delivered, Nurse N legally cannot be held liable for her conduct.

	True	*False*
	☐	☐

3-43 ☐	**3-44** ☑	**3-45** *False*
☑	☐	
☐	☐	*If you checked the wrong answer, turn to p. 190, Note A.*

EXPLANATORY NOTES

Note A (from Frame 3-30)

What happens if the nurse discreetly challenges the physician's order but the physician nevertheless chooses to proceed with the treatment? Should the nurse simply remain silent? Not if the nurse really cares about the patient and at the same time wants to protect both himself or herself and the hospital from possible liability. In this situation—assuming that the nurse still has substantial reason to believe that harm will result to the patient if the order is carried out—the nurse should delay executing the order and seek immediate guidance from the supervisor. All hospitals have written procedures for dealing with situations like this when a nurse believes an error has been made in a physician's order prescribing specific drugs or treatment, and nursing administrators are taught to anticipate and know how to deal with these situations.

The reasonably prudent nurse, therefore, will not simply challenge the physician but will follow through with a prompt report to the nursing supervisor or other hospital authority if there is substantial reason to believe that carrying out an order, *even after it is confirmed by the physician*, will cause harm to the patient. In short, simply "going through the motions" of challenging an order will not protect either the nurse or the hospital from legal liability when a physician's course of conduct is clearly calculated to be detrimental to the patient's welfare. For an excellent recent case demonstrating the correct way to challenge a physician's potentially harmful order, see *NKC Hospitals, Inc.* v. *Anthony*, 849 S.W. 2d 564 (Ky. 1993).

Proceed to Frame 3-31.

EXPLANATORY NOTES

Note B (from Frame 3-38)

It is well established that in an emergency situation a nurse may perform any medical act deemed necessary to preserve life or limb. The reasonableness of the nurse's conduct in such a situation is always gauged by the surrounding circumstances, and the nurse is not held to the standard of nursing care expected under more normal circumstances. In all cases involving emergency care it is expected that the nurse will summon medical assistance as soon as possible, and the legal privilege of making medical judgments and undertaking medical acts in an emergency is limited to those immediate, at-the-scene measures deemed absolutely necessary to save life or limb.

If the nurse is a clinical specialist in emergency nursing and is employed in a hospital ER or other emergency care setting, the legal situation is different. Many nurses who work in the ER and/or cover ambulance services are qualified Emergency Medical Technicians (EMTs) who are prepared to provide Basic Life Support, and most have also had training in Advanced Cardiac Life Support. Accordingly, they are well equipped to manage trauma and emergency stabilization of the patient until the physician can be accessed. Nurse-specialists in emergency care typically function within guidelines (protocols) established with the hospital's medical staff. In recognition of emergency nursing as a specialty, some states are revising their nurse practice acts to permit nurses who are certified in emergency nursing to make diagnoses and implement procedures that would otherwise be deemed the practice of medicine. We will cover these "scope-of-practice" issues in Part 5 of this course.

Proceed to Frame 3-39.

EXPLANATORY NOTES

Note C (from Frame 3-40)

The RN and LPN share the common objective of rendering skillful nursing care to the ill, injured, or infirm, but the LPN's legal status, as determined by state and provincial licensure laws, is considerably more restricted because of the more limited educational background of the LPN. Both the RN and the LPN are required to have the same basic concepts of nursing care (including the necessary manual skills), but the RN has a much greater responsibility for (1) assessing the nursing needs of patients, (2) evaluating the incapacities of patients, (3) judging how much the patient can do for himself or herself and how much assistance he or she needs, and (4) understanding and observing the effects of the treatments and medications administered. The RN, by training, has been prepared to structure a comprehensive nursing care plan to fit the needs of the individual patient.

The LPN, by contrast, is authorized to perform *selected* nursing acts, and then only under the direction of a physician, dentist, or RN. In the traditional institutional setting, the LPN is the bedside nurse whose normal activities center on meeting the patient's basic physical needs for hygiene and comfort. In carrying out these activities, the LPN works in a close relationship with the RN and under the RN's direct supervision. The nurse practice acts in some states fairly clearly define the limitations of LPNs in terms of scope of practice—for example, prohibiting them from inserting IV lines. Because of the continuing shortage of RNs, however, at least 30 states have recognized the right of LPNs to perform in an expanded role, such as administering drugs, performing venipuncture, and withdrawing IV fluids, provided the LPN is properly trained for the task. In the managed care/case management model of health care set forth in recent health care reform proposals (described more fully in Part 8), the RN typically is the case manager while the LPN is designated as the case associate, working under the direction of the RN.

Unquestionably, the LPN's concern for proper patient care is every bit as great as that of the RN, and while the LPN may perform many of the same nursing functions performed by RNs, he or she must be constantly aware of the limitations imposed by law, specifically the state nurse practice act. With shortages of RNs in all parts of the nation likely to continue for some time, it can be expected that increasing numbers of states will enact laws that further expand the patient care role of the LPN.

Proceed to Frame 3-41.

FAILURE TO COMMUNICATE

3-46 Nurses must continually evaluate a mass of information and findings, and as soon as they become aware of significant medical data, dangerous circumstances, or a dramatic worsening of the patient's condition, they are required to communicate this information to the treating physician at once. Their failure to communicate these observations can have disastrous consequences and will certainly increase the chances for malpractice litigation.

■ A mother brings her two young boys to the hospital's emergency department for treatment of rashes and fever. She specifically mentions to Nurse N that she had taken several ticks from the body of one of the children, but Nurse N fails to communicate this information to Doctor D, the emergency department physician. As a result, Doctor D diagnoses measles rather than Rocky Mountain spotted fever, and the condition of both children deteriorates rapidly, with one child dying several days later. Doctor D eventually makes the correct diagnosis and is able to treat the second child successfully.

In a lawsuit brought by the parents of the deceased child against the hospital, Doctor D, and Nurse N, whom would a jury most likely find *primarily* liable for the child's wrongful death?

☐ Nurse N, because the nurse failed to communicate the vital information that could have saved the child's life

☐ Doctor D, because it was the physician's responsibility to make an accurate diagnosis and prescribe accordingly

☐ the hospital, because it is legally responsible for the quality of care provided to all patients seeking care in its emergency department

---

3-47 If Nurse N is held liable, is it likely that N's hospital employer will also be held liable?

Yes	No
☐	☐

3-46 *Nurse N, because the nurse failed to communicate the vital information that could have saved the child's life*

3-47 *Yes*

3-48 With respect to the matter of communication, indicate whether the conclusions set forth below are true or false.

True	*False*	
☐	☐	It is the nurse's legal duty to observe and report to the treating physician all significant changes in the patient's condition.
☐	☐	It is the nurse's legal duty to communicate abnormal data about a patient to the physician only when the nurse believes the physician will take appropriate action based thereon.
☐	☐	In deciding whether to communicate significant data to the treating physician, it is the nurse's responsibility to determine what is significant and what is not.
☐	☐	A nurse cannot be held liable for failing to contact a physician about a patient's worsening condition if the nurse knows from past experience the physician is not likely to respond to the call.
☐	☐	When a nurse cannot locate the patient's physician to report vital information about the patient's worsening condition, the nurse should communicate the information to a supervisor.

3-49 The fundamental reason why a nurse should communicate essential facts and information about a patient's worsening condition to the treating physician is

☐ to avoid personal liability in case of a lawsuit

☐ to comply with specific medical orders or hospital protocols

☐ to reduce the risk of harm to the patient

3-48	*True*	*False*	**3-49**	*to reduce the risk of harm to the patient*
	☑	☐		
	☐	☑		
	☑	☐		
	☐	☑		
	☑	☐		

BREAKDOWNS IN COMMUNICATION

Breakdowns in communication between physician and nurse can result from a multitude of causes, and the differences are important even though the consequences may be the same. As already noted, communicating significant changes in the patient's status to the treating physician (or nursing supervisor, if the physician is not immediately available) is a fundamental component of good nursing practice, yet we continue to see case after case involving the nurse's failure to notify the physician of such changes.

A recent review of litigated malpractice cases revealed a failure on the part of nurses to notify or advise treating physicians of the following significant medical conditions: changes in a casted leg resulting from circulatory compromise; fetal tachycardia and meconium; pain and vaginal bleeding; increased pulse rate and lack of response to stimulation in an ICU patient; dehydration and general seriousness of the patient's condition; jaundice; and excessive oxygen levels.

A second form of communication breakdown is more closely linked to unusual situational or environmental factors, although nursing judgment is almost always involved. For example, in *White* v. *Methodist Hospital South*, 844 S.W. 2d 642 (Tenn. 1992), a nurse-anesthetist was informed by the patient immediately before tubal ligation surgery that she had a history of hypertension and that she was experiencing a severe headache following administration of the preoperative medication. Since vital signs appeared to be within normal limits, however, the patient was taken to the operating room. Shortly thereafter, the patient's pulse rate skyrocketed to 212 beats per minute, but the administration of additional drugs brought it down to 120 beats per minute. When the surgeon arrived to begin the procedure, the nurse-anesthetist failed to mention the earlier spike in pulse rate. Immediately after the initial incision, the patient's pulse rate again spiked to over 200 beats per minute, and even though additional medications brought it down again, the patient experienced cardiac arrest, with consequent hypoxic encephalopathy. At trial, expert witnesses testified that had the nurse-anesthetist apprised the surgeon of the abnormal vital signs before the operation began, he would have been alerted to the fact that the abnormal vital signs might have been "masked" by the additional medication given immediately before and during the surgery, and in all probability he would not have proceeded. Emergency department care, as noted in Part 1, also lends itself to many communication breakdowns because of the general hubbub in the ER and the urgent nature of the care provided there.

A third—and most unfortunate—form of communication breakdown may occur when a nurse *knows* she should communicate important information about a patient to the treating physician but decides not to because she is convinced that the physician will not act thereon. That is what occurred in the highly-publicized tragic case of *Goff* v. *Doctors Hospital of San Jose*, 333 P. 2d 29 (Cal. 1958), the facts of which were outlined in Frame 3-41.

Analyses of litigated malpractice suits indicate that most failures in communication are preventable. The reasonable and prudent nurse should always be on guard against possible foulups in communication, especially in a busy, super-charged atmosphere like the ER. The prompt, complete, and accurate recording of data in patients' charts is essential to the communication process, as is the need for nurses to sharpen their assessment skills and improve their ability to judge when a patient's condition clearly needs a physician's attention. Communicating effectively is a vital part of the nurse's primary responsibility to protect the patient from harm.

IMPROPER SUPERVISION

3-50 Negligence in supervision is a growing cause of malpractice claims against registered professional nurses. The registered nurse who is a supervisor, unlike other categories of nurses, is legally and professionally responsible for directing and supervising the activities of practical nurses, nurse's aides, and other nurses involved in direct patient care. Ordinarily, supervisors are held liable only for their *own* negligence in caring for a patient, but they can also be held liable, under certain circumstances, for the negligence of someone they are supervising.

Which of the following classes of nurses can be held liable for negligence in supervision?

☐ practical nurses

☐ RNs

☐ all categories of nurses

3-51 Why would a practical nurse ordinarily not be held liable for negligence in supervision?

☐ because practical nurses are generally prudent and careful

☐ because practical nurses are not competent to supervise others

☐ because practical nurses are not legally or professionally responsible for supervising others

---

NOTE: Although LPNs do not ordinarily supervise or manage nursing units, in certain settings, such as nursing homes, they are sometimes given these responsibilities. Notwithstanding this fact, the National Labor Relations Board has long held that LPNs were not "supervisors" within the strict meaning of that term in the National Labor Relations Act (NLRA). However, in *NLRB* v. *Health Care and Retirement Corporation of America*, 987 F. 2d 1256 (Ohio 1993), the Sixth Circuit Court of Appeals ruled otherwise. Because of conflicts between judicial circuits on this issue, the U.S. Supreme Court granted review of the case, and in May, 1994— in a 5 to 4 decision with a vigorous dissenting opinion by Justice Ginsberg—the Court agreed with the Sixth Circuit Court of Appeals and held that the LPNs in question were "supervisors" within the meaning of the NLRA and could not, therefore, avail themselves of the protection accorded to employees (but not to supervisors) under the statute (114 S. Ct. 1778).

3-50 *RNs*   **3-51** ☐
                                  ☐
                                  ☑

3-52 In general, a nursing supervisor's potential liability is   ☐ greater than   ☐ the same as   ☐ less than   that of other hospital-based nurses.

3-53 A nursing supervisor, as a specialist, is held to the standard of care of the reasonably prudent nursing supervisor in carrying out professional and administrative responsibilities. This responsibility includes not only the making of staff assignments, but his or her conduct in other supervisory situations.

■ Supervisory Nurse S was informed by staff Nurse N that one of his patients who was recovering from major surgery showed clear signs of advancing tetanus. Supervisor S chose not to call the patient's physician because he knew the physician was out of town at a medical conference, nor did S summon any other physician for a period of 3 days. By that time, the patient's condition had so deteriorated that all efforts to save him were futile.

Nurse S's liability, if any, in this case would be based on

☐ her negligence in supervising Nurse N

☐ the doctrine of *respondeat superior*

☐ the rule of personal liability

3-54 The supervisor who assigns duties to an otherwise competent nurse cannot be held liable for the latter's negligence in carrying out those duties *simply because he or she is the nurse's supervisor.* Under the rule of personal liability, every person is legally responsible for his or her own negligent conduct.

■ Nurse S is a supervisory nurse in a general hospital and Nurse N is S's subordinate. Both are RNs with several years of experience in all phases of nursing. Nurse S assigns Nurse N to a pediatric unit, and while there, Nurse N negligently administers an overdose of a medication to an infant.

Nurse S   ☐ will   ☐ will not   be held liable for Nurse N's conduct because

☐ her liability as a supervisor extends only to administrative responsibilities

☐ the assignment was well within N's degree of competence

☐ the hospital assumes liability for all medication errors by nurses

---

3-52	*greater than*	3-53	*the rule of personal liability*	3-54	*will not*
					☐
					☑
					☐

3-55 Liability for negligence in supervision is generally based on (1) failure of the supervisor to determine which of the patient's needs he or she can safely assign to a subordinate nurse or (2) failure of the supervisor to give closer personal supervision to a subordinate who requires such supervision.

- A malpractice suit is filed against Supervisory Nurse S for injuries resulting from a nursing student's negligence in catheterizing a patient. At the trial it is shown that Nurse S was aware of the student's limited experience with catheterization procedures at the time she made the assignment. The jury finds Nurse S negligent and holds her liable for the injuries to the patient.

Which one or more of the following actions on Nurse S's part might have shielded her from liability in this situation?

☐ She could have performed the procedure herself in a safe manner.

☐ She could have directed the nursing student in the performance of the procedure, to ensure it was done safely in her presence.

☐ She could have assigned the procedure to a nurse she knew to be capable of carrying it out safely.

3-56 On what grounds (if any) might the nursing student in the previous frame also be held liable?

☐ He could be held liable for failing to meet the standard of care expected of his supervisor.

☐ He could be held liable for attempting to carry out a procedure clearly beyond his capabilities.

☐ He could not be held liable, since he was only a nursing student.

3-55	☑	3-56	*He could be held liable*
	☑		*for attempting to carry*
	☑		*out a procedure clearly*
			beyond his capabilities.

3-57 Which of the following expresses the general rule regarding the legal liability of a supervisory nurse?

☐ The supervisory nurse cannot be held liable for acts of negligence on the part of registered nurses he or she supervises, but can be held liable for acts of negligence on the part of practical nurses or nurse's aides whom he or she supervises.

☐ The supervisory nurse is not automatically liable for all acts of negligence on the part of those whom he or she supervises, but may be held liable where he or she is negligent in supervising others.

☐ The supervisory nurse cannot be held liable for acts of negligence on the part of nurses whom he or she supervises, since each nurse is liable for his or her own negligent conduct.

3-58 It should be noted that even though a supervisory nurse may be held liable for the negligence of subordinates, this liability is not based on the doctrine of *respondeat superior*, since this doctrine is applicable only to persons or legal entities who are in a master-servant or principal-agent relationship. Supervisory nurses are not the employers (masters) of the nurses who work under their supervision, even though they exercise their authority on behalf of their hospital or nursing home employer.

■ Patient P, injured while being treated in Hospital H, files suit against Supervisory Nurse S for the negligent acts of Nurse N, who had been assigned by Nurse S to care for him.

If P is to prevail in his suit against Nurse S, he will have to prove

☐ that Nurse S stood in the same legal position as Nurse N's employer because of the authority to supervise granted to Nurse S

☐ that Nurse S was negligent in his own right and not because of any secondary or derivative liability imposed on him

☐ that Nurse S is liable because the law holds a supervisor responsible for the negligent acts of all subordinates

---

3-57   ☐   3-58   *that Nurse S was negli-*
       ☑   *gent in his own right . . .*
       ☐

SUPERVISORS AND SHORT-STAFFING PROBLEMS

Whatever the title—head nurse, charge nurse, patient care supervisor, or other comparable designation—the nursing supervisor is the person legally in charge. This means he or she is not only directly responsible for supervising the work of floor-duty nurses, but the services of special-duty nurses, nursing students, nurses' aids, orderlies, and technicians as well. In short, the nursing supervisor is responsible for ensuring that all medical orders on his or her unit are executed promptly and skillfully, and that all appropriate measures are taken to ensure patient safety.

As noted earlier (in Part 2), under the doctrine of hospital corporate liability a hospital is obligated to provide its patients with such reasonable care and attention for their safety as their known physical and mental condition may require, and may be held liable for injury resulting to a patient caused by the negligent conduct of its employees. Due to the shortage of nurses, however, many hospitals today are understaffed and the available nurses are overworked—a situation that greatly increases the risk of injury to patients and consequent legal liability. In *HCA Health Services of Midwest, Inc.* v. *National Bank of Commerce*, 745 S.W. 2d 120 (Ark. 1988), for example, the court held that a hospital could be held liable for brain damage sustained by a newborn infant when the nurses in its understaffed nursery failed to discover timely that the baby had stopped breathing. The nursery had 18 babies and only three nurses, and the evidence at trial showed that the infant's area had not been checked by any of the nurses for at least 30 minutes before he was found lying face down with no pulse or respiration.

Although it is the hospital's prime responsibility to provide adequate staffing for the safe care of patients, there are circumstances in which a nursing supervisor can be held personally liable in a short-staffing situation. In *Horton* v. *Niagara Falls Memorial Medical Center*, 380 N.Y.S. 2d 116 (N.Y. 1976), a patient was admitted for treatment of pneumonitis and was confused, uncoordinated, weak, and had difficulty seeing. Throughout the afternoon, his wife stayed with him in his second floor room that had an adjoining balcony. Shortly after his wife left, construction workers nearby saw the patient on the balcony calling to them for a ladder, and they notified the charge nurse. She called the patient's doctor, who ordered restraints for the patient and told the charge nurse to keep an eye on him, and if further trouble developed, to move him to a safer room.

The charge nurse also phoned the wife and suggested she return to the hospital to sit with her husband. The wife agreed, but asked the nurse to have someone watch her husband until her mother, who lived only 10 minutes away, could get there. The charge nurse responded, "We can't possibly do that" because the hospital was understaffed. By the time the patient's mother-in-law arrived, he had fallen from the balcony and suffered serious injuries. Suit was brought against the charge nurse as well as the hospital, alleging failure to provide continuous supervision of the patient.

At the trial, the jury was given evidence indicating that the hospital had enough trained personnel to provide continuous supervision for the 10 to 15 minutes necessary before the mother-in-law arrived. Moreover, the aide assigned to the patient's room was allowed to go to supper, while the remaining nursing staff were carrying out routine nursing duties. Based on this evidence, the court held the charge nurse negligent for "failing to use the available staff in a reasonable manner."

The *Horton* case illustrates the point that, while short-staffing problems will be considered in determining whether a nursing supervisor acted reasonably in any given fact situation, short-staffing alone will not excuse the supervisor who fails to do what a reasonable nursing supervisor would have done under the same or similar circumstances.

As we discussed earlier, floating nurses to understaffed hospital units presents legal problems for all parties concerned, but they can be especially troublesome to the nursing supervisor who has to make such assignments, since she has to make on-the-spot decisions that can have a significant impact on patient safety. For example, the supervisor who is forced to float a nurse to a specialty unit (pediatrics, intensive care, coronary care, emergency department) with full knowledge of the nurse's limitations in that specialty will be held legally liable for any consequent injury to patients who suffer harm because of the floated nurse's negligence.

TIPS FOR SUPERVISORS FORCED TO MAKE FLOAT ASSIGNMENTS

The conscientious nursing supervisor who must make staffing assignments with inadequate numbers of trained nurses should not permit the situation to get out of hand. Here are some tips for dealing with chronic understaffing problems.

- Make hospital administration fully aware of the potential harm to patients resulting from inadequate staffing and your greatly increased risk of personal liability if injury occurs.

- Be sure to follow all appropriate channels of communication—up to and including the hospital board of trustees, if necessary.

- Document your concerns in writing and maintain records of all communications (oral and written) to the appropriate hospital authorities.

- Know (or ascertain) the experience and capabilities of nurses before you float them to hospital specialty units with which they may be unfamiliar.

- Supervise all float-nurse assignments meticulously, always mindful of the legal consequences if their negligent conduct causes injuries to patients.

POINTS TO REMEMBER

1. Except in an emergency, or when specifically authorized by statute, a nurse may not lawfully make a *medical* diagnosis of a patient's condition for the purpose of instituting treatment.

2. A professional nurse is legally authorized to make a *nursing* diagnosis to determine appropriate steps necessary to prevent complications or a worsening of the patient's condition.

3. A nursing diagnosis is one that involves the evaluation of all physical, mental, sociological, and economic factors that have an influence on the patient's recovery.

4. In a life-threatening emergency a nurse may make a medical diagnosis and undertake whatever treatment is necessary before a physician can be summoned and arrives.

5. A fundamental legal responsibility of the nurse is to keep accurate records of the patient's physical and mental condition.

6. Because of additional training, the professional nurse is held to a higher standard of care than the practical nurse in *evaluating* the patient's reactions and symptoms.

7. Although supervisory nurses ordinarily are held liable only for their own negligent acts, under certain circumstances they can also be held liable for negligence in supervising others.

8. Negligence arising out of supervision applies only to professional nurses since a practical nurse has neither the legal authority nor the responsibility to exercise professional supervision over subordinates.

9. Supervisory negligence may result from assigning a task to a subordinate that is clearly beyond the latter's capabilities and from failing to give closer supervision to someone who requires such supervision.

10. Even though a supervisor may be held liable for supervisory negligence, the negligent subordinate is not thereby relieved of liability for his or her own negligent conduct.

MEDICATION ERRORS

3-59 Mistakes in administering medications are among the most common causes of malpractice suits against nurses. Liability of the nurse may result from administering the wrong drug, or for administering the correct drug either at the wrong time, in the wrong dosage, or through the wrong route of administration. Obviously, liability may result from administering drugs to the wrong patient. A frequent cause of medication errors by nurses is misreading a doctor's order or failing to check with the doctor or hospital pharmacist when the order is questionable.

■ In a hurry, a physician writes an incomplete and partially illegible medication order. Nurse N, in an effort to be efficient and in order not to bother the physician with questions, decides which drug was intended, the dosage form, and the route of administration of the drug. Nurse N's judgment proves wrong, and the patient suffers serious harm.

On what basis could Nurse N be held liable for failing to have exercised reasonable care?

☐ for failing to question the physician concerning the incomplete and partially illegible medication order

☐ for showing more concern for the doctor than for the patient

☐ for prescribing a drug without proper legal authority

3-60

■ Patient P goes to Doctor D's office for treatment of a dislocated thumb, and Doctor D asks the office nurse, Nurse N, to secure Novocain for local anesthesia. Nurse N orders a medical technician (also employed by Doctor D) to get the drug, but the latter, by mistake, hands Nurse N a bottle labeled Adrenalin. Nurse N does not check the label and prepares the hypodermic for Doctor D. Thirty minutes after receiving the injection, Patient P dies from a systemic reaction to the Adrenalin.

What conduct on the part of Nurse N would legally constitute unreasonable care in this case?

☐ requesting a technician to get the drug

☐ failing to check the label on the drug

☐ preparing the hypodermic before showing the drug to the doctor

---

3-59 ☑ *Amplification of the nurse's*
☐ *responsibilities in drug admin-*
☐ *istration can be found on p.*
190, Note B.

3-60 *failing to check the label on the drug*

3-61 Would Doctor D have a right to assume that the hypodermic prepared by Nurse N contained the proper drug in the proper dosage?

Yes	*No*
☐	☐

3-62 Who could be held liable to P's estate in this case?

- ☐ only Nurse N
- ☐ only Doctor D
- ☐ only the technician
- ☐ both Nurse N and Doctor D
- ☐ Nurse N, Doctor D, and the technician

3-63 Many medication errors involve faulty technique in giving injections, usually resulting in nerve injury to the patient. Certainly, not every nerve injury following an injection is attributable to faulty technique on the part of the nurse, but where the onset of nerve injury is immediate and not otherwise explainable, the nurse generally is held liable for negligence in giving the injection.

■ Practical Nurse N gives a 5-year-old patient an intramuscular injection in his left buttock. Immediately thereafter the child experiences a painful, burning reaction at the site of the injection. A hematoma, ecchymosis, and sloughing soon develop at the site of the injection, necessitating additional medical care and surgery.

The facts as stated prove that Nurse N was negligent in giving the injection.

True	*False*
☐	☐

3-61 *Yes*	**3-62** ☐	**3-63** *False*
As a general rule the answer is "yes." The facts in a specific case might prove otherwise, however.	☐ ☐ ☐ ☑	If you checked True, turn to p. 191, Note C.

NOTE: It serves no useful purpose to detail the multitude of cases involving medication errors of one type or another. From a statistical standpoint, they continue to rank among the top causes of malpractice claims against nurses, undoubtedly because medication errors frequently have serious consequences. A review of malpractice cases involving nursing care as reported in the *Association of Trial Lawyers of America (ATLA) Law Reporter* for 1985 included the following examples of medication errors: gave wrong medication on discharge; failed to discontinue oxytocin as required by hospital policy when obstetrician was absent; administered morphine without notifying physician; failed to give diazepam (Valium) as ordered; gave excessive dose of disulfiram (Antabuse); allowed inappropriate use of IV equipment, causing extensive infusing of fluids extravascularly into leg and foot; administered potassium chloride improperly; and mishandled infusion pump (Northrop CE, "Nursing Actions in Litigation," *Quality Review Bulletin* 13[10]:343-8, 1987).

TIPS FOR PREVENTING MEDICATION ERRORS

We're all human, so mistakes are going to be made when nurses administer drugs. Doctors and pharmacists will make their share of mistakes as well. The intelligent nurse will take all this for granted, and will go out of his or her way to reduce errors as much as possible by taking the following precautions.

■ Keep current on new drugs by reading about them in nursing magazines, by attending drug seminars, and by having discussions with the hospital pharmacist.

■ Before you use it, know a drug's safe dosage limits, toxicity, potential adverse reactions, and contraindications for use.

■ Prevent errors by reading container labels three times.

■ When in doubt about a drug, have a second nurse check your work, i.e., the drug itself, the proper dosage, route of administration, and so forth.

■ If a doctor gives you a verbal drug order over the phone, write it down exactly as he gives it, and note the date and time. Then, repeat the order back to him to confirm its accuracy.

■ Be sure to document all verbal drug orders as soon as possible, and get the doctor to cosign them.

■ Refuse to accept illegible, confusing, or otherwise unclear drug orders. Seek clarification from your nursing supervisor, the doctor, or the hospital pharmacist before administering any unclear or confusing orders.

■ Delay administering any drug that you think has been misprescribed (dosage too high, contraindicated because of drug interactions, etc.) until you have had a chance to discuss it with your supervisor and/or the prescribing doctor.

EXPLANATORY NOTES

Note A (from Frame 3-45)

Throughout this course it has been stressed that every professional person is liable for his or her own negligent conduct (malpractice), and this frame illustrates this principle once again. The fact that the physician is held liable for personal negligent conduct does not mean that the nurse is free from liability for his or her negligent conduct. As a matter of fact, many of the more recent malpractice cases have involved both the physician and the nurse, and in a number of these cases both parties have been held liable for their concurrent acts of negligence. Remember: The rule of personal liability is always operative, and it should serve as a constant warning to nurses that they must act with reasonable care at all times.

Proceed to Frame 3-46.

Note B (from Frame 3-59)

Perhaps no aspect of nursing care is fraught with more risk than that relating to the administration of drugs. It has been reliably estimated that nearly one out of every seven medication orders in hospitals is erroneously carried out, emphasizing the extreme caution that must be exercised by all nurses who handle drugs. In no other area of nursing practice is there a greater need for independent and intelligent judgment, and the wise nurse will *always* question an ambiguous or incomplete medication order. The courts are not as lenient and forgiving as they once were, and more and more nurses are being held liable for medication errors as the number and potency of new drugs continue to increase.

Many physicians permit their office nurses to authorize prescription refills by telephone without direct orders from the physician. While this practice is permissible, since the nurse is merely acting as a conduit for information, it should be clearly noted that a nurse is not permitted to *prescribe* and will be held personally liable for the untoward consequences of advising a patient what medication to take, *even though the drug may be purchased without a physician's prescription.* This type of activity is to be deplored since it involves the area of medical diagnosis, and the office nurse would be well advised to refrain from giving gratuitous advice concerning medications over the telephone.

Proceed to Frame 3-60.

EXPLANATORY NOTES

Note C (from Frame 3-63)

There have been cases in which the very fact of nerve injury following an injection has been submitted as proof of negligence, but most courts do not accept this proposition and require *some* proof of negligence on the part of the nurse. Most medical practitioners would agree that unforeseen and undesirable reactions from an injection can result from causes other than negligence, including the emotions and allergies of the patient, non-traumatic arthritis associated with the injection (but not due to negligence), and the internal condition of the patient before or after an operation. Nurses administering injections are not held liable where the resulting injury is not directly related to improper technique in administering the injection. For this reason, the correct response to this frame is a negative answer.

Proceed to Frame 3-64.

POOR NURSING JUDGMENT OR IMPROPER MANAGEMENT

In every nursing malpractice case the defendant nurse's conduct is measured against that of a reasonably prudent nurse under the same or similar circumstances. As mentioned earlier with regard to patient safety, the nurse's duty is to anticipate all reasonably foreseeable risks; this sometimes boils down to a simple matter of exercising ordinary common sense or good nursing judgment. Two relatively recent cases illustrate what can happen when good nursing judgment flies out the window.

In *Manning* v. *Twin Falls Clinic & Hospital*, 830 P. 2d 1185 (Idaho 1992), 67-year-old Daryl Manning was suffering from chronic obstructive pulmonary disease (COPD) when he was admitted to the hospital with marked hypoxia and increased CO_2 retention. At the time of admission, his physician advised the family that the patient's death was imminent and they, in turn, requested that he be classified as a "no code" patient. For the next 3 days, Manning was placed on 24-hour-a-day supplemental oxygen, which was administered through a nasal canula, and during this period virtually all of his strength and energy was needed simply to breathe. As the patient's condition worsened, a decision was made by the hospital staff to move Mr. Manning to a private room, and preparatory to making the move his supplemental oxygen was temporarily disconnected despite the pleas of family members present who strenuously urged that he be placed on a portable oxygen unit during the move. The nurses refused to do so, ostensibly because of the relatively short distance of the transfer and because it was not their practice to do so. In the few seconds that the supplemental oxygen was disconnected, Manning suffered extreme respiratory distress and stopped breathing. Because of the family's prior "no code" instructions, no resuscitation was attempted and he died.

The family brought suit against the hospital and the staff nurses involved in the move, claiming negligence in Mr. Manning's care. During the trial, the director of nursing testified that nurses at the hospital regularly moved patients from room to room without supplemental oxygen. One of the hospital's doctors testified, however, that it was a breach of the standard of care for a patient in Manning's condition to be moved without his prescribed oxygen. The doctor further testified that death was caused by a sudden plummet of the patient's already terribly low oxygen level and that the plummet was the direct result of Manning's prescribed oxygen being removed. On appeal, both the hospital and the cited nurses were held liable for compensatory and emotional distress damages. The poor nursing judgment exercised in this case was unpardonable, especially in light of the family's pleas while the room transfer was being made.

Harmon v. *Patel*, 617 N.E. 2d 183 (Ill. 1993), was another case in which good nursing judgment was sorely lacking. Here, a female patient injured in an automobile accident was admitted to the hospital suffering considerable pain in her right knee and leg, but because the x-rays failed to show any broken bones, her physician's diagnosis was that the leg was "merely bruised." Despite this diagnosis, the leg began to swell and change color over the next 4 days and, apart from an increase in pain medication, the patient's pleas for more aggressive medical attention went unheeded.

On the ninth night, the patient begged her nurses to call her mother or a doctor, but the attending nurse refused because, in her opinion, the patient was "hallucinating." When she attempted to reach the telephone on the side of her bed, *nurses actually wrestled it away from her.* Eventually, she was able to call her sister, who immediately came to the hospital and demanded that the nurse call Dr. Patel, the treating physician. Dr. Patel delayed coming for 4 hours, and when he arrived—accompanied by an orthopedic surgeon—the latter diagnosed a fulminating necrotizing fascitis requiring immediate and drastic surgery to release the pus accumulated in her leg.

Although the malpractice suit that followed focused on the negligence of Dr. Patel, who was found liable for damages by the jury, the actions of the nurses in this case were nothing short of outrageous and certainly contributed to the delayed diagnosis of the serious infection sustained by the patient. Nurses should listen to and evaluate patients' complaints in a professional manner, and not be too quick to draw the conclusion that they are hallucinating merely because they are in deep pain.

NEGLIGENCE IN CARING FOR MENTALLY ILL PATIENTS

3-64 Earlier it was pointed out that the nature and quality of nursing care legally required to protect patients from harm are based on the patients' physical conditions and on their ability to contribute to their own safety and security. This rule assumes particular importance when the patients are suffering some form of mental illness that prevents them from appreciating the risk of harm to which they may be exposed.

Which of the following factors is the most legally significant in determining the degree of care required to protect a patient from harm?

☐   the patient's physical and mental condition

☐   the patient's age and occupation

☐   the patient's health history

3-65 Why is the nurse held to a higher standard of care in safeguarding a mentally ill patient?

☐   because mentally ill patients are more likely to bring lawsuits

☐   because a mentally ill person frequently does not appreciate his or her exposure to potential harm

☐   because state and provincial statutes generally impose a higher standard of care with respect to the treatment of mentally ill persons

3-66 Rank the following patients in order of the relative quality and degree of nursing care necessary to protect each of them from any foreseeable harm (use 1, 2, and 3, placing a 1 in the box before the patient requiring the most care):

☐   a 41-year-old woman about to undergo a hysterectomy

☐   a 72-year-old alcoholic with a schizophrenic syndrome

☐   a 10-year-old girl convalescing with a fractured leg

3-64   *the patient's physical*   **3-65** ☐   **3-66** ③
           and mental condition   ☑   ①
                                                   ☐   ②

3-67 When there is neither historical nor present indication that the patient is dangerous to others or to himself or herself, the degree of care and watchfulness expected of the nurse is less. Correspondingly, the degree of alertness must be heightened where suicide has been threatened or the patient has known assaultive tendencies.

Indicate whether the nurse would be expected to exercise normal care or special care in supervising each of the following patients, basing your answer solely on the characteristics noted.

Normal care	*Special care*	
☐	☐	The patient has a violent temperament.
☐	☐	The patient is scheduled for a brain scan.
☐	☐	The patient is mentally retarded.
☐	☐	The patient is a paranoid schizophrenic.

3-68

■ Patient P is convalescing from leg surgery and is permitted to move about in a wheelchair. He has exhibited erratic and somewhat violent behavior on several occasions, and on one occasion four attendants were required to subdue him. When Nurse N comes on duty on P's floor, Supervisory Nurse S issues no special orders with respect to P's supervision.

Yes	*No*	
☐	☐	Is P's described conduct such that it is reasonably foreseeable he may cause injury to someone?
☐	☐	If P causes injury to someone, can Nurse S be held liable for failing to order closer supervision of him?
☐	☐	If P injures someone during Nurse N's tour of duty, could N be held liable for not taking extra precautions?

3-67	*Normal care*	*Special care*	**3-68**	*Yes*	*No*
	☐	☑		☑	☐
	☑	☐		☑	☐
	☐	☑		☑	☐
	☐	☑			

3-69 The prudent nurse must learn how to assess the suicidal potential of a patient before the act is committed. The nurse should know that the older patient is much more likely to commit suicide than the younger or middle-aged patient; that although women make more suicide attempts than men, men successfully commit suicide at a rate twice that of women; and that almost all successful suicides have a history of at least one prior attempt.

- Patient P, a 39-year-old woman, was suffering from cancer and had undergone a left mastectomy, followed shortly by a right pleural effusion and oophorectomy. After being informed that the cancer had metastasized, P became severely depressed and, while at her daughter's home, attempted suicide by strangling herself with a towel. She was admitted to the psychiatric ward of Hospital H, where she openly expressed the desire to commit suicide and even asked members of the nursing staff to assist in this process.

Although P was ordered to be placed under "constant supervision" by the staff physician, 1 week after being admitted, and while under the direct care of Nurse N, she was permitted to prepare her own bath. Forty minutes elapsed before Nurse N checked on her again, at which time she found the bathroom door locked. When it was finally opened, P was found fully clothed submerged in the water-filled bathtub. The medical examiner ruled drowning as the cause of P's death.

P's estate sues Nurse N for malpractice, claiming negligence in N's supervision of P.

What was Nurse N's legal duty in this case?

☐ to exercise sufficiently close supervision over P to protect her from harming herself or others

☐ to make sure that P did not take a bath without an express order from the patient's physician

☐ to stay with P every minute of the day

3-70 The fact that P had attempted suicide on one prior occasion ☐ would ☐ would not indicate a sufficiently self-destructive intent to require extra care on the part of the nurses assigned to care for Patient P.

3-69 *to exercise sufficiently close supervision over P to protect her from harming herself or others*

3-70 *Would*

3-71   Which of the following would have afforded Nurse N a plausible legal defense in the law-suit?

- ☐ the testimony of experts that not all persons who threaten suicide actually carry out their threat(s)

- ☐ proof that N monitored P several times while P was taking her bath

- ☐ proof that the hospital was extremely understaffed on the day of the patient's suicide

---

NOTE: Can a mentally disturbed person who is known to be prone to self-damaging acts be held to have contributed to his or her own injury, thereby absolving the hospital and its nursing personnel from liability? The modern trend in the law appears to favor application of a capacity-based standard for the contributory negligence of mentally disturbed plaintiffs. Under this standard, a mentally disturbed plaintiff is deemed incapable of adhering to a reasonable person's standard of self-care but is nevertheless held responsible for the consequences of conduct that is found to be unreasonable in light of the plaintiff's diminished capacity. See Keeton W, Doobs D, Keeton R, Owen D, *Prosser and Keeton on the Law of Torts*, ed 5, § 32, 178, 1984; Annotation, *Civil Liability for Death by Suicide*, 11 A.L.R. 2d 751.

Despite the law's recognition of some degree of responsibility on the part of a mentally disturbed person, when a hospitalized patient is *known* to be suicidal, the duty of care on the part of the hospital and its nursing personnel to prevent self-inflicted harm is clearcut and absolute because of the dire foreseeable consequences of not meeting that duty of care. Thus, the defense of contributory negligence simply won't be allowed where the plaintiff committed the very act that the defendant hospital and its nurses were under a duty to prevent. We will discuss the issue of contributory negligence more fully in Part 6.

3-71   *proof that N monitored P several times while P was taking her bath*

3-72   Reasonable care in treating suicidal patients requires prompt recognition of the frequently overlooked warning clues to suicide—whether verbal, behavioral, or otherwise. One of the most widespread myths about suicide is: "People who talk about it won't actually do it." In fact, almost all suicidal patients give verbal clues to those around them. Evidence of depression, disorientation, and deeply emotional dependency patterns are particularly associated with suicidal tendencies, and reasonable care requires the nurse to recognize and cope with these symptoms *promptly*, to forestall the possibility of suicide before the idea gets too firmly rooted in the patient's mind.

Which of the following remarks made to a nurse by a patient would be indicative of a suicidal intent?

☐   "I give up. I can't take the pain much longer."

☐   "If I can't walk again, what's the point of going on like this?"

☐   "I won't be a problem much longer. Anyway, I'm worth more dead than alive."

3-73   Which of the following statements is the *most accurate*?

☐   Suicidally inclined persons almost always exhibit some overt signs of their suicidal tendencies.

☐   Suicidally inclined persons generally give clues to their suicidal tendencies which, if recognized by the nurse in time, may permit the nurse to prevent the suicide from occurring.

☐   Suicidally inclined persons are easily identified by their depression, disorientation, and emotional dependence.

> **NOTE:**   Nearly all suicidal patients have ambivalent feelings, so they cry out for help before they attempt to kill themselves. Seizing upon this ambivalence, the concerned nurse will reinforce the part of the patient who wants to live by emphasizing the patient's importance to family and friends; by discussing the effects of suicide on any surviving dependents; and by discussing other hard times in the past, and how the patient coped with them. The wise nurse also will involve the patient's family, friends, co-workers, and clergy in the process of support through this crisis period. In the final analysis, sensitivity, warmth, concern, and consistency are probably the most meaningful help a nurse can give a suicidal patient.

3-72	☑	3-73	*Suicidally inclined persons generally give clues to their suicidal tendencies which, if recognized by the nurse in time . . .*
	☑		
	☑		

TIPS FOR DEALING WITH SUICIDAL PATIENTS

Bearing in mind that the concept of patient safety takes on added significance where the patient is known to be suicidally inclined, here are some tips for preventing suicides from occurring in the institutional setting.

- Your first obligation is to provide extremely close supervision, sometimes even one-on-one, until the immediate threat of harm has passed.

- Assess the physical environment for all possible dangers and be sure to remove all potentially dangerous objects from the patient's room, such as belts, ties, bed linens, glassware, and eating utensils.

- Make absolutely sure the patient swallows all pills that you give, to prevent his or her attempt to accumulate them for later ingestion *en masse*.

- Check to make sure the patient can't easily open or break his or her room windows to escape undetected. If necessary, move the patient to a seclusion room.

POINTS TO REMEMBER

1. Medication errors are a common cause of malpractice claims against nurses and usually involve misreading of a medication order or failing to check with the physician when the order is ambiguous or incomplete.

2. Another major cause of malpractice claims is faulty technique in giving injections.

3. While not all nerve injuries due to injections are due to negligence, where the onset of pain, ecchymosis, and sloughing is immediate, the likelihood of malpractice is great.

4. Unless legally sanctioned by statute, a nurse is not authorized to *prescribe* medications and may be held personally liable for the untoward consequences of advising a patient what medications to take.

5. When there is no historical or present indication that the patient is dangerous to self or others, only the normal degree of reasonable care is expected of the nurse to safeguard the patient.

6. When patients are suffering some form of mental illness, their ability to contribute to their own safety and security is considerably diminished. This situation requires the exercise of a higher degree of care with respect to the safety of mentally ill persons.

7. Most patient with suicidal tendencies give verbal or behavioral clues to their destructive intent, and the careful nurse will always be alert to these clues to prevent suicide from occurring.

SELECTED REFERENCES–PART THREE

Patient Safety Errors

Clark MD, "Toward Safer Nursing Practice," *Nurs Management* 22(3):88, 1991.

Varga K, "How to Protect Yourself Against Malpractice," *Imprint* 36(5):33, 1989-1990.

"Lawsuits: An Ounce of Prevention," *Nursing '90* 20(5):146, 1990.

Knight M, "Our Safety Net Keeps Patients from Falling," *RN* 48(12):9, 1985.

Greenlaw J, "Failure to Use Siderails: When Is It Negligent?" *Law Med Health Care* 10(6):125, 1982.

Annotations: 9 ALR 4th 149, "Hospital's Liability for Patient's Injury or Death as Result of Fall from Bed"; 51 ALR 2d 970, "Nurse's Liability for Her Own Negligence or Malpractice."

Beverly Enterprises—Virginia v. *Nichols*, 441 S.E. 2d 1 (Va. 1994)

Atkins v. *Pottstown Medical Center*, 634 A. 2d 258 (Pa. 1993)

Beckham v. *St. Paul Fire & Marine Ins. Co.*, 614 So. 2d 760 (La. 1993)

Landes v. *Women's Christian Association*, 504 N.W. 2d 139 (Iowa 1993)

Manning v. *Twin Falls Clinic & Hospital, Inc.*, 830 P. 2d 1185 (Idaho 1992)

McDonald v. *Aliquippa Hospital*, 606 A. 2d 1218 (Pa. 1992)

Pierce v. *Mercy Medical Health Center, Inc.*, 847 P. 2d 822 (Okla. 1992)

Scribner v. *Hillcrest Medical Center*, 866 P. 2d 437 (Okla. 1992)

Stacy v. *Truman Medical Center*, 836 S.W. 2d 911 (Mo. 1992)

Robison v. *Micheline Faine and Catalano's Nurse Registry*, 525 So. 2d 903 (Fla. 1987)

Wooten v. *United States*, 574 F. Supp. 200 (Tenn. 1983)

Thomas v. *St. Joseph's Hospital*, 618 S.W. 2d 791 (Texas 1981)

Beaches Hospital v. *Lee*, 384 So. 2d 234 (Fla. 1980)

University Community Hospital v. *Martin*, 328 So. 2d 858 (Fla. 1976)

Duty to Follow or Question Physicians' Orders

70 *Corpus Juris Secundum*, PHYSICIANS & SURGEONS, § 54, p. 976.

Note, "Nurses Intervening in Patient's Improper Treatment Protected from Discharge," *J Health & Hosp L*, 26:244, 1993.

Creighton H, "Nurse's Failure to Follow Physician's Orders," *Nurs Management* 20(1):18, 1989.

Benninger Barbara R, "Nursing Malpractice—The Nurse's Duty to Follow Orders," *W. Va. L Rev* 90:1291, 1988.

Regan W, "When Nurses Fail to Follow Doctors' Orders: Disaster," *Regan Rep on Nurs L* 26(7):1, 1985.

Guariello D, "When Doctor's Orders Aren't the Best Medicine," *RN* 47(5):19, 1984.

Tammelleo A and Gill D, "When Following Orders Can Cost You Your License," *RN* 47(7):13, 1984.

Roach WH, "Responsible Intervention: A Legal Duty to Act," *J Nurs Admin* 10(7):18, 1980.

Bremmer v. *Charles*, 859 P. 2d 1148 (Ore. 1993)

Frank v. *South Suburban Hospital Foundation*, 628 N.E. 2d 953 (Ill. 1993)

Kirk v. *Mercy Hospital Tri-County*, 851 S.W. 2d 617 (Mo. 1993)

Sullivan v. *Sumrall by Ritchley*, 618 So. 2d 1274 (Miss. 1993)

Navarro v. *George*, 615 A. 2d 890 (Pa. 1992)

Treinis v. *Deepdale General Hospital*, 570 N.Y.S. 2d 188 (N.Y. 1991)

Hoffson v. *Orentreich et al.*, 543 N.Y.S. 2d 242 (N.Y. 1989)

Koeniguer v. *Eckrich*, 422 N.W. 2d 600 (S.D. 1988)

Nelson v. *Trinity Medical Center*, 419 N.W. 2d 886 (N.D. 1988)

Hurlock v. *Park Lane Medical Center*, 709 S.W. 2d 872 (Mo. 1986)

Jarvis v. *St. Charles Medical Center*, 713 P. 2d 620 (Ore. 1986)

Bleiler v. *Bodnar*, 489 N.Y.S. 2d 885 (N.Y. 1985)

Wickliffe v. *Sunrise Hospital, Inc.*, 706 P. 2d 1383 (Nev. 1985)

Bivins v. *Detroit Osteopathic Hospital*, 258 N.W. 2d 527 (Mich. 1981)

Young v. *Department of Health*, 405 So. 2d 1209 (La. 1981)

Physicians' Assistants

Schaft G and Cawley J, *The Physician Assistant in a Changing Health Care Environment*, Aspen Systems, Rockville, Md, 1987.

U.S. Congress, Office of Technology Assessment, *Nurse Practitioners, Physician Assistants, and Certified Nurse-Midwives: A Policy Analysis*, (OTA-HCS-37), Washington, D.C., U.S. Government Printing Office, 1986.

Bullough B and Winter C, "Physicians' Assistants and the Law." In Bullough B, editor: *The Law and the Expanding Nurse Role*, Appleton-Century-Crofts, New York, 1980.

Bliss A and Cohen ED, *The New Health Professionals: Nurse Practitioners and Physician Assistants*, Aspen Systems, Germantown, Md., 1977.

Fowkes V and McKay D, "A Profile of California's Physician Assistants," *West J. Med* 153:328, 1990.

Gara N, "State Laws for Physician Assistants," *J Am Acad Phys Assts* 2:303, 1989.

Bottom WD and Echevarria E, "Regulatory Changes Regarding Physician's Assistant Clinical Practice," *J Fla Med Assn* 75(7):437, 1988.

Central Anesthesia Associates v. *Worthy*, 325 S.E. 2d 819 (Ga. 1985)

Polischek v. *United States*, 533 F. Supp. 1261 (Pa. 1982)

Washington State Nurses' Association v. *Board of Medical Examiners*, 605 P. 2d 1269 (Wash. 1980)

Reynolds v. *Medical and Dental Staff, etc.*, 382 N.Y.S. 2d 618 (N.Y. 1976)

Diagnosis, Observation, and Monitoring Errors

North American Nursing Diagnosis Association, *Classification of Nursing Diagnoses: Proceedings of the Ninth Conference*, J.B. Lippincott, Philadelphia, 1991.

Campbell C, *Nursing Diagnosis and Intervention in Nursing Practice*, John Wiley & Sons, New York, 1978.

Fiesta J, "Failure to Assess," *Nurs Management* 24(9): 16, 1993.

Dolan MB, "Why Nurses and Doctors Should be Partners in Diagnosis," *Nursing '90* 20(11):41, 1990.

Florek C, "The Nurse's Role in Diagnosing and Prescribing—Legal Boundaries of the Registered Nurse Under California's 1974 Nursing Practice Act," *U West LA L Rev* 19:73, 1987.

Fadden T, "Nursing Diagnosis, A Matter of Form," *Am J Nurs* 84(4):470, 1984.

Warren J, "Accountability and Nursing Diagnosis," *J Nurs Admin* 13(10):34, 1983.

Bruce J and Snyder M, "The Right and Responsibility to Diagnose," *Am J Nurs* 82(4):645, 1982.

Booth v. *Silva*, 626 N.E. 2d 903 (Mass. 1994)

Glassman v. *St. Joseph Hospital*, 631 N.E. 2d 1186 (Ill. 1994)

Carey v. *Lovett*, 622 A. 2d 1279 (N.J. 1993)

Dent v. *Perkins*, 629 So. 2d 1354 (La. 1993)

Feeney v. *New England Medical Center, Inc.*, 615 N.E. 2d 585 (Mass. 1993)

Porter v. *Lima Memorial Hospital*, 995 F. 2d 629 (Ohio 1993)

Scott v. *Capital Area Community Health Plan*, 594 N.Y.S. 2d 370 (N.Y. 1993)

Tye v. *Wilson*, 430 S.E. 2d 129 (Ga. 1993)

Vincent by Staton v. *Fairbanks Memorial Hospital*, 862 P. 2d 847 (Alaska 1993)

Eyoma v. *Falco*, 589 A. 2d 653 (N.J. 1991)

Pirkov-Middaugh v. *Gillette Children's Hospital*, 479 N.W. 2d 63 (Minn. 1991)

Ewing v. *Aubert*, 532 So. 2d 876 (La. 1988)

Cignetti v. *Camel*, 692 S.W. 2d 329 (Mo. 1985)

Metsaris v. *73rd Corp.*, 482 N.Y.S. 2d 792 (N.Y. 1985)

Poor Sisters of St. Francis v. *Catron*, 435 N.E. 2d 305 (Ind. 1982)

Vasey v. *Burch*, 262 S.E. 2d 865 (N.C. 1980)

Utter v. *United Hospital Center, Inc.*, 236 S.E. 2d 213 (W.Va. 1977)
Hiatt v. *Groce*, 523 P. 2d 370 (Kan. 1974)

Failure to Communicate

Fiesta J, "Duty to Communicate—'Doctor Notified,'" *Nurs Management* 24(1):24, 1994.
Bernzweig E, "How a Communication Breakdown Can Get You Sued," *RN* 48(2):47, 1985.
Cushing M, "Failure to Communicate," *Am J Nurs* 82(8):1597, 1982.
Greenlaw J, "Communication Failure: Some Case Examples," *Law Med Health Care* 10(2):77, 1982.
Glassman v. *St. Joseph Hospital*, 631 N.E. 2d 1186 (Ill. 1994)
Baptist Medical Center v. *Wilson*, 618 So. 2d 1335 (Ala. 1993)
Cassandra P. v. *Center for Women's Health*, 25 Cal. Rptr. 2d 667 (Cal. 1993)
White v. *Methodist Hospital South*, 844 S.W. 2d 642 (Tenn. 1992)
Major v. *North Valley Hospital*, 759 P. 2d 153 (Mont. 1988)
Lambert v. *Sisters of Mercy Health Corp.*, 369 N.W. 2d 417 (Iowa 1985)
Ramsey v. *Physicians' Memorial Hospital*, 373 A. 2d 26 (Md. 1977)
Krestview Nursing Home v. *Synowiec*, 317 So. 2d 94 (Fla. 1975)
Thomas v. *Corso*, 288 A. 2d 379 (Md. 1972)

Improper Supervision

Pozgar G, *Legal Aspects of Health Care Administration*, Aspen Systems, Germantown, Md., 1983, pp. 80–81.
Bernzweig E, "When a Nurse Doesn't Fit the Job," *RN* 48(1):13, 1985.
Regan W, "Nursing Supervisors and Careless RNs," *Regan Rep on Nurs L* 21(9):1, 1981.
McMillan v. *Durant*, 439 S.E. 2d 829 (S.C. 1993)
Raicevich v. *Plum Creek Medical P.C.*, 819 F. Supp. 929 (Colo. 1993)
Salas by Salas v. *Wang*, 846 F. 2d 897 (N.J. 1988)
Carter v. *Anderson Memorial Hospital*, 325 S.E. 2d 78 (S.C. 1985)
Metsuris v. *73rd Corp.*, 482 N.Y.S. 2d 792 (N.Y. 1985)
Macy v. *Presbyterian Intercommunity Hospital*, 612 P. 2d 769 (Ore. 1980)

Inadequate-Staffing Problems

Fiesta J, "Staffing Implications: A Legal Update," *Nurs Management* 25(6):34, 1994.
Fiesta J, "Legal Update for Nurses, Part II: Assigning, Delegating and Staffing," *Nurs Management* 24(2):14, 1993.
Fiesta J, "The Nursing Shortage: Whose Liability Problem?" *Nurs Management* 21(2):22, 1990.
Rosen LF, "Liability for Understaffing: Who Is Responsible?" *Today's OR Nurse* 12(1):36, 1990.
Huff D, "Liability Issues Arising From Hospitals' Use of Temporary Supplemental Staff Nurses," *Loyola U Chi L J* 21:1141, 1990.
Hollowell EE and Eldridge JE, "The Nursing Shortage: The Increased Risk of Legal Liability and How to Avoid It," *J Pract N* 39(2):28, 1989.
ECRI, "The Nursing Shortage: A Liability Threat," *Hosp Risk Control Update*, Oct. 1988.
Annotation, 2 ALR 5th 286, "Hospital's Liability for Injury Resulting From Failure to Have Sufficient Number of Nurses on Duty."
St. Paul Medical Center v. *Cecil*, 842 S.W. 2d 809 (Texas 1992)
HCA Health Services of Midwest, Inc. v. *National Bank of Commerce*, 745 S.W. 2d 120 (Ark. 1988)
Horton v. *Niagara Falls Memorial Medical Center*, 380 N.Y.S. 2d 116 (N.Y. 1976)

Medication Errors

Cohen MR, Senders J, and Davis NM, "12 Ways to Prevent Medication Errors," *Nursing '94* 24(2):34, 1994.

Parisi SB, "What to Do After a Med Error," *Nursing '94* 24(6):59, 1994.

Senders J, "Theory and Analysis of Typical Errors in a Medical Setting," *Hosp Pharm* 28(6):505, 1993.

McGovern K, "10 Golden Rules for Administering Drugs Safely," *Nursing '92* 22(3):49, 1992.

Carr DS, "New Strategies for Avoiding Medication Errors," *Nursing '89* 19(8):38, 1989.

Wolf ZR, "Medication Errors and Nursing Responsibility," *Holistic Nurs Prac* 4(1):8, 1989.

Annotation, 23 ALR 3d 1288, "Mistakenly-Administered Drugs."

Nowak v. High, 433 S.E. 2d 602 (Ga. 1993)

Navarro v. George, 615 A. 2d 890 (Pa. 1992)

Peters v. Judd Drugs, Inc., 602 N.E. 2d 162 (Ind. 1992)

Montgomery v. Opelousas General Hospital, 529 So. 2d 52 (La. 1988)

Serota v. Kaplan, 511 N.Y.S. 2d 667 (N.Y. 1987)

Brooks v. Memphis & Shelby County Hospital Authority, 717 S.W. 2d 292 (Tenn. 1986)

Tripp v. Humana, Inc., 474 So. 2d 88 (Ala. 1985)

Keefer v. C.R. Bard, 313 N.W. 2d 151 (Mich. 1982)

Dessauer v. Memorial General Hospital, 628 P. 2d 337 (N.M. 1981)

Leavitt v. St. Tammany Parish Hospital, 396 So. 2d 406 (La. 1981)

Schmidt v. Intermountain Health Care, Inc., 635 P. 2d 99 (Utah 1981)

Story v. McCurtain Memorial Medical Management, Inc., 634 P. 2d 778 (Okla. 1981)

Negligence in Treating Mentally Disturbed Patients

Moore GM, "Surviving a Malpractice Lawsuit: One Nurse's Story," *Nursing '93* 23(10):55, 1993.

Reid W, "The Role of the Nurse Providing Therapeutic Care for the Suicidal Patient," *J Advanced Nurs* 18(9):1369, 1993.

Stewart KB, "Attempted Suicide," *Nursing '93* 23(12):25, 1993.

Coleman P and Shellow RA, "Suicide: Unpredictable and Unavoidable—Proposed Guidelines Provide Rational Test for Physicians' Liability," *Nebr L Rev* 71:643, 1992.

Parker BA, "When Your Medical/Surgical Patient Is Also Mentally Ill," *Nursing '92* 22(5):66, 1992.

Fiesta J, "Liability Issues: Patients with Psychiatric Problems," *Nurs Management* 22(9):14, 1991.

Note, "Suicide Liability," *NJ Med* 88(6):387, 1991.

Reubin, R, "Spotting and Stopping the Suicide Patient," *Nurs '79* 9(4):82, 1979.

Schneidman E, "Preventing Suicide," *Am J Nurs* 65:11, 1965.

Annotation, 11 ALR 2d 751, "Civil Liability for Death by Suicide."

Hatley v. Kassen, 859 S.W. 2d 367 (Texas 1992)

Brandvain v. Ridgeview Institute, Inc., 372 S.E. 2d 265 (Ga. 1988)

Cowan v. Doering, 545 A. 2d 159 (N.J. 1988)

Keebler v. Winfield Carraway Hospital, 531 So. 2d 841 (Ala. 1988)

Nally v. Grace Community Church of the Valley, 747 P. 2d 527 (Cal. 1988)

Robison v. Micheline Faine and Catalano's Nurse Registry, 525 So. 2d 903 (Fla. 1987)

Bennett v. Winthrop Community Hospital, 489 N.E. 2d 1032 (Mass. 1986)

Rosemont, Inc. v. Marshall, 481 S. 2d 1126 (Ala. 1986)

Stokes v. Leung, 651 S.W. 2d 704 (Tenn. 1983)

North Miami General Hospital v. Krakauer, 393 So. 2d 57 (Fla. 1981)

Delicata v. Bourlesses, 404 N.E. 2d 667 (Mass. 1980)

Abile v. United States, 482 F. Supp. 703 (Cal. 1980)

Pisel v. Stamford Hospital, 430 A. 2d 1 (Conn. 1980)

Horton v. Niagara Falls Medical Center, 380 N.Y.S. 2d 116 (N.Y. 1976)

Miscellaneous Acts of Negligence, Improper Management, Etc.

Fiesta J, *20 Legal Pitfalls for Nurses to Avoid*, Delmar Publishers, Inc., Albany, N.Y., 1994.

Fiesta J, "Liability Issues for the Office Nurse," *Nurs Management* 23(1):17, 1992.

Clark MD, "Toward Safer Nursing Practice," *Nurs Management* 22(3):88, 1991.

Harmon v. *Patel*, 617 N.E. 2d 183 (Ill. 1993)

Wheeler v. *Yettie Kersting Memorial Hospital*, 866 S.W. 2d 32 (Texas 1993)

Manning v. *Twin Falls Clinic & Hospital*, 830 P. 2d 1185 (Idaho 1992)

Bacon v. *Mercy Hospital of Fort Scott, Kansas*, 756 P. 2d 416 (Kan. 1988)

Berry v. *Rapides General Hospital*, 527 So. 2d 583 (La. 1988)

Lambert v. *Sisters of Mercy Health Corp.*, 369 N.W. 2d 417 (Miss. 1985)

Hughes v. *St. Paul Fire & Marine Insurance Co.*, 401 So. 2d 448 (La. 1981)

Variety Children's Hospital v. *Perkins*, 382 S. 2d 331 (Fla. 1980)

PART FOUR

INTENTIONAL WRONGS AND CONSENT TO TREATMENT

Part 4

INTRODUCTORY NOTE

The prime focus of this course is nursing malpractice in which the nurse's liability is based on some negligent act or omission to act that causes injury to the patient. There are, however, related areas of nursing practice that involve acts of an intentional nature, and these frequently create legal problems for nurses. Because of the close relationship of these intentional acts to the unintentional (negligent) acts discussed in this course, we will devote this part to a brief explanation of them. In the material that follows we will discuss several intentional torts and the problem of consent to the medical or nursing treatment.

ASSAULT AND BATTERY

4-1   In Part 1 we pointed out that a tort may be either an intentional wrong or an unintentional wrong, but that in either case the wrong is vindicated by way of a civil action for damages against the person who caused it. We also noted that some *intentional* wrongs represent antisocial behavior that is also punishable under the criminal law. Assault and battery are examples of two intentional torts that often result in criminal charges, even though a civil action also may result.

True	*False*	
☐	☐	An act that constitutes an intentional tort also may constitute a crime.
☐	☐	An intentionally wrongful act may be either a tort or a crime, but cannot be both.
☐	☐	All torts involve intentionally wrongful behavior.
☐	☐	Assault and battery are torts based on intentional conduct.

4-2   We begin our discussion of intentional torts with the torts of assault and battery and will concern ourselves with the use of these terms in the civil law context only.

While the words *assault* and *battery* are often used synonymously, they are quite different in the legal sense. A *battery* is the unconsented and unlawful touching of another's person. (A touches B without B's consent.) An *assault* is the act of placing another person in fear of being touched without his consent—or, a threatened battery. (A tells B: "If you don't keep quiet, I'm going to give you an injection to calm you down.")

A patient who has been civilly assaulted

☐   has a legal basis for suing even if not physically touched

☐   has a legal basis for claiming assault and battery in a lawsuit

☐   has no legal basis for suing unless he or she has suffered some bodily harm

---

4-1	*True*	*False*		4-2	*has a legal basis for suing even if not physically touched*
	☑	☐			
	☐	☑			
	☐	☑			
	☑	☐			

4-3   What legal element is necessary for a civil assault to take place?

☐   the physical ability to cause harm

☐   the threat of harm

☐   actual harm

4-4   In the civil law context assault and battery refer to

☐   a single legal act

☐   two distinct legal acts

☐   equivalent legal acts

4-5   A battery (unauthorized or unconsented touching) may result even in the absence of intent to do harm. As a matter of fact, even a touching that is beneficial may constitute a battery if it was not authorized or consented to by the person physically touched.

What would be necessary for a doctor's successful defense in a civil action for battery arising out of his or her treatment of a patient?

☐   proof that the patient's condition was benefited by the treatment

☐   proof that no harm resulted to the patient or that the harm was trivial

☐   proof that the patient authorized or consented to the treatment in question

---

4-3   *the threat of harm*   **4-4**   *two distinct legal acts*   **4-5**   ☐
                                                                                             ☐
                                                                                             ☑

4-6 A patient's consent to treatment has no legal effect on the doctor's or nurse's liability for negligence in carrying out the authorized procedure. No patient ever consents to negligent treatment.

Indicate in which of the following cases a patient's suit claiming battery would probably be successful or unsuccessful.

Successful *Unsuccessful*

☐ ☐ A patient consents to treatment with a diathermy machine. The diathermy is carelessly administered and the patient suffers extensive burns.

☐ ☐ A patient agrees orally to the taking of a blood sample. In the process, the nurse's hand slips and the needle injures the patient.

☐ ☐ In the course of a routine examination, without saying anything to the patient, the doctor lances a large boil on the patient's back.

☐ ☐ A patient agrees to removal of a polyp in his right ear. The doctor successfully removes a polyp from the patient's left ear instead.

4-7 In considering a nurse's liability for battery, the question of whether the specific nursing act benefited the patient

☐ is always legally relevant

☐ may sometimes be legally relevant

☐ is always legally irrelevant

4-6 *Successful* *Unsuccessful*
☐ ☑
☐ ☑
☑ ☐
☑ ☐

4-7 *is always legally irrelevant*

If you have any problem with this answer, turn to p. 222, Note A.

POINTS TO REMEMBER

1. Assault and battery, in addition to being the basis of criminal action, are recognized by the law as intentional torts that may give rise to civil actions for damages.

2. A civil assault is the act of placing another person in fear of being touched without his or her authorization or consent.

3. A civil battery is the actual unconsented touching of another's person.

4. A battery may result even if there is no assault, and an assault may result without any battery.

5. Even though an unauthorized touching may prove beneficial, it is nevertheless considered unlawful and will give rise to legal liability in a civil action.

6. A patient's consent to a particular form of treatment has no effect on the doctor's or nurse's liability for negligence in providing that treatment.

THE CONCEPT OF CONSENT TO TREATMENT

An area of professional conduct that has become increasingly troublesome to physicians and nurses stems from the legal requirement that a physician obtain a patient's consent to treatment. The doctrine of consent to medical treatment has been with us since the turn of the century. It is based on the notion that every person of adult years and sound mind has the fundamental right to decide whether (and the extent to which) he or she will allow another person to violate his or her bodily integrity. Thus, in the absence of emergency or extenuating circumstances, a physician or surgeon must first obtain the consent of the patient (or of someone legally authorized to give such consent) before treating or operating on the patient. The physician's failure to obtain such consent will give rise either to a possible legal action for battery, based on the unauthorized touching of the patient, or—as is more often the case—a legal action for negligence.

In recent years, there has been a strong trend in the law for informed consent cases to be dealt with as negligence claims rather than claims based on alleged battery. In most modern cases, some form of patient "consent" is generally present, thus the issue usually addressed is whether that consent contained all the elements necessary to make it legally effective. Thus, a patient alleging negligence (as opposed to battery) must show that the health care professional was negligent—that is, unintentionally failed to perform according to acceptable professional standards—in fulfilling his or her duties toward the patient.

Much confusion has arisen in the legal literature with regard to the matter of consent resulting from a failure to distinguish between various consent-to-treatment issues. Often, the problem is less related to the scope or quality of the patient's consent than the fact that *no consent was obtained at all*. The material that follows begins with this basic issue and its relationship to battery or unauthorized treatment. Then other important consent issues are discussed, including the types of consents needed in emergency situations, when treating minors and incompetents, and in surgical procedures that extend beyond the specifically consented to procedure.

4-8   An individual may, of course, give consent to the touching of his or her person, and if he or she does so, there is no legal battery. Sometimes this consent is given *expressly* (either by words or in writing), and sometimes it is *implied* by the surrounding circumstances. By way of illustration, when a person engages a physician to treat an ailment, he or she implicitly consents to all procedures that form a reasonable and customary part of that treatment.

A patient goes to her doctor's office for a routine annual physical. Which of the following procedures would she implicitly consent to merely by presenting herself for examination?

- ☐   testing her knee jerk reflex
- ☐   removal of a plantar wart discovered during the examination
- ☐   taking of a blood sample

4-9   In the eyes of the law, the patient's consent to a particular type of treatment

- ☐   may be implied by the circumstances
- ☐   must be obtained in writing
- ☐   must be given expressly

> **NOTE:**   The common law does not require a patient's *written* consent to treatment, but rather, his or her voluntary and informed consent, whether in writing or not.* The written consent form is merely proof of the fact that the patient signed a document presented to him or her that purportedly reflects the patient's consent to the treatment proposed. While its value in an evidentiary sense cannot be minimized, neither should the mere signing of the form lull the doctor or nurse into a false sense of security. Informed consent cases are proliferating at an amazing pace, and the prudent doctor and nurse will not naively assume that a consent form is a guarantee against liability.

---

*In Canada, several provincial legislatures have long made it a *statutory* requirement to obtain the patient's consent in writing where a surgical procedure is involved. More recently, several U.S. states have enacted similar laws. Notwithstanding these statutory enactments, a patient may still sue the physician on the theory that he or she was not adequately informed concerning the proposed procedure, the written consent representing merely a rebuttable presumption that true consent was obtained, as under the common law.

4-8   ☑
         ☐
         ☑

4-9   *may be implied by the circumstances*

4-10 Even when a patient consents to a particular type of treatment, the consent extends only to all procedures that form a reasonable and customary part of that treatment or are otherwise necessary to repair unforeseen consequences of the treatment to which consent was given. Even an express verbal or written consent does not extend to wholly unrelated or unnecessary procedures.

- P enters the hospital for a cholecystectomy, and gives his written consent to the operation.

For which of the following might the operating surgeon be held legally liable for battery?

☐ for extending the incision 3 inches because of the unusual location of the gallbladder

☐ for removing the patient's normal appendix

☐ for removing a mole on the patient's abdomen

4-11

- P goes to her doctor for treatment of an infection, and the doctor gives her a penicillin injection. On receiving the injection, P develops symptoms of anaphylaxis, whereupon the doctor gives an injection of epinephrine.

Why would the doctor not be held liable for committing battery in this situation?

☐ because penicillin and epinephrine are both injectable substances

☐ because the injection of epinephrine was a reasonably necessary procedure for dealing with the life-threatening circumstances

☐ because the doctor can always choose to employ any therapeutic procedure he or she deems best, once a patient's consent is obtained

---

4-10 ☐   4-11 *because the injection of*
     ☑   *epinephrine was a rea-*
     ☑   *sonably necessary pro-*
                   cedure . . .

                   The emergency rule
                   applies here. It will be
                   discussed again, shortly.

4-12

- P requests an immunization before going overseas, and Nurse N gives a typhoid injection. In the process, the needle breaks off in the patient's arm, requiring the physician-employer of Nurse N to remove the needle surgically, leaving a scar.

A later lawsuit by P against the physician and Nurse N alleging battery

☐   will probably be successful

☐   will probably be unsuccessful

☐   may or may not be successful, depending on the degree of negligence proved

---

NOTE: Although it has been discussed before, it is worth repeating that merely obtaining a proper consent from the patient does not make the health care professional immune from liability if substandard care is rendered. A patient *never* consents to receive substandard care; thus, if the care provided falls below the acceptable standard, the patient's consent is no defense to a claim of malpractice brought against the negligent physician or nurse.

4-12   *will probably be unsuccessful*

If you checked the wrong box, turn to p. 222, Note B.

4-13   It is not always appreciated that a person who has given his or her free and voluntary consent has the legal right to revoke or withdraw that consent at any time before the commencement of treatment. The physician or nurse who proceeds with treatment in reliance on the original consent will be held liable for battery if it is shown that the patient withdrew his or her consent before treatment began.

■ P enters the hospital for a series of radiation therapy treatments. He gives his consent to the proposed treatment in writing. After the first treatment he experiences intense discomfort and pain and tells the physician and nurse he does not want to proceed with further treatment. Nevertheless, the physician orders the second treatment and the nurse (with the aid of an orderly) forcibly takes P to the radiation therapy room. In the course of this second treatment, P sustains radiation burns and he later sues the physician and nurse claiming battery and negligence.

Indicate whether the following statements are true or false.

True	False	
☐	☐	P's consent to the treatment terminated the moment he told the physician and nurse he did not want to proceed.
☐	☐	P can recover damages either for battery or negligence, but not both in the same case.
☐	☐	P will not prevail in his battery claim unless he can prove his consent was withdrawn in writing.
☐	☐	P's claim alleging negligence can succeed even if he fails to prove his claim alleging battery.

4-13   True   False
       ☑   ☐
       ☐   ☑
       ☐   ☑
       ☑   ☐

"DO NOT RESUSCITATE" (DNR) ORDERS

The concept of battery occasionally arises in the context of implementing "do not resuscitate" (DNR) orders, hence their importance to all nurses who work with elderly or terminally ill patients. As noted in the preceding material, a competent adult patient has the right not only to consent to specific medical treatment but the companion right to withdraw that consent and decline any further treatment. The physician or nurse who disregards the patient's wishes not to have further treatment runs the risk of a lawsuit claiming battery.

In addition to the right to withdraw from treatment, a competent adult patient may decide in advance not to undergo life-sustaining treatment or medical intervention in clearly specified circumstances, and these wishes must be respected. This right is especially important where the patient informs the physician that he or she does not wish heroic resuscitation and life-sustaining efforts to be employed in the event of sudden cessation of breathing. If the patient and physician are in agreement on this matter, the physician will write a DNR order in the patient's chart for the benefit of all nursing and other personnel who later may be called upon to initiate or participate in cardiopulmonary resuscitation. The case discussed next shows the legal risks of failing to respect the patient's advance directive not to resuscitate.

In *Anderson* v. *St. Francis-St. George Hospital*, 614 N.E. 2d 841 (Ohio 1992), an elderly adult patient was admitted to the hospital suffering chest pain. After receiving initial care in the ER, he was transferred to the CCU where, in a discussion with his family and his private physician concerning the proposed course of treatment, a DNR order was requested and was subsequently placed in the patient's medical record. Three days after admission, the patient went into ventricular fibrillation and, despite the DNR order, a nurse resuscitated the patient by shocking his heart with an electric current. Following the defibrillation, the patient suffered a paralyzing stroke, as well as pain, emotional distress, and disability, along with additional medical expenses. After his death, the administrator of his estate filed suit against the hospital alleging battery, negligence, and "wrongful life." A motion for summary judgment in favor of the hospital was overturned on appeal. The appellate court held, among other things, that the patient had a right to expressly refuse treatment even in an emergency, and that medical treatment rendered in violation of a DNR order constitutes battery, for which damages can be awarded. Accordingly, the case was remanded for trial.

Nurses should be keenly aware of the patient's right to make his or her own medical treatment decisions, including the right to refuse treatment entirely. It is the nurse's obligation to follow DNR orders on patients' charts notwithstanding any personal beliefs regarding the necessity or advisability of resuscitative efforts. If a nurse is not disposed to follow DNR orders because they conflict with the nurse's personal moral beliefs, he or she should make this fact known to the charge nurse or unit supervisor *in advance* to ensure removal from situations that might require implementation of DNR orders. In the absence of such request, the patient's decision to accept or reject medical treatment must be implemented without interference.

Finally, under no circumstances is a patient's living will a substitute for the express wishes of a competent adult, who has the absolute right to refuse medical treatment for any reason. A patient's living will comes into play only when the patient is seriously ill and is no longer physically or mentally competent to make his or her wishes known. This subject and related matters are discussed in detail in Part 5 of this course.

POINTS TO REMEMBER

1. If a person consents to the touching of his or her person, no civil battery has been committed.

2. Consent to medical treatment may be given expressly or implicitly. Consent given either way will be legally effective.

3. Consent given to a particular medical procedure is generally limited to the procedure in question and those related procedures necessary to repair unforeseen consequences of the authorized procedure.

4. Consent, once validly given, may be revoked by the patient either orally or in writing at any time before commencement of the procedure in question.

5. Written consent, in and of itself, is no more legally effective than oral consent or consent implied by law or the patient's actions.

4-14

True	False	
☐	☐	To be binding, a DNR order must be placed in the patient's chart by the treating physician.
☐	☐	Once a DNR order has been placed in the patient's chart, all nursing personnel are legally obliged to follow it.
☐	☐	Failure to implement a DNR order is ground for an action alleging battery even if the patient is successfully resuscitated.
☐	☐	Once issued, a DNR cannot be withdrawn by the patient.

CONSENT IN EMERGENCY SITUATIONS

4-15   The principles we have been discussing up to this point concern treatment of an elective or nonemergency nature. In an emergency, however, where the patient's life is threatened, and it is impossible to obtain the consent of the patient or someone legally authorized to act on the patient's behalf, the law permits the necessary treatment to be undertaken without obtaining consent. In this specific situation the law *implies* the patient's constructive consent to all procedures necessary to save the patient's life.

The law implies a patient's constructive consent to treatment when

☐   the patient's condition has taken a turn for the worse

☐   the patient is unconscious and cannot give consent

☐   the patient's life is in danger and consent cannot be obtained from anyone authorized to give such consent

4-16   In an emergency situation, the law permits the doctor or nurse to proceed with treatment

☐   only if the patient is mentally incompetent

☐   only if the consent cannot otherwise be obtained

☐   only if the patient is an adult

4-14	*True*	*False*	**4-15**	☐	*If you checked the 2d box, turn*	**4-16**	☐
	☑	☐		☐	*to p. 222, Note C.*		☑
	☑	☐		☑			☐
	☑	☐					
	☐	☑					

EXPLANATORY NOTES

Note A (from Frame 4-7)

Whether an unconsented procedure proves to be beneficial to a patient is legally irrelevant. The law recognizes the absolute fundamental right of adult, competent patients to refuse any unauthorized invasion of their persons, even for admittedly beneficial procedures or essential surgery. Hence, knowing that a patient has categorically refused to undergo a certain procedure or course of treatment, a nurse must not risk legal liability by proceeding or participating in carrying out the procedure; this applies even if a doctor orders the nurse to do so. The proper course of action for the nurse in these circumstances is to call the matter to the attention of the nursing supervisor or a responsible hospital official.

Proceed to Frame 4-8.

Note B (from Frame 4-12)

It should be noted that P consented to the immunization, and no later adverse result would alter the legal effect of this consent. Moreover, the surgical removal of the needle would be considered a medically necessary concomitant of the immunization procedure and thereby encompassed within the original consent. The point to remember is that in a suit alleging *battery*, the critical element is proof of an unauthorized touching—not whether harm resulted from the procedure. Obviously, where harm does result, the patient is more likely to bring suit alleging *negligence* (malpractice) rather than *battery*. The example was intended to illustrate the distinction between the legal bases for these two causes of action.

Proceed to Frame 4-13.

Note C (from Frame 4-15)

Unconsciousness does not necessarily signify that a patient is in immediate danger of death or other serious harm. Thus, under the given facts there may be no emergency at all. On the other hand, even if a true emergency exists, and the patient is unconscious, an attempt should be made to locate the patient's spouse, a close relative, or other authorized legal representative before proceeding with treatment. However, under no circumstances should treatment be delayed unduly in order to locate such a person. The law presumes "constructive consent" in this situation, and the nurse should have little fear of liability if he or she proceeds with treatment.

Proceed to Frame 4-16.

4-17   In which of the following situations would an ER nurse be justified in proceeding with treatment without obtaining consent, verbal or otherwise?

☐   An unconscious, profusely bleeding auto accident victim is brought in by ambulance.

☐   A 13-year-old child is brought to the ER after suffering a fractured arm while at school.

☐   A construction worker comes to the ER to have a boil lanced.

4-18   The rule permitting treatment without obtaining anyone's consent in an emergency situation applies whenever (1) there is immediate danger of death or serious bodily harm, and (2) the patient is physically or legally incapable of giving consent.

True	*False*
☐	☐

4-19

- A patient is under general anesthesia for removal of cancerous tissue in her stomach. During the operation, the surgeon discovers that the patient has a dangerously inflamed appendix.

Yes	*No*	
☐	☐	May the surgeon remove the appendix without obtaining anyone's consent?
☐	☐	Would this situation fall within the emergency (constructive consent) rule?
☐	☐	Could the surgeon be held liable for battery if he or she is negligent in removing the appendix?

4-17   *An unconscious, profusely bleeding auto accident victim . . .*   **4-18**   *True*   **4-19**   Yes   No
                                                                                                ☑   ☐
                                                                                                ☑   ☐
                                                                                                ☐   ☑

NOTE: The given example illustrates the variation of the emergency rule exception known as the "extension" doctrine. We touched on it briefly in Frame 4-10. This doctrine applies when unanticipated conditions are discovered during a surgical procedure. It justifies the physician in extending the operation beyond the scope of the patient's original expressed consent when the extension is necessary to cope with an immediate threat to life or a permanent impairment of health.

THE DOCTRINE OF THERAPEUTIC PRIVILEGE

The common law has long recognized another exception to the informed consent doctrine, known as the doctrine of therapeutic privilege. It is a doctrine that has it origins in the common law defense of necessity—where a defendant's actions, even though in violation of law, are excused because they are aimed at achieving a greater good. For example, an individual may break into a burning house in order to save the occupants from perishing in the fire, without becoming liable for trespassing, unlawful entry, and so on.

In the medical context, the doctrine of therapeutic privilege comes into play when, in the good faith judgment of a physician, disclosure of material information about a patient's diagnosis, prognosis, or treatment is likely to (1) hinder or complicate necessary treatment, (2) cause severe psychological harm, or (3) be so upsetting as to render a rational decision by the patient impossible. In such circumstances, the physician is permitted to proceed with the necessary treatment without making the disclosures normally required and obtaining the patient's informed consent.

The doctrine of therapeutic privilege, although codified in the statutes of several states, is not favored in the law, for obvious reasons, and is therefore narrowly construed by the courts. Generally, it applies only when the patient is severely and emotionally unstable and where some dread disease presents an imminent peril to the patient's life. Under no circumstances is it permitted merely to support a physician who believes an operation or treatment modality is desirable or necessary and that the patient probably would decline the surgery or treatment if given all the facts. This would be a complete perversion of the doctrine.

It is the physician's responsibility to document in the patient's record what the detrimental effects probably would be if the information he or she has decided to withhold were to be given to the patient. Once the decision has been made to proceed without making the normally required disclosures and obtaining the patient's informed consent, it is the nurse's duty to respect the physician's decision and act in accordance therewith. Thus, if the patient repeatedly asks probing questions regarding his or her condition, prognosis, treatment, and the like, the questions should be parried and the physician promptly notified so that he or she may take whatever steps are deemed appropriate under the circumstances.

CONSENT FOR TREATING MINORS AND MENTAL INCOMPETENTS

4-20   The law considers minors (i.e., persons legally under age) and mentally incompetent persons incapable of giving consent to treatment. Before treating a minor or a person of doubtful mental capacity, the necessary consent should be obtained from a duly authorized person—generally a parent, spouse, legal guardian, or person standing *in loco parentis* ("in place of the parent").

In a situation involving the treatment of a child or a person of doubtful mental competence, liability for unauthorized treatment will be avoided if

- ☐   the individual requesting treatment agrees to assume all responsibility for any possible harm

- ☐   the treatment in question is relatively simple in nature

- ☐   an authorized person consents to the treatment in question

---

4-21   Before undertaking nonemergency treatment on a minor child, the physician or nurse should first make sure that the person who requests such treatment for the child is the child's

- ☐   next of kin

- ☐   parent, legal guardian, or person standing *in loco parentis*

- ☐   teacher or closest adult friend

4-22   In the previous frame, does the physician or nurse risk being held liable for battery if he or she assumes the adult has the necessary legal authority to give consent to the treatment proposed without inquiring into the latter's authority or relationship to the patient?

	Yes	*No*
	☐	☐

4-20   *an authorized person consents to the treatment in question*

4-21   *parent, legal guardian, or person standing* in loco parentis

4-22   *Yes*

See Note A, p. 246.

TREATING MATURE MINORS

Physicians, nurses, and other health care professionals are faced with the continuing problem of determining whether a minor patient can give valid legal consent to nonemergency medical treatment, either over the objection of, or without the knowledge of, his or her parents. Their concern stems from the fact that in most states, the age of majority is 18 years, and persons under that age are considered legally incapable of giving or withholding consent to medical treatment. Indeed, the common law has long held that, with the exception of emergency care, treatment of a child under the legal age of adulthood without parental consent—even without professional negligence and even if the result is satisfactory—will give rise to an action for battery by the parents against the treating health care professional.

In addition to vast changes in societal values over the past several decades, particularly those relating to matters of sex, reproduction, and child abuse, public attitudes toward the rights of children have dramatically changed. Because of the increasing number of legal problems in this area, the courts have not only eased the requirements for obtaining parental consent, but most states have enacted so-called "minor treatment statutes" that give greater legal recognition to the rights of minors. The statutes vary widely in their age limits and substantive provisions, but for the most part recognize the right of young persons between 14 and 17 years of age to consent to ordinary, nonemergency treatment without parental approval.

Emancipated Minors

All jurisdictions have carved out areas in which some minors are allowed to make medical decisions for themselves. For example, 23 states have laws permitting minors who are "emancipated" to consent to general medical treatment without parental approval. An emancipated minor is generally held to be one who is no longer dependent on parents for support or otherwise subject to parental control. Although the precise definition varies from jurisdiction to jurisdiction, nearly all define an emancipated minor as one who is not living at home and is self-supporting. Married minors are considered emancipated in all jurisdictions and may consent to treatment for themselves as well as their children. In addition, in many jurisdictions, minors are considered to be emancipated if they are in military service or are college students living away from home.

Mature Minors

Apart from the concept of emancipation from parental control, another legal doctrine that is finding increasing acceptance in the legal community concerns the legality of consent given by a mature minor—someone who can and does make his or her own decisions on daily affairs, is independent, and intellectually able to appreciate the risks and benefits of proposed medical treatment. Thus far only four states have incorporated the doctrine into their statutes, but even in the absence of a statute that gives specific legal recognition to mature minors, health care professionals should not be unduly concerned about providing treatment to minor patients who are 15 or older and who appear able to understand and appreciate the risks of treatment that is for their own benefit and is medically indicated.

Section 59a of the American Law Institute's *Restatement of the Law of Torts* gives additional legal support to the mature minor doctrine. It provides, in part:

> If a child . . . is capable of appreciating the nature, extent and consequences of the invasion [of his body] his assent prevents the invasion from creating liability, though the assent of the parent, guardian, or other person [in loco parentis] is not obtained or is expressly refused.

Obviously, a rule of reason must apply when it comes to treating even so-called mature minors. What may be reasonable to treat without parental consent in one case, such as providing routine medical care, may be decidedly unreasonable in another, such as undertaking major, life-threatening surgery. It should be some comfort to know, however, that there are no reported decisions within the past 25 years in which a parent has recovered damages against a health care provider for failure to obtain parental consent to treating a mature minor.

A few states have taken a different approach to the consent issue. Rather than establishing criteria for determining whether a minor is emancipated or sufficiently mature to consent to treatment, they have set a statutory age of consent that limits the authority or situations in which a minor can consent to treatment. For example, the Rhode Island statute restricts consent to "routine emergency or medical care" to individuals 16 years of age or over, or who are married (R.I. Gen. Laws §§ 23-4.6-1 [1979]). South Carolina and Kansas have also made 16 years of age the determinative age for minors seeking medical or surgical treatment without parental consent.

Consent by a Minor Parent

Children are sexually active much earlier than in previous years, with increasing teenage pregnancy the consequence. Health care providers have been understandably reluctant to accept authorization for treatment of such infants by their minor parents on grounds that minors in general are legally barred from giving valid consent. However, there is nothing in the common law that distinguishes minor parents from adult parents; traditional rules requiring parental consent for treatment of an unemancipated minor apply in both instances. In addition, a number of state legislatures have enacted laws specifically authorizing minor parents to give legally valid consent to treatment on behalf of their infant children. Even in the absence of such legislation, it would seem legally incorrect to require consent from the minor parent's father, mother, or other relative. An exception would apply, of course, if it is shown that the minor parent is incapable of giving a knowing and informed authorization to treatment because of mental incapacity or other infirmity.

Treating Specific Conditions Affecting Minors

Finally, every state has enacted legislation that enables minors to consent to treatment for specific medical conditions, such as sexually transmitted diseases, alcohol and drug abuse, birth control information, pregnancy care, and communicable disease. A common element running through many of these statutes is a grant of immunity to physicians against a claim of battery for treating the minor without parental consent. They also typically state that the minor's authorization for care is not subject to disaffirmance because of the child's minority. Some statutes include specific prohibitions against certain procedures, such as abortion, blood donation, or donation of an organ, in the absence of parental consent if the child has not attained a specified age.

4-23 As just noted, in some jurisdictions a minor is authorized to give valid consent to medical treatment without parental approval if he or she is considered a mature minor or legally emancipated. This determination can only be made by careful questioning of the minor.

Choose from the brief facts presented below those situations *clearly* indicating the minor is capable of giving a valid consent to surgery or other nonroutine medical treatment.

- ☐ Bill is 16 and a student at a military prep school.

- ☐ Janice is 13, lives at home with her parents, and shows symptoms of being pregnant.

- ☐ Irene is 15, has a steady boyfriend, and is the school's top math student.

- ☐ Hank is 17, has his own apartment, and works full time as a gardener.

4-24

- ■ A 17-year-old woman, recently graduated from high school, comes to the office of a plastic surgeon for the purpose of having cosmetic surgery to remove a birthmark on her cheek. Before undertaking to treat this patient in any matter, the physician (or office nurse acting on the physician's behalf) should

- ☐ make sure the patient is intelligent enough to comprehend all the risks of the surgery before proceeding

- ☐ determine whether the patient is emancipated or otherwise capable of giving proper consent before proceeding

- ☐ insist on obtaining the consent of the patient's parents before proceeding

---

	4-23 ☐	4-24	*determine whether the*
	☑		*patient is emancipated*
	☐		*or otherwise capable . . .*
	☑		

4-25   Check each of the situation(s) below in which the physician or nurse may assume adequate legal consent for treatment of the minor patient.

☐   A father brings his 10-year-old son to a clinic for a routine physical. While undergoing the physical, the boy objects to having his blood taken for analysis.

☐   A married, 17-year-old college student goes to a private physician for treatment of a disabling arthritic condition.

☐   Neither of the above.

NOTE: Obtaining proper legal consent where a minor patient claims to be legally emancipated or sufficiently mature to consent to treatment on his or her own can present a problem to busy medical/nursing personnel who seldom have the time to corroborate the minor's claim of independence from parental control. When in doubt, the wisest course of action is to temporarily postpone undertaking any clearly "elective" treatment until it is determined that the minor actually is emancipated or is sufficiently mature to be able to consent thereto under state law. If treatment is not purely elective but is clearly indicated or necessary, hospital-based nurses should consult with the hospital's legal counsel on the current status of consent laws in their respective states. Once the decision is made to proceed with treatment on the basis of the minor's consent alone, this decision and the surrounding circumstances should be fully documented in the patient's medical record.

After valid legal consent has been given, all the usual rules relating to consent apply. Thus, a minor can always withdraw his or her consent after it has been given, and the physician or nurse can be held liable for battery if he or she continues treatment thereafter. Note also that the rules relating to consent for minors in nonemergency cases do not apply where the minor patient's injury is life threatening and no person with authority to give valid legal consent (i.e., parent, legal guardian, or person standing *in loco parentis*) is readily available. In that situation, the law implies the necessary consent.

4-25   ☑   *If you did not check the*
        ☑   *2d box, turn to p. 246,*
        ☐   *Note B.*

Types of Consent to Treatment

Form of Consent	Example
Express Consent—Oral	After having a relatively minor therapeutic procedure explained to him, the patient says to the physician, "That's fine with me, doctor, let's get on with it."
Express Consent—Written	After having an operative procedure fully explained to her, the patient reads and then signs a hospital consent form for the procedure in question.
Implied Consent—By Actions	After being told that free flu shots are being given in the allergy clinic, the patient goes to the clinic, waits his turn, and when the nurse says, "Next person," he rolls up his sleeve and exposes his arm to the nurse to receive the shot.
Implied Consent—Emergency	A patient is brought to the ER after suffering a blow on the head and is bleeding profusely from nose, ears, and mouth. He is conscious but in deep shock. The law implies his consent to be treated in these circumstances.
Consent Implied in Law	The patient is a minor and the parent, guardian, or other person standing *in loco parentis* brings the patient to the physician's office for an examination. The law implies the minor's consent to the examination.

4-26 Every adult is presumed to be *legally* competent, and this presumption is rebutted (over-ruled) only when a judge adjudicates the individual to be incompetent in a formal competency proceeding. The legal presumption of competency is clearly applicable to persons seeking medical treatment, even though occasionally the physician or nurse may have strong clinical reasons to doubt the mental competency of a patient.

- A physician is confronted with a patient of adult years whose behavior raises a question concerning his competence to appreciate the risks involved in a proposed course of treatment.

Which of the following statements expresses the correct position with respect to the patient's competency to consent to the proposed treatment?

☐ The physician can assume the patient's mental competence to understand the nature of the proposed treatment.

☐ The physician can assume the patient is legally competent to give valid consent to the proposed treatment.

☐ Both assumptions are correct.

☐ Neither assumption is correct.

4-26   *The physician can assume the patient is legally competent to give valid consent to the proposed treatment.*

4-27 When it is apparent to the physician and/or nurse that the patient is clinically incompetent—that is, unable to understand the true nature of the proposed treatment, whether surgery, nursing care, or some other form of therapy—the treatment should be postponed until interested and available family members can be consulted and involved in the decision-making process as much as possible. Generally, the views of the patient's spouse are given highest priority, although the views of other family members are also commonly given consideration.

■ An elderly patient whose mental faculties appear to be affected by senility comes to a physician's office accompanied by his adult son. Cancer is diagnosed and the physician normally would recommend the prompt commencement of chemotherapy by his nurse-specialist. The physician asks the son in private whether his father has been declared mentally incompetent, and the son replies in the negative, but urges the physician to proceed with the treatment proposed. The father tells the doctor he is unwilling to undergo the chemotherapy.

Indicate whether the following statements are true or false.

True	False	
☐	☐	The physician or nurse would be on legally safe ground if they were to proceed with treatment with the son's authorization despite the patient's objections.
☐	☐	The physician or nurse would be on legally safe ground if they were to postpone treatment until the legal status of the patient's competence is resolved in a competency proceeding.
☐	☐	The physician or nurse could not rely on the son's authority to consent to his father's treatment without knowing more about the family's handling of the father's affairs.

4-27	True	False
	☐	☑
	☑	☐
	☑	☐

4-28   The physician and nurse in the previous example would be justified in honoring the son's request to begin treatment at once only if, on making inquiry, they determined that

☐   the patient invariably refused to follow his son's advice on all types of matters, not just medical treatment

☐   the son was a licensed physician himself

☐   the son was the father's duly appointed legal guardian

4-29   Assuming the patient in the previous example had been declared legally incompetent, his written consent to the proposed treatment would be

☐   legally valid, provided he was lucid at the time consent was given

☐   legally invalid, and therefore of no consequence

☐   legally valid, provided he agreed to pay all treatment costs

4-28   *the son was the father's duly appointed legal guardian*

4-29   *legally invalid, and therefore of no consequence*

SURROGATE DECISION MAKING FOR ELDERLY INCOMPETENT PATIENTS

It is estimated that by the year 2000, there will be 36.3 million Americans over the age of 65, which is 13.2% of the population. In 1975, 38% of the elderly (people over 65) were 75 or older; by the year 2000, it is estimated that fully 45% of the elderly population will be over the age of 75. These statistics are significant because the incidence of two of the most prevalent forms of dementia, Alzheimer's disease and multiinfarct dementia, increases with age. In light of these statistics, the issue of the patient's mental and legal competence to make critical treatment decisions becomes a matter of paramount importance for doctors and nurses alike.

At present, there are no universally accepted standards for determining a patient's incompetency. Although the courts are always available to make such determinations, in practice it is customary for the patient's attending physician to make a judgment concerning the patient's competence while discussing the risks and benefits of the proposed course of treatment. In his or her dialogue with the patient, the physician tries to obtain answers to one or more of the following: (1) is the patient capable of making a definitive decision one way or another, (2) does the patient appear to understand the information disclosed about the treatment being proposed, (3) does the patient demonstrate the ability to engage in decision making in a rational way with an appreciation of the potential outcomes, or (4) can the patient make a decision about treatment that is reasonable in itself?

If the patient is judged to be clinically incompetent by reference to one or more of the above standards, the physician's obligation to obtain consent from the patient is legally suspended, although the decision as to whether and how the patient is to be treated from that point on may require initiation of formal legal proceedings to have someone appointed the patient's legal guardian. As a practical matter, however, physicians and nurses cannot be expected to suggest formal guardianship every time they have some doubt about the clinical competency of an elderly patient. This action would not only impose an unnecessary financial and emotional burden on the patient and the patient's family but would place unwarranted burdens on the health professionals as well.

Once the patient is determined to be clinically incompetent in accordance with the informal standards noted above, the widespread practice in current health care delivery is to consult the patient's family as soon as possible and have them participate in the health care decision-making process. Such family involvement usually works out well for the patient, since, in the vast majority of cases, family members can be counted on to act in a manner that is consistent with the patient's own values and preferences and in the patient's best interests.

Although obtaining consent from relatives on behalf of an elderly patient who has not been judicially declared incompetent creates some degree of legal risk, it is better than relying totally on the clinically incompetent patient's consent alone. Recently the law has begun to recognize the family's legitimate surrogate decision-making power both in statutes and judicial decisions, provided the family acts in good faith. Doctors and nurses should be willing to tolerate whatever legal uncertainty may still exist in dealing with clinically incompetent patients, and should urge formal competency/guardianship proceedings only when there is obvious dissension in the patient's family or where they have substantial reason to doubt the decision-making motives or abilities of the family.

POINTS TO REMEMBER

1. Consent is not legally required where immediate treatment is necessary to save the patient's life and consent cannot be obtained either from the patient or from a duly authorized legal representative.

2. The type of consent recognized in a medical emergency situation is called constructive consent, or consent implied by law.

3. Persons who are considered minors under state law* or who are adjudged mental incompetents are not legally capable of giving valid consent to medical treatment.

4. Minors who live apart from their parents, or are married, frequently are considered in the eyes of the law to be emancipated and capable of giving consent to medical treatment.

5. A number of states have enacted special laws pertaining to the rights of minors to give legal consent to specific types of medical treatment.

6. The law presumes every adult person to be mentally competent until adjudicated otherwise in a judicial competency and guardianship proceeding.

7. An individual who has been declared mentally incompetent in a judicial proceeding cannot give a valid consent to medical and/or nursing treatment.

8. Where a patient is deemed to be clinically incompetent, but has not been declared legally incompetent, the physician and nurse should seek the participation of the patient's next-of-kin in the decision-making process.

9. If family members cannot agree on the treatment regimen for their mentally incompetent relative, treatment should be postponed until such time as a legal guardian is appointed with authority to make the necessary medical decisions.

---

*In most states, a minor is anyone below the age of 18 (below the age of 21 in a few states) who has not been emancipated by marriage or some other special circumstance.

INFORMED CONSENT

4-30   The underlying concept of informed consent is a simple one: A patient's consent to a particular medical procedure is not legally effective unless the patient fully understands to what he or she is consenting. The mere signing of a consent form (valuable though this may be) does not necessarily mean the patient fully understood to what he or she was consenting. Failure to obtain the patient's informed consent will give rise to either a possible legal action for battery, based on the unauthorized touching of the patient, or an action alleging negligence, based on failure to adequately disclose the risks of treatment.

The doctrine of informed consent recognizes the fundamental right of   ☐   the doctor ☐   the patient   to decide what course of treatment to undertake.

4-31   A patient's consent to treatment is said to be informed when

    ☐   the patient consents to the procedure in writing

    ☐   the patient's physician has spoken to him or her about the proposed treatment

    ☐   the patient fully understands the nature of the treatment

---

4-32   The failure to obtain a patient's informed consent is legally classified as

    ☐   tortious conduct

    ☐   unethical professional conduct

    ☐   criminal conduct

4-33   If a patient's informed consent to treatment has not been obtained, he or she is likely to prevail in a suit filed against all who participated in the treatment if the patient alleges

    ☐   assault and battery

    ☐   negligence or battery

    ☐   willful misconduct or battery

4-30 *the patient*	**4-31** *the patient fully understands the nature of the treatment*	**4-32** *tortious conduct*	**4-33** *negligence or battery* *For amplification of this response, turn to p. 246, Note C.*

4-34   Under what circumstances would a patient's informed consent to treatment not be necessary?

☐   when at least two physicians agree that the patient's condition is terminal in nature

☐   under no circumstances, since the doctrine is rigidly applied to all medical situations

☐   only when the patient is unable to give consent and a medical emergency exists

---

4-35

True	*False*	
☐	☐	From the legal standpoint, obtaining the patient's written consent to a particular course of treatment is considered legal proof that he or she understands the nature of the proposed treatment.
☐	☐	The fundamental purpose of the informed consent requirement is to encourage the practice of getting patients to consent to treatment in writing.
☐	☐	The law makes no distinction between a patient's consent that is informed and one that is uninformed.
☐	☐	From the legal standpoint, the signing of a consent form has no legal value as evidence of the patient's consent.

NOTE: The nurse becomes legally concerned—and sometimes enmeshed—in informed consent cases not because of any primary responsibility to obtain the patient's consent, but because he or she is generally present at the time the proposed course of treatment is explained to the patient. Every nurse should understand that the law places the duty of informing the patient concerning the proposed treatment on the treating physician, not the nurse.

Getting the patient's signature on a consent form is no guarantee that he or she understands what is to happen, nor will it prevent the patient from later alleging that he or she was not adequately "informed" about the nature of the treatment or its alternatives. As a matter of fact, in nearly all malpractice cases alleging lack of informed consent, a document with the patient's signature on it has been offered as proof of the patient's legal consent. The courts invariably ignore these *pro forma* consent forms and ask instead, "What did the doctor actually tell the patient? What questions did the patient ask? How was consent really manifested?" These and other consent issues relevant to nursing practice are discussed in the material that follows.

4-36 As noted earlier, there are occasions when the patient's consent to treatment can be *implied* (such as when the patient needs immediate treatment in an emergency but is unable to consent, or when the patient's consent is clearly indicated by his or her actions). The patient may, of course, give his or her consent *expressly*, either verbally or in writing, and either way is considered legally effective as long as it can be later proved that he or she fully understood the nature of the proposed treatment.

Indicate the type of legal consent demonstrated in the described situations.

Express	*Implied*	
☐	☐	An unconscious accident victim is treated for a cranial fracture.
☐	☐	A patient rolls up his or her sleeve to receive a vitamin injection.
☐	☐	A patient signs a consent form for a vasectomy.
☐	☐	A patient needing minor surgery tells the doctor to "go ahead."

4-36	*Express*	*Implied*
	☐	☑
	☐	☑
	☑	☐
	☑	☐

4-37 In the eyes of the law, a patient's oral consent to treatment does not have the same legal effect as a consent given in writing.

True   *False*
☐   ☐

4-38 Neither express consent nor implied consent to treatment is legally effective when the patient is mentally incompetent.

True   *False*
☐   ☐

4-39 For his or her consent to be effective, the patient must understand what is to be done and the essential nature of the choices available. Liability will result if the physician withholds any facts that are necessary to form the basis of an intelligent choice by the patient, or if the physician minimizes the known dangers of a procedure in order to induce the patient's consent.

As a general proposition, consent will be legally *ineffective* when

- ☐ the patient is given information that is ambiguous or vague
- ☐ the doctor denies the patient information because he or she believes it might cause the patient to refuse the treatment
- ☐ the doctor does not discuss the available options with the patient

4-37   *False*   4-38   *True*   4-39   ☑
                                                      ☑
                                                      ☑

4-40 A blanket consent form used by Hospital H authorizes the carrying out of "any medical or surgical procedure the treating physician deems necessary for the patient's welfare."

This type of consent form is

☐ generally upheld as a valid consent provided it is signed by the patient and properly witnessed

☐ generally held to be invalid, since it does not adequately describe the proposed treatment

☐ generally considered the most effective way to obtain the patient's consent

4-40 *generally held to be invalid, since it does not adequately describe the proposed treatment*

STANDARDS OF DISCLOSURE IN INFORMED CONSENT CASES

The law is in a state of flux as to *how much* information must be given to a patient to obtain a legally effective consent. Currently, three different standards of disclosure have been adopted by the courts. The majority of American jurisdictions adhere to either the "community" or "reasonable physician" standard, under which the adequacy and amount of disclosure to the patient is judged against the amount and type of information that a reasonable health care professional would have disclosed to that patient under similar conditions.

Generally, the patient must be told all the *inherent* risks of the proposed procedure but need not be told about the *unexpected* risks that may arise after the procedure is underway. Disclosure must always be made when the nature of the procedure is such that serious injuries may result (e.g., as in electroshock therapy or insulin shock therapy). In general, the tendency of the courts in the more recent cases has been to require *more* rather than *less* disclosure.

A growing minority of jurisdictions has accepted a more expansive standard of disclosure, the "reasonable patient" or "material risk" standard, under which the physician is required to communicate the type and amount of information that a theoretically "reasonable patient" would need to make an intelligent decision regarding treatment. Material risks are considered those factors that might make a significant difference to a reasonable and prudent patient (e.g., the risk of death or permanent loss of use of any major body organ); hence, this standard, although objective in nature, is decidedly oriented toward the patient's informational needs.

The third disclosure standard, referred to as the "individual patient" standard, is clearly a subjective one. This standard, which has not been adopted by any significant number of courts, asks what the *particular* patient, rather than a *reasonable* patient, would have wanted to know under the circumstances.

Most legal commentators are inclined toward the reasonable patient or material risk standard because it gives appropriate recognition to patient autonomy, enhances physician-patient and nurse-patient communications, encourages better health awareness, and appears to result in less malpractice litigation.

There is little doubt that most patients and their families today *do* want more information than most physicians are willing to disclose. For this reason, physicians (and their associated nursing personnel) who take pains to provide more rather than less information about the proposed treatment regimen are on firmer legal ground than those who choose to reveal only the minimum of facts.

In the final analysis, the problem of informed consent is simply a communication problem. It stands to reason that physicians and nurses who maintain good rapport with their patients in all other aspects of treatment are not likely to get into legal difficulty because of a failure to disclose essential information about specific procedures or modes of therapy.

4-41

■ Doctor D chooses not to tell a terminal cancer patient of the risk of burns involved in cobalt irradiation, knowing the patient probably will decline the treatment. Based on the information given, the patient gives her written consent to the treatment and thereafter sustains painful burns and scarring of her skin.

The patient sues the doctor for damages, alleging lack of informed consent.

What is the likely result?

☐ The doctor will prevail because a patient with a terminal condition is deemed legally incapable of giving an effective consent.

☐ The patient will prevail because the doctor withheld information essential for her to give an informed consent.

☐ The doctor will prevail because the patient gave her consent to the treatment in writing.

4-42   In the previous example the patient's consent to the cobalt treatment

☐ was legally insufficient because she failed to ask about the risks involved

☐ was legally insufficient because it was obtained through deception on the doctor's part

☐ was legally insufficient because no patient ever consents to being injured

---

4-43   The result of the previous lawsuit might be different if, in the physician's professional opinion, the risk of burns was too insignificant to bring to the patient's attention.

	True	*False*
	☐	☐

4-41   *The patient will prevail because the doctor withheld . . .*

4-42   *was legally insufficient because it was obtained through deception on the doctor's part*

4-43   *True*

For additional discussion, turn to p. 247, Note D.

Basic Requirements for Obtaining a Patient's Informed Consent

To be informed, a patient must receive, in terms he or she understands, all the information that would affect a reasonable person's decision to consent to or refuse a proposed course of treatment or medical/surgical procedure. The information, which should be given to the patient by the treating physician, should include:

- A brief but straightforward description of the treatment or procedure

- The name and qualifications of the person who will perform the procedure, if that person is someone other than the physician

- An explanation of the potential for death or serious harm, (e.g., brain damage, paralysis, permanent scarring) or discomforting side effects during or after the treatment or procedure

- An explanation and description of alternative treatments or procedures

- A discussion of the possible effects of not undergoing the proposed treatment or procedure

- Advice to the effect that he or she has a right to refuse the treatment or procedure without having alternative care or support withdrawn

- Advice to the effect that he or she can withdraw consent previously given even if the treatment or procedure has already begun

THE NURSE'S ROLE IN OBTAINING THE PATIENT'S CONSENT

Although a nurse may be capable of explaining a proposed medical or surgical procedure to a patient in such a manner that the patient will be fully "informed" about what is to be done, that is not the nurse's legal responsibility—it is the responsibility of the physician. This was the holding in the case of *Petriello* v. *Kalman et al.*, 576 A. 2d 474 (Conn. 1990), where a nurse, contrary to hospital policy, administered preoperative medication to a patient before checking to see if the hospital's informed consent form had been signed by the patient. When the surgeon arrived, he was told by the OR supervisor of the absence of the patient's signature on the form, whereupon the surgeon—despite the fact that the patient was already under the effect of the medication—had the plaintiff sign the form and then began the procedure, a dilatation and curettage to remove a dead fetus from the patient's womb. During the course of the D&C procedure, the patient suffered injuries when her uterus was perforated by a suction device, and she subsequently sued the surgeon and the hospital.

At trial, the plaintiff argued that the hospital and its nurses owed her a duty to ensure that the consent form was signed before the preoperative medication was given and that the breach of this duty was a violation of the hospital's own policy. The court ruled, however, that the hospital had no duty with respect to obtaining a patient's informed consent for a surgical procedure to be performed by a nonemployee physician. The court further ruled that, notwithstanding the admitted violation of its own policy, the hospital owed no legal duty to ensure that its consent form was signed by the patient before surgery, stating, "This contention is unsound, because it equates the signing of the form with the actuality of informed consent, which is the sole responsibility of the attending physician to obtain." On appeal, the court affirmed the verdict against the physician and the trial court's directed verdict in favor of the hospital.

The fact that it is the physician's fundamental legal responsibility to obtain the patient's informed consent to treatment does not mean that the nurse has absolutely no responsibility with respect to the matter of consents. Quite the contrary, both the hospital and its nurse-employees have a duty to use reasonable care to ascertain whether the patient's consent (not just a signed consent form) has, in fact, been obtained. Thus, if the nurse becomes aware that a patient who has signed a consent form, or is being asked to sign one, (1) has been told nothing about the proposed procedure, (2) has not been adequately informed of all the material risks of the procedure by the physician or does not appear to comprehend the significance of the information provided, or (3) indicates a genuine change of heart about proceeding with treatment, *the nurse has a legal obligation to notify the patient's physician or the nursing supervisor as soon as possible.*

Nurses sometimes are asked to "get the patient's signature" on a surgical consent form, often just before surgery, which can present some tactical and legal problems where the operating surgeon has not adequately discussed the risks of surgery with the patient. From a practical standpoint, when a nurse asks a patient to sign a surgical consent form and it is clear that the patient has been given little or no information about the procedure or its risks by the operating surgeon, the nurse should immediately cease all efforts to get the patient's signature on the form. The nurse should also decline to answer the patient's questions about the procedure and its risks and instead advise the patient that this is the doctor's responsibility and that he or she will bring the matter to the doctor's attention, using language such as, "I'll tell Dr. Thompson about our conversation, and I'm sure he will want to talk with you about these matters." Obviously, the nurse should proceed to speak with the physician *promptly*.

Also, bear in mind that it is the nurse's continuing legal duty to observe the patient and recognize all critical factors relating to the treatment, including the patient's emotional state and degree of comprehension of what is about to be done with his or her body. Thus, even when a patient has been fully informed about a surgical procedure and has given written consent thereto, if there is any indication the patient does not want to proceed with the surgery, the nurse must bring this fact to the attention of the surgeon or nursing supervisor at once, and, if necessary, the surgical procedure should be postponed until the issue is satisfactorily resolved.

EXPLANATORY NOTES

Note A (from Frame 4-22)

The technically correct response to this frame is "yes," although as a practical matter physicians and nurses frequently make assumptions about the identity, relationship, and legal authority of persons who accompany and request nonemergency treatment for minors. The law does not expect or require doctors or nurses to routinely initiate formal inquiries into the legal authority of adults to act on behalf of the minors they bring in for treatment. From the legal standpoint, as long as the doctor or nurse acts on a good faith belief in the apparent or ostensible authority of the person or persons making the request for treatment, it is unlikely that a court would find such conduct either unreasonable or contrary to currently accepted medical and nursing practice.

Proceed to Frame 4-23.

Note B (from Frame 4-25)

The second fact situation was given to illustrate the legal concept of emancipation. As noted in Frame 4-23, an emancipated minor is one who—though legally a minor because of age—either is married or has otherwise taken steps to emancipate himself or herself from parental control. Merely being a college student living away from home would not be sufficient proof of legal emancipation in all states, but a married college student certainly would be considered emancipated and capable of giving legal consent to treatment. In a number of states, laws have been enacted authorizing or validating consents by legal minors in specific situations (e.g., blood donation, abortion, receipt of contraceptive information, obstetrical care, etc). Prudent nurses should become familiar with the relevant laws in their states.

Proceed to Frame 4-26.

Note C (from Frame 4-33)

While a patient may bring a suit alleging battery, more and more suits alleging lack of informed consent are being predicted on a theory of negligence—failure on the part of the physician to disclose to a patient what other reasonably prudent practitioners would normally disclose under the same or similar circumstances. The choice of legal theory can have a significant effect on the type of proof necessary, as well as the amount of damages that may be recovered. Although Frame 4-33 indicates the action can be one of negligence or battery, the reader should be aware that the trend of the law is toward viewing informed consent cases as a problem of negligence in physician-patient communications, rather than one of battery.

Proceed to Frame 4-34.

EXPLANATORY NOTES

Note D (from Frame 4-43)

Frames 4-41 to 4-43 illustrate the overall problem of informed consent. The mere fact that a patient may have a terminal condition does not vitiate the fundamental legal principle that *every* person has a right to decide what will or will not be done to his or her body, provided the patient is legally competent to make such a decision. No physician can usurp this basic right, and the physician who uses deceptive tactics to gain a patient's consent will be held legally liable for so doing in a later lawsuit alleging lack of informed consent. The courts invariably side with the patient in cases of this nature.

Proceed to Frame 4-44.

POINTS TO REMEMBER

1. An informed consent is one that is given by a patient who fully understands to what he or she is consenting.

2. The mere signing of a consent form does not represent legal proof that the patient fully understood the nature of the proposed course of treatment.

3. In a medical emergency, where consent cannot be obtained from the patient or an authorized legal representative, formal consent to treatment is not necessary. The law implies constructive consent in these situations.

4. Informed consent may be reflected either orally or in writing, and both ways are legally effective. For purposes of proving that consent was given, however, it is generally considered advisable to obtain the patient's consent in writing.

5. For a consent to be an informed one, the patient must be told the nature of the proposed treatment, the alternative treatments possible, and the relative risks of the proposed and alternative treatments.

6. The majority of American jurisdictions follow the "reasonable physician" standard as to the type and amount of information that must be disclosed to a patient. This standard gauges the effectiveness of the disclosure by comparing it to what a reasonable and prudent physician would have disclosed to the patient under the circumstances.

7. Liability for battery or negligence will result if a physician minimizes the dangers of a procedure in order to obtain the patient's consent.

8. Blanket consent forms are a poor way of obtaining consent and rarely stand up in cases in which the issue of informed consent is involved.

CONSENT TO ABORTION, STERILIZATION, RECEIPT OF BIRTH CONTROL INFORMATION, AND TREATMENT OF SEXUALLY TRANSMITTED DISEASES

It is not within the scope or purpose of this programmed course on malpractice law to discuss the underlying philosophical, moral, and religious issues pertaining to abortion, sterilization, birth control, and the like. However, since these matters directly affect the professional activities of nurses and nursing students—primarily in the area of consent to treatment—they deserve brief mention at this point.

Abortion

The landmark Supreme Court decisions of *Doe* v. *Bolton*, 410 U.S. 179 (1973), and *Roe* v. *Wade*, 410 U.S. 113 (1973), held that during the first trimester of pregnancy (12 weeks) the state is without power to restrict or regulate abortions; hence, during this period the decision to undergo an abortion is strictly a matter between the pregnant woman and her physician. The Court further held that the consent of the pregnant woman's spouse to an abortion during the first trimester is not necessary and any state law requirement of such consent is unconstitutional.

The Supreme Court also ruled that during the second trimester (fourth to sixth month) the state may regulate the medical conditions under which an abortion is performed, but only to the extent that such regulations reasonably relate to the preservation and protection of the mother's health. Thus, the state may regulate the qualifications of the person who is to perform the abortion, the licensure of that person, the type of facility in which the abortion is to be performed, and the licensure of that facility. Beyond these limited matters, the state cannot otherwise interfere in the regulation of abortions, and later court cases have confirmed this position. In the third trimester the Supreme Court held that a state may prohibit all abortions except those deemed necessary to protect the mother's life or health.

The decisions in *Doe* v. *Bolton* and *Roe* v. *Wade* were based on the concept that every woman's right to privacy and control over her body gives her the right to decide whether to bear a child without interference by the state. The Court noted the medical and psychological harm of denying abortion, as well as the distress and adverse consequences associated with bringing an unwanted child into a family unable or unwilling to care for it.

Since those two Supreme Court decisions in 1973, many state legislatures have tried to impose various limitations on the availability of abortions both before and after the fetus has become viable. Most of those efforts were invalidated by the Court, even though the Court in the mid-80s—now reconstituted with a decidedly more conservative bias—showed signs of retreating from its fundamental holdings in *Roe* v. *Wade* and *Doe* v. *Bolton*. Thus, while it reaffirmed those holdings in 1983 in *City of Akron* v. *Akron Center for Reproductive Health, Inc.*, 462 U.S. 416, in the same year it upheld a Missouri statute that required either parental consent or judicial approval (i.e., court-ordered authorization) before a minor could obtain an abortion (*Planned Parenthood Association of Kansas City, Missouri* v. *Ashcroft*, 462 U.S. 476 [1983]).

In July 1989, the Supreme Court decided *Webster* v. *Reproductive Health Services, Inc.*, 109 S. Ct. 3040, probably the most controversial decision issued by the Court during its 1988-89 term. Although it did not categorically overrule *Roe* v. *Wade*, the Court gave a clear signal in *Webster* that it was no longer firmly committed to the proposition that women have a constitutional right to abortion.

Moreover, it clearly opened the door to further state governmental regulation of abortion that previously would have been prohibited. *Webster* involved the Court's interpretation of several sections of a Missouri abortion statute aimed at barring public employees from assisting in abortions and prohibiting abortions from being performed in state hospitals or other publicly owned facilities. The Court not only upheld those sections but also upheld the provision of the Missouri statute requiring doctors to perform whatever fetal viability tests are necessary before being allowed to perform an abortion on a woman believed to be ≥20 weeks pregnant.

Unquestionably, the abortion issue will be a major source of litigation for some time to come. Many states have enacted laws within the past several years designed to circumvent the criteria for allowing abortions outlined in *Roe*, as was expected. The most recent challenge to *Roe* was *Planned Parenthood of Southeastern Pennsylvania* v. *Casey*, 112 S. Ct. 2791 (1992), which involved provisions of a Pennsylvania statute that required spousal notification and clearcut informed consent from all women seeking to have abortions. Although *Casey* did not overturn *Roe*, the Supreme Court made it clear in its decision that *Roe* was not unalterable in some respects. *Casey* held that spousal notification cannot be demanded of a woman seeking an abortion, but the Court also held that a woman's constitutional right to an abortion was not violated by those provisions of the Pennsylvania law that required medical disclosure of the nature and risks of the abortion procedure, including very specific details regarding the gestational age of the fetus and a description of the fetus, in addition to informing the patient of alternatives to pregnancy termination.

It is extremely doubtful that the ruling in *Casey* will mark the end of abortion litigation, and in light of the nationwide uproar and controversy spawned by *Roe* and subsequent abortion cases, including the *Casey* decision just discussed, nurses should have little difficulty in keeping abreast of developments in their respective states. Obviously, before participating in any questionable abortion procedure, the prudent nurse should seek the advice of the nursing supervisor or the hospital's legal counsel.

In any event, it should be noted that the Supreme Court has specifically recognized the right of physicians, nurses, and other hospital personnel to refuse to participate in abortion procedures, because of religious, moral, or personal reasons, without incurring any occupational redress or civil liability. Virtually all states now have a "conscience clause" in their statutes relating to abortion. In addition, the federal Health Program Extension Act now forbids requiring medical or nursing personnel to perform or assist in abortion or sterilization procedures if to do so would be contrary to the individual's religious beliefs or moral convictions (42 U.S.C. § 300a-7).

To the extent that nurses or nursing students choose not to participate in abortion proce-dures on grounds of conscience, they should make their position known in advance to their clin-ical instructor, head nurse, or other supervisory official. On the other hand, if they do not so object, they can feel secure in the knowledge that their participation in abortion procedures legally sanctioned by the Supreme Court will not subject them to civil or criminal liability sim-ply by assisting therein.

Sterilization

When a pregnancy might seriously endanger a woman's life or health, it may be medically necessary to terminate her ability to conceive or her husband's ability to impregnate. Because of the medical necessity involved in these cases, the resulting sterility is deemed incidental to the basic medical objective. Therapeutic sterilizations of this nature have never been against public policy, and accordingly they raise no unique legal questions for the medical and nursing person-nel involved.

In the past, legal questions have arisen when there was no therapeutic reason for remov-ing a reproductive organ or for preventing impregnation. In fact, several states had enacted spe-cial laws regulating elective contraceptive sterilizations, generally aimed at ensuring that both husband wife fully comprehended the consequences thereof, and requiring the informed consent of *both*.

The law is clear, however, that state statutes requiring spousal consent as a precondition to voluntary sterilization are unconstitutional (*Ponter* v. *Ponter*, 342 A. 2d 574 [N.J. 1975]). *Murray* v. *Vandevander*, 522 P. 2d 302 [Okla. 1974]. In *Ponter*, the New Jersey Superior Court noted that the sterilization issue is closely related to the abortion issue; accordingly, the rationale for giving women the constitutional right to control their reproductive functions—as set forth in *Roe* and subsequent cases—is equally applicable to their right to make unilateral decisions with respect to elective sterilization.

From the nurse's vantage point, the only real concern will be the effectiveness of the con-sent obtained for an elective sterilization. Although it is the physician's responsibility to explain the procedure and its consequences, everyone who participates in the patient's care has a stake in the matter because the patient (or spouse) generally sues all the health care personnel who were involved in the procedure and follow-up care. It goes without saying that legal liability can always result if the sterilization procedure or follow-up care is performed negligently.

Birth Control Information

The Supreme Court has ruled that many medical decisions, and especially those relating to procreation, involve the constitutionally protected right to privacy. As far back as 1965, the court held that a state law making the use of contraceptives a criminal offense was unconstitu-tional (*Griswold* v. *Connecticut*, 381 U.S. 479 [1965]). Although *Griswold* involved adults, minors also have the constitutional right of privacy in the area of obtaining contraceptive information. That issue was decided by the Supreme Court in *Carey* v. *Population Services International*, 431 U.S. 678 (1977). (See also, *Doe* v. *Irwin*, 615 F. 2d 1162 [Mich. 1980], *cert. denied* 449 U.S. 829 [1980]). As matters now stand, parents do not have a constitutional right to receive prior notice that their minor children are getting birth control information and supplies from family planning clinics or other authorized medical sources. Indeed, when the federal government sought to impose a regulatory requirement on clinics and other entities receiving federal funds for family planning services to notify within 10 days the parents of minors who had received contraceptive services, federal courts in New York and the District of Columbia declared the regulations unconstitutional (*State of New York* v. *Heckler*, 719 F. 2d 1191 [N.Y. 1983]; *Planned Parenthood Federation of America* v. *Heckler*, 712 F. 2d 650 [D.C. 1983]; *accord: Planned Parenthood Association of Utah* v. *Matheson*, 582 F. Supp. 1001 [Utah 1983]; *Jane Does* v. *State of Utah Department of Health*, 776 F. 2d 253 [Utah 1985]).

Treatment for Sexually Transmitted Diseases and Drug Abuse

Currently, all 50 states and the District of Columbia have laws allowing a minor to consent to diagnosis and treatment of venereal disease without prior parental consent. As mentioned earlier, some of these statutes give the physician discretionary authority to notify the parents, even over the minor's objection. Although fewer states have laws allowing treatment of alcohol or drug abuse problems without parental consent, proceeding with treatment on the basis of the minor's consent alone is not likely to create any significant liability. As one legal commentator has wisely observed, "Even in the absence of a statute, a child with a drug problem who refuses to tell his parents that he needs treatment, or to permit the physician to do so, undoubtedly would be held competent by a court to give [his] consent to such treatment, since the social and personal consequences to the child of the addiction are so profound and since continuing to make illegal purchases of drugs will subject the child to serious risks of arrest and punishment" (Holder AR, *Legal Issues in Pediatrics and Adolescent Medicine*, Yale University Press, New Haven, 1985, p. 131).

FALSE IMPRISONMENT

4-44 In legal terms, false imprisonment is the unlawful restraint or detention of another person against his or her wishes. Actual force is not necessary to constitute a false imprisonment. All that is required is that there be a reasonable fear of force to restrain or detain the threatened individual. The potential to carry out the threat can be implied by words or gestures.

A charge of false imprisonment will not lie unless

☐ A threatens physical harm to B

☐ A threatens to harm B if B leaves a specified confined area

☐ A places B in a confined area

4-45

■ P, a 25-year-old man of Arab extraction who cannot speak English, is brought by ambulance to the hospital ER after receiving a stab wound while being mugged. After the wound is treated, P attempts to leave, but Nurse N quickly calls a uniformed security guard and tells him, "Watch this character for me until we find out who's going to pay his bill." P is detained for 3 hours in this manner until N finally gets around to calling an interpreter. Through the interpreter it is learned that P is the son of a Kuwaiti diplomat who, upon being called, agrees to pay the bill at once.

The fact that would lend the greatest legal support to a later claim of false imprisonment brought by P against Nurse N would be

☐ N's assignment of the security guard to watch over P

☐ N's determination not to let P leave until his bill was paid

☐ N's delay in calling for an interpreter

4-44 *A threatens to harm B if B leaves a specified confined area*

4-45 *N's assignment of the security guard to watch over P*

4-46 Which of the following is *not* necessary for a charge of false imprisonment to be successfully made?

☐ actual force

☐ fear of bodily injury

☐ physical confinement

4-47 The nurse may be subject to legal liability for false imprisonment if he or she locks a patient in a room against the patient's will and with the threat of force. Most often, cases of this type relate to mentally ill persons, and the nurse engaged in psychiatric care should be particularly alert to his or her liability for false imprisonment.

Which of the following statements most accurately summarizes the foregoing?

☐ False imprisonment is a charge that is likely to be brought whenever a patient is locked in a room.

☐ Liability for false imprisonment is a legal hazard only for nurses engaged in psychiatric care.

☐ Most false imprisonment lawsuits are brought by mentally ill patients.

4-48 What is the common element in the intentional torts of assault and false imprisonment?

☐ physical injury

☐ threatened physical injury

☐ violent and abusive language

4-46 *actual force*   **4-47** *Most false imprisonment lawsuits are brought by . . .*   **4-48** *threatened physical injury*

4-49

■ P had been a surgical patient at Hospital H. The day of her scheduled discharge she was asked to pay her bill, but she steadfastly declined, claiming that her postoperative care was terrible and that she would sue the hospital unless her bill was reduced. Supervisory Nurse S was sent to P's room to "persuade" her to make payment. After a fruitless discussion, Nurse S finally remarked: "If you think you're going to leave here without paying your bill, you're sadly mistaken. I'll give you just 5 minutes more to reconsider, and if you haven't changed your mind by the time I return, I'm going to sedate you with a needle and keep you sedated until you *do* change your mind." In fact, Nurse S had no intention of carrying out this threat, but P believed she would and remained in her room for nearly 5 additional hours until relatives came to get her.

P later brings a suit against S, charging false imprisonment. Which of the following will be the most likely result?

☐ S will be held liable for false imprisonment even though she never came near P with a hypodermic needle.

☐ S cannot be held liable for false imprisonment since P was not locked in her room.

☐ S cannot be held liable for false imprisonment because she had no intention of carrying out her threat.

4-50   If sued, Hospital H could not be held liable for Nurse S's conduct in this case.

True	*False*
☐	☐

4-51   The legal basis of Nurse S's liability in this case would be

☐ the doctrine of *respondeat superior*

☐ the rule of personal liability

☐ the supervisor's liability for the acts of others

4-49 *S will be held liable for false imprisonment even though she . . .*   **4-50** *False*   **4-51** *the rule of personal liability*

4-52   On what legal theory or rule of law would Hospital H be held liable, if at all, for Nurse S's conduct?

☐   A hospital is liable for all harms caused by its supervisory personnel.

☐   A hospital is liable for harm resulting from the acts of its employees within the scope of their employment.

☐   A hospital is liable for harms caused by employees, but only if related to the care and treatment of patients.

☐   None of the above

4-53   If Nurse S actually had given P a sedative in the manner threatened

☐   S could be held liable for assault and battery, but not false imprisonment

☐   S could be held liable only for false imprisonment, as charged

☐   S could be held for assault and battery, as well as false imprisonment

---

4-54   Being charged with false imprisonment is a professional hazard most likely to be faced by

☐   supervisory nurses

☐   ER nurses

☐   psychiatric nurses

4-52   *A hospital is liable for harm resulting from the acts of its employees within the scope of . . .*

4-53   *S could be held liable for assault and battery, as well as false imprisonment*

4-54   *psychiatric nurses*

OTHER TYPES OF INTENTIONAL WRONGS

Although this course relates primarily to the nurse's liability for *negligent* (i.e., unintentional) conduct, the preceding discussion has dealt with several *intentional* torts—battery and false imprisonment—that also can have a direct effect on the nurse's daily activities. Although they are not covered in this part, there are several other intentional wrongs of which the reader should be aware, including intentional infliction of emotional distress, defamation of character (libel and slander), malicious prosecution of a civil proceeding, violation of another's civil rights under federal or state law, invasion of privacy, and breach of confidentiality. One distinction between intentional and unintentional torts is the nature of damages recoverable. Punitive damages, which are not normally recoverable in a malpractice claim, *are* recoverable in claims involving intentional tortious conduct in order to punish and deter those who engage in such conduct.

Part 8 includes brief discussion of several intentional torts not covered in this part, as well as selected references to other source materials.

POINTS TO REMEMBER

1. False imprisonment is the unlawful restraint or detention of another person against his or her will.

2. Force is not essential to hold an individual liable for false imprisonment. The law merely requires proof of a reasonable fear of force on the part of the person restrained or detained.

3. Most false imprisonment cases in the medical setting involve locking up mentally ill patients in their rooms. For this reason, nurses engaged in psychiatric nursing should be alert to their exposure to false imprisonment claims by their patients.

4. Under the doctrine of *respondeat superior*, a hospital can be held liable for the conduct of a nurse-employee who unlawfully confines or detains a patient against his or her will.

5. Other intentional torts that may affect the nurse's activities include intentional infliction of emotional distress, libel, slander, invasion of privacy, breach of confidentiality, and interference with civil rights.

6. Punitive damages are rarely recoverable in malpractice suits but are often recoverable in actions involving intentional torts.

SELECTED REFERENCES—PART FOUR

Unauthorized Touching or Treatment—Battery

Louisell D and Williams H, *Medical Malpractice*, Matthew Bender & Co., New York, 1988, §§ 22.04.

Smith L, "Battery in Medical Torts," *Cleveland-Marshall L Rev* 16:22, 1967.

Note, "Surgery Without Consent—Malpractice or Battery?" *Albany L Rev* 29:342, 1965.

Comment, "Physicians and Surgeons—Liability for Unauthorized Treatment," *North Dakota L Rev* 38:334, 1962.

McCoid G, "A Reappraisal of Liability for Unauthorized Medical Treatment," *Minn L Rev* 41:381, 1957.

Anderson v. *St. Francis-St. George Hospital,* 614 N.E. 2d 841 (Ohio 1992)

Lounsbury v. *Capel,* 836 P. 2d 188 (Utah 1992)

Foflygen v. *R. Zemel,* 615 A. 2d 1345 (Pa. 1992)

Fox v. *Smith,* 594 So. 2d 596 (Miss. 1992)

Young v. *Oakland General Hospital,* 437 N.W. 2d 321 (Mich. 1989)

Kozup v. *Georgetown University,* 851 F. 2d 437 (D.C. 1988)

People v. *Coe,* 501 N.Y.S. 2d 997 (N.Y. 1986)

Kahoutek v. *Hafner,* 366 N.W. 2d 633 (Minn. 1985)

Skripek v. *Bergamo,* 491 A. 2d 1336 (N.J. 1985)

Spikes v. *Heath,* 332 S.E. 2d 889 (Ga. 1985)

Hillbrook v. *Schatten,* 299 S.E. 2d 128 (Ga. 1983)

Lojuk v. *Quandt,* 706 F. 2d 1456 (Ill. 1983)

Nelson v. *Patrick,* 293 S.E. 2d 829 (N.C. 1982)

Kinikin v. *Heupel,* 305 N.W. 2d 589 (Minn. 1981)

Need for Competent Patient's Informed Consent to Treatment

Rozovsky FA, *Consent to Treatment: A Practical Guide*, ed 2, Little, Brown & Co., Boston, 1990.

Applebaum PS, Lidz CW, and Meisel A, *Informed Consent, Legal Theory and Clinical Practice*, Oxford University Press, New York, 1987.

Faden RR and Beauchamp T, *A History and Theory of Informed Consent*, Oxford University Press, New York, 1987.

Louisell D and Williams H, *Medical Malpractice*, Matthew Bender & Co., New York, 1983, § 22.

President's Commission for the Study of Ethical Problems in Medicine and Biomedical and Behavioral Research, *Making Health Care Decisions, The Ethical and Legal Implications of Informed Consent in the Physician-Patient Relationship*, Vol. 1, U.S. Government Printing Office, Washington, 1983.

"Informed Consent," Chapter 3 in *Hospital Liability and Risk Management*, Practicing Law Institute, New York, 1981.

Prosser W. *Handbook of the Law of Torts*, ed 4, West Publishing, St. Paul, 1971, pp. 165-166.

61 *Am Jur 2d*, PHYSICIANS, SURGEONS & OTHER HEALERS, §§ 152-161.

Annotations, 42 ALR 4th 543, "Medical Malpractice Liability Based on Misrepresentation of the Nature and Hazards of Treatment."; 38 ALR 4th 900, "Medical Malpractice: Liability for Failure of Physician to Inform Patient of Alternative Modes of Diagnosis or Treatment."; 89 ALR 3d 32, "Malpractice: Questions of Consent in Connection with Treatment of Genital or Urinary Organs."; 88 ALR 3d 1008, "Modern Status of Views as to General Measure of Physician's Duty to Inform Patient of Risks of Proposed Treatment."; 69 ALR 3d 1223, "Malpractice: Physician's Duty to Inform Patient of Nature and Hazards of Radiation or X-ray Treatments under the Doctrine of Informed Consent."; 69 ALR 3d 1250, "Malpractice: Physician's Duty to Inform Patient of Nature and Hazards of Treatment in Pregnancy and Childbirth Cases under the Doctrine of Informed Consent."

Note, "Power, Knowledge, Consent: Medical Decision-Making," *Mod L Rev* 24(3):1, 1988.

Mazur DJ, "What Should Patients Be Told Prior to a Medical Procedure?" *Am J Med* 81(6): 1051, 1986.

Weissbard L, "Informed Consent: The Law's Uneasy Compromise with Ethical Theory," *Nebr L Rev* 65:749, 1986.

Youngner S, "Patient Autonomy, Informed Consent, and the Reality of Critical Care," *Critical Care Clinics* 2(1):41, 1986.

Foflygen v. *R. Zemel,* 615 A. 2d 1345 (Pa. 1992)

Pedersen v. *Vahidy,* 552 A. 2d 419 (Conn. 1989)

Crawford v. *Wojnas,* 754 P. 2d 1302 (Wash. 1988)

Cole v. Wiggins, 487 So. 2d 203 (Miss. 1986)

Moser v. *Stallings,* 387 N.W. 2d 599 (Iowa 1986)

Lipsius v. *White,* 458 N.Y.S. 2d 928 (N.Y. 1983)

Canterbury v. *Spence,* 464 F. 2d 772 (D.C. Cir. 1972)

Cobbs v. *Grant,* 502 P. 2d 1 (Cal. 1972)

Wilkinson v. *Vesey,* 295 A. 2d 676 (R.I. 1972)

Patient's Right to Withdraw Consent

Rozovsky FA, *Consent to Treatment: A Practical Guide,* ed 2, Little, Brown & Co., Boston, 1990, § 1.11.

"Changing Her Mind," *Nursing '92* 22(10):106, 1992.

Rodriguez v. *Pino,* 634 So. 2d 681 (Fla. 1994)

Fox v. *Smith,* 594 So. 2d 596 (Miss. 1992)

Busalacchi v. *Vogel,* 429 So. 2d 217 (La. 1983)

Mims v. *Boland,* 138 S.E. 2d 902 (Ga. 1964)

Competent Patient's Right to Refuse Treatment, Including DNR Orders

Emanuel EJ, *The Ends of Human Life: Medical Ethics in a Liberal Policy,* Harvard University Press, Cambridge, 1991.

Meisel A, *The Right to Die,* John Wiley & Sons, New York, 1989.

Annotation, 93 ALR 3d 67, "Patient's Right to Refuse Treatment Allegedly Necessary to Sustain Life."

Curtin LL, "DNR in the OR: Ethical Concerns and Hospital Policies," *Nurs Management* 25(2):29, 1994.

Kass LR, "Is There a Right to Die?" *Hastings Center Rep,* Jan-Feb 1993.

Fiesta J, "Refusal of Treatment," *Nurs Management* 23(11):14, 1992.

"Documenting Discharge A.M.A.," *Nursing '92* 22(9):30, 1992.

Salladay S and McDonnell M, "Facing Ethical Conflicts," *Nursing '92* 22(2):44, 1992.

"Guidelines for the Appropriate Use of Do-Not-Resuscitate Orders," *JAMA* 265(14):1868, 1991.

Maltz A, "When a Patient Doesn't Want to Be Resuscitated," *RN* 54(2):65, 1991.

Wear AN and Brahams D, "To Treat or Not to Treat: The Legal, Ethical and Therapeutic Implications of Treatment Refusal," *J Med Ethics* 17:131, 1991.

Kramer RS, "Effect of New York State's Do-Not-Resuscitate Legislation on In-Hospital Cardiopulmonary Resuscitation Practice," *Am J Med* 88:108, 1990.

Weiss FS, "The Right to Refuse: Informed Consent and the Psychosocial Nurse," *J Psychosoc Nurs and Mental Health Serv,* 28(8):25, 1990.

Wainess L, "Physician's Duty to Inform Patients Who Refused Treatment: Truman v. Thomas in Perspective," *Med Trial Tech Q* 12:444, 1986.

Schwartz IM, "Patients' Rights to Refuse Treatment: Legal Aspects, Implications and Consequences," *Med Trial Tech Q* 32:430, 1986.

Frey LO, "The Right to Treat a Competent Adult Who Refuses Treatment to Prolong Life," *Med Trial Tech Q* 29:432, 1981.

Rodriguez v. *Pino,* 634 So. 2d 681 (Fla. 1994)

Thor v. *Superior Court,* 855 P. 2d 375 (Cal. 1993)

Anderson v. *St. Francis-St. George Hospital,* 614 N.E. 2d 841 (Ohio 1992)

Norwood Hospital v. *Munoz*, 564 N.E. 2d 1017 (Mass. 1991)
Cruzan v. *Director, Missouri Department of Public Health*, 497 U.S. 261 (1990)
Fosmire v. *Nicoleau*, 551 N.E. 2d 77 (N.Y. 1990)
Elbaum v. *Grace Plaza of Great Neck, Inc.*, 544 N.Y.S. 2d 840 (N.Y. 1989)
Public Health Trust v. *Wons*, 541 So. 2d 96 (Fla. 1989)
In re Milton, 505 N.E. 2d 255 (Ohio 1987), *cert. denied* 484 U.S. 820 (1987)
Estate of Leach v. *Shapiro*, 469 N.E. 2d 1047 (Ohio 1984)

Implied or Constructive Consent to Treatment

Kozup v. *Georgetown University*, 851 F. 2d 437 (D.C. 1988)
Estate of Leach v. *Shapiro*, 469 N.E. 2d 1047 (Ohio 1984)
Hernandez v. *United States*, 465 F. Supp. 1071 (Kan. 1979)
Banks v. *Wittenberg*, 266 N.W. 2d 788 (Mich. 1978)
Cobbs v. *Grant*, 502 P. 2d 1 (Cal. 1972)

Patient's Implied Consent in Emergency Situations

Keeton WP et al, *Prosser and Keeton on The Law of Torts*, ed 5, West Publishing, St. Paul, 1993, §§ 18, 32.
Lounsbury v. *Capel*, 836 P. 2d 188 (Utah 1992)
Kasenetz v. *Vieta*, 568 N.Y.S. 2d 383 (N.Y. 1991)
Bendiburg v. *Dempsey*, 707 F. Supp. 1318, *aff'd* 909 F. 2d 463 (Ga. 1989)
Douget v. *Touro Infirmary*, 537 So. 2d 251 (La. 1988)
Shinn v. *St. James Mercy Hospital*, 675 F. Supp. 94, *aff'd* 847 F. 2d 836 (N.Y. 1987)
Stafford v. *Louisiana State University*, 448 So. 2d 852 (La. 1984)
Plutshack v. *University of Minnesota Hospitals*, 316 N.W. 2d 1 (Minn. 1982)
Charter Medical Corp. v. *Curry*, 262 S.E. 2d 568 (Ga. 1979)

Doctrine of Therapeutic Privilege

Rozovsky FA, *Consent to Treatment: A Practical Guide*, ed 2, Little, Brown & Co., Boston, 1990, § 2.4.
Somerville D, "Therapeutic Privilege: Variation on the Theme of Informed Consent," *L Med & Health Care* 12:4, 1984.
Louisell D and Williams H, *Medical Malpractice*, Matthew Bender & Co., New York, 1988, § 22.04.
Lindquist v. *Ayerst Laboratories*, 607 P. 2d 1339 (Kan. 1980)
Wooley v. *Henderson*, 418 A. 2d 1123 (Me. 1980)
Carman v. *Dippold*, 379 N.E. 2d 1365 (Ill. 1978)
Sard v. *Hardy*, 379 A. 2d 1014 (Md. 1977)
Canterbury v. *Spence*, 464 F. 2d 772 (D.C. 1972), *cert. denied*, 409 U.S. 1064 (1972)
Cobbs v. *Grant*, 502 P. 2d 1 (Cal. 1972)
Nishi v. *Hartwell*, 473 P. 2d 116 (Hawaii 1970)
Roberts v. *Woods*, 206 F. Supp. 579 (Ala. 1962)

Minor Patient's Legal Capacity to Consent to Medical Treatment or Abortion

Rozovsky FA, "Minors' Consent to Treatment." In *Consent to Treatment, A Practical Guide*, ed 2, Little, Brown & Company, Boston, 1990, Ch. 5.
Keeton WP et al, *Prosser and Keeton on the Law of Torts*, ed 5, West Publishing, St. Paul, 1993, §§ 18 and 32.
Holder AR, *Legal Issues in Pediatrics and Adolescent Medicine*, ed 2, Yale University Press, New Haven, 1985.
Melton GB, Koocher GP, and Saks MJ, editors, *Children's Competence to Consent*, Plenum Press, New York, 1983.
Note, "Minors, Medical Treatment and Interspousal Disagreement," *De Paul L Rev* 41:841, 1992.

Cohn R, "Minor's Right to Consent to Medical Care, *Med Trial Tech Q* 31:286, 1985.

Ewald LS, "Medical Decision-Making for Children: An Analysis of Competing Interests," *St. Louis LJ* 25:689, 1982.

Munson CF, "Toward a Standard of Informed Consent by the Adolescent in Medical Treatment Decisions," *Dickinson L Rev* 8:431, 1981.

Wilkins J, "Children's Rights: Removing the Parental Consent Barrier to Medical Treatment of Minors," *Ariz St. L J* 1975:31, 1975.

Hodgson v. Minnesota, 110 S. Ct. 2926 (1990)

Ohio v. Akron Center for Reproductive Health, 110 S. Ct. 2972 (1990)

In the Matter of Anonymous, a Minor, 515 So. 2d 1254 (Ala. 1987)

Planned Parenthood of Central Missouri v. Danforth, 428 U.S. 52 (1976)

Ballard v. Anderson, 484 P. 2d 1345 (Cal. 1971)

Lacey v. Laird, 139 N.E. 2d 25 (Ohio 1956)

Tabor v. Scobee, 254 S.W. 2d 474 (Ky. 1952)

Consents Given by Emancipated and/or Mature Minors

Rozovsky FA, *Consent to Treatment, A Practical Guide,* ed 2, Little Brown & Company, Boston, 1990, §§ 5.2.2, 5.2.3.

Holder AR, *Legal Issues in Pediatrics and Adolescent Medicine,* ed 2, Yale University Press, New Haven, 1985.

The Legal Status of Adolescents, U.S. Department of Health and Human Services, Washington, D.C., 1981.

Annotation, 32 ALR 3d 1055, "What Voluntary Acts of Child, Other Than Marriage or Entry Into Military Service, Terminate Parent's Obligation to Support."

Wilkins J, "Children's Rights: Removing the Parental Consent Barrier to Medical Treatment of Minors," *Ariz St. L J* 1975:31, 1975.

Comment, "Medical Care and the Independent Minor," *Santa Clara Lawyer* 10:334, 1970.

Cardwell v. Bechtol, 724 S.W. 2d 739 (Tenn. 1987)

In the Matter of Anonymous, a Minor, 515 So. 2d 1254 (Ala. 1987)

Carter v. Cangello, 164 Cal. Rptr. 361 (Cal. 1980)

Planned Parenthood of Central Missouri v. Danforth, 428 U.S. 52 (1976)

Younts v. St. Francis Hospital & School of Nursing, 469 P. 2d 330 (Kan. 1970)

Minor's Right to Receive Birth Control Information

42 U.S.C. § 602(a)15

Holder AR, *Legal Issues in Pediatrics and Adolescent Medicine,* ed 2, Yale University Press, New Haven, 1985.

Thompson J, "The Rights of the Child," *Nurs Times* 86(10):67, 1990.

Benshoof J and Pilpel H, "Minors' Rights to Confidential Abortions: The Evolving Legal Scene." In Butler J and Walbert D, editors, *Abortion, Medicine and the Law,* Facts on File Publications, New York, 1986.

Hosek N, "Minors' Rights of Privacy: Access to Contraceptives Without Parental Notification," *J Juvenile L* 7:99, 1984.

Morano AL, "The Right of Minors to Confidential Access to Contraceptives," *Albany L Rev* 47:214, 1982.

Jane Does v. State of Utah Department of Health, 776 F. 2d 253 (Utah 1985)

Planned Parenthood Federation of America v. Schweiker, 559 F. Supp. 658, 712 F. 2d 650 (N.Y. 1983)

Doe v. Irwin, 615 F. 2d 1162 (Mich. 1980), *cert. denied,* 449 U.S. 829 (1980)

Carey v. Population Services, International, 431 U.S. 678 (1977)

Eisenstadt v. Baird, 405 U.S. 438 (1972)

Griswold v. Connecticut, 381 U.S. 479 (1965)

Consent Required for Treating Incompetent Persons

Rozovsky FA, *Consent to Treatment, A Practical Guide,* ed 2, Little, Brown & Company, Boston, 1990, § 1.6.

Jordan SM, *Decision Making for Incompetent Persons,* Charles Thomas, Springfield, Ill., 1985.

Emanuel E and Emanuel L, "Proxy Decision Making for Incompetent Patients," *JAMA* 267(15):2067, 1992.

Yuen M, "Letting Daddy Die: Adopting New Standards for Surrogate Decision-Making," *UCLA L Rev* 39:581, 1992.

Fentiman LC, "Privacy and Personhood Revisited: A New Framework for Substitute Decisionmaking for the Incompetent Incurably Ill Patient," *Geo Wash L Rev* 57:801, 1989.

Shaver E, "Do Not Resuscitate: The Failure to Protect the Incompetent Patient's Right of Self-Determination," *Cornell L Rev* 75:218, 1989.

Areen J, "The Legal Status of Consent Obtained From Families of Adult Patients to Withhold or Withdraw Treatment," *JAMA* 258:229, 1987.

Drane DF, "The Many Faces of Incompetency," *Hastings Center Rep* 15(2):17, 1985.

In the Matter of Harvey "U," 501 N.Y.S. 2d 920 (N.Y. 1986)

Aponte v. *United States,* 582 F. Supp. 65 (Puerto Rico 1984)

Davis v. *Hubbard,* 506 F. Supp. 915 (Ohio 1980)

Matter of Quackenbush, 383 A. 2d 785 (N.J. 1978)

Northern v. *State of Tennessee,* 575 S.W. 2d 946 (Tenn. 1978)

In re Schiller, 372 A. 2d 360 (N.J. 1977)

Dale v. *State of New York,* 355 N.Y.S. 2d 485 (N.Y. 1974)

Long Island Jewish-Hillside Medical Center v. *Levitt,* 342 N.Y.S. 2d 356 (N.Y. 1973)

Consent for Abortion or Sterilization

Cohn SD, *Malpractice and Liability in Clinical Obstetrical Nursing,* Aspen Publishers, Rockville, Md., 1990, Ch. 3.

Niswander K and Porto M, "Abortion Practices in the United States: A Medical Viewpoint." In Butler JD and Walbert D, editors, *Abortion, Medicine and the Law,* Facts on File Publications, New York, 1986.

David H, "Abortion Policies." In Hodgson J, editor, *Abortion and Sterilization: Ethical and Social Issues,* Grune & Stratton, New York, 1981.

Baron C, "Abortion and the Legal Process in the United States: An Overview of the Post-Webster Legal Landscape," *L Med and Health Care* 17:368, 1989.

George BJ, "State Legislation Versus the Supreme Court: Abortion Legislation in the 1980s," *Pepperdine L Rev* 12:427, 1984.

Annotations, 89 ALR 3d 32, "Malpractice: Questions of Consent in Connection with Treatment of Genital or Urinary Organs."; 62 ALR 3d 1097, "Woman's Right to Have Abortion Without Consent of, or Against Objections of, Child's Father."; 27 ALR 3d 906, "Medical Malpractice, and Measure and Element of Damages in Connection with Sterilization or Birth Control Procedures."

Planned Parenthood of Southeastern Pennsylvania v. *Casey,* 112 S. Ct. 2791 (1992)

Hodgson v. *Minnesota,* 110 S. Ct. 2926 (1990)

Ohio v. *Akron Center for Reproductive Health,* 110 S. Ct. 2972 (1990)

Webster v. *Reproductive Health Services, Inc.,* 492 U.S. 490 (1989)

In the Matter of Anonymous, a Minor, 515 So. 2d 1254 (Ala. 1987)

Thornburgh v. *American College of Obstetricians and Gynecologists,* 476 U.S. 747 (1986)

City of Akron v. *Akron Center for Reproductive Health,* 462 U.S. 416 (1983)

Flateau v. *Thom,* 393 So. 2d 392 (La. 1980)

Bellotti v. *Baird,* 428 U.S. 132 (1979)

Beck v. *Lovell,* 361 So. 2d 245 (La. 1978)

Rothenberger v. *Doe,* 374 A. 2d 57 (N.J. 1977)

The Nurse's Right of Conscience

42 U.S.C. § 300a-7

"Statement Regarding Risk Versus Responsibility in Providing Nursing Care," *Ethics in Nursing: Position Statements and Guidelines*, American Nurses Association, Kansas City, Mo., 1988.

Rosen L, "The Right to Refuse," *Today's OR Nurse* 6(12):29, 1984.

Comment, "Accommodation of Conscientious Objection to Abortion: A Case Study of the Nursing Profession," *Brigham Young L Rev* 1982:253, 1982.

Kenny v. Ambulatory Centre of Miami, 400 So. 2d 1262 (Fla. 1981)

Swanson v. St. John's Lutheran Hospital, 597 P. 2d 702 (Mont. 1979)

Who Has the Duty to Obtain the Patient's Consent?

Rozovsky FA, *Consent to Treatment: A Practical Guide*, ed 2, Little, Brown & Company, Boston, 1990.

Fiesta J, "Informed Consent Process—Whose Legal Duty?" *Nurs Management* 22(1):17, 1991.

Rozovsky FA, "A Risk Management Approach to Consent," *Hosp Risk Management*, July 1990.

Bernzweig E, "Don't Cut Corners on Informed Consent," *RN* 47(12):15, 1984.

Lysman M, "Informed Consent and the Nurse's Role," *RN* 42(9):50, 1972.

Barbee G, "Consents: The Nurse's Role in Obtaining and Using Them," *Hosp Forum* 9:23, 1966.

Foflygen v. Zemel, 615 A. 2d 1345 (Pa. 1992)

Patriello v. Kalman, 576 A. 2d 474 (Conn. 1990)

Hoffson v. Orentreich et al., 543 N.Y.S. 2d 242 (N.Y. 1989)

Mele v. Sherman Hospital, 838 F. 2d 925 (Ill. 1988)

Wilson v. Lockwood, 711 S.W. 2d 545 (Mo. 1986)

Porter v. Sisters of St. Mary, 756 F. 2d 669 (Mo. 1985)

Roberson v. Menorah Medical Center, 588 S.W. 2d 134 (Mo. 1979)

Liability for False Imprisonment

"Patient Sues Hospital for Unnecessary Restraint, Seclusion," *Mental Disease L Rep* 4:93, 1980.

Rogers v. Bruntrager, 841 F. 2d 853 (Mo. 1988)

Patrick v. Menorah Medical Center, 636 S.W. 2d 134 (Mo. 1982)

Pounders v. Trinity Court Nursing Home, 576 S.W. 2d 934 (Ark. 1979)

Big Town Nursing Home v. Newman, 461 S.W. 2d 195 (Texas 1970)

Meier v. Combs, 263 N.E. 2d 194 (Ind. 1970)

Bailie v. Miami Valley Hospital, 221 N.E. 2d 217 (Ohio 1966)

PART FIVE

REGULATION OF NURSING AND SCOPE OF NURSING PRACTICE

Part 5

INTRODUCTORY NOTE

Occasionally, significant conflicts occur when nurses are asked by their employers to perform tasks that extend beyond those permitted by the state nursing authority. Nurses who carry out such tasks run the risk of severe penalty, including license revocation, in addition to incurring liability for any injury caused the patient.

In this part we discuss the issue of nurse licensure and the range of tasks a nurse is permitted to perform without exceeding the scope of practice authorized by law. We will also address the question of how much responsibility the nurse can assume without incurring legal liability when attempting more specialized functions in the treatment curriculum.

REGULATION OF THE PRACTICE OF NURSING

In this part we will be discussing an issue of great importance—the legal scope of the nurse's authority to practice as a nurse. Before doing so, however, it would be appropriate to outline briefly the manner in which nurses are licensed and how their professional activities are regulated by statute.

Every state requires that anyone who wishes to practice nursing within its jurisdiction shall be appropriately licensed before being permitted to do so. The state's authority to license nurses (as well as other professionals) includes the authority to define nursing practice, establish qualifications for obtaining such license, collect license fees, establish standards of nursing practice, exercise disciplinary authority over licensees and suspend or revoke their licenses, and address other responsibilities relating to the practice of nursing deemed to be in the public interest. The statutory authority to carry out these responsibilities is given to the state nurse licensing board, an official body usually consisting of about 10 persons appointed by the governor of the state.

State nurse practice acts commonly have provisions exempting nursing students from application of the act. Accordingly, allegations of practicing nursing without a license cannot be brought against nursing students because the state statute allows them to practice nursing while learning to become nurses. Nevertheless, nursing students can be held liable for negligence in carrying out their patient care responsibilities, as discussed more fully in Part 1 of this course.

Under all the state nurse practice acts, an applicant for a nursing license must pass a written examination and meet statutory educational requirements. Many state licensing boards have been using the national, standardized licensing examination, which is administered twice a year. Nurses already licensed in one state are generally allowed to obtain their licenses in another state without the necessity of taking a second examination, in accordance with so-called reciprocity statutes between the states. While graduates of Canadian nursing schools are accorded the same rights as graduates of U.S. schools, nurses graduated from schools in other foreign countries generally must meet special educational and experience requirements before being allowed to apply for licensure in the United States.

One thing should be made clear: the state's nurse practice act plays a major role in defining the term *nursing* or the *practice of nursing*, which, in turn, defines (i.e., sometimes expands and sometimes limits) the scope of the nurse's legal authority within the state. The state nurse practice acts differ considerably in their definitions of acceptable nursing practice. These differences make it difficult to determine whether a particular procedure in patient care falls within nursing or medical practice. With the movement toward expanding the role of nurses, many states have revised their nurse practice acts to legitimize nursing functions previously restricted to licensed physicians. This trend has not gone unnoticed by the courts, as evidenced by the following observation in a California case: "The changes taking place in nursing reflect increasing emphasis on high standards for nurses; those with superior education and experience often exercise independent judgment as to the care of patients whether in a hospital setting or elsewhere" (*Fraijo* v. *Hartland Hospital*, 99 Cal. App. 3d 342 [Cal. 1979]).

State nurse practice acts invariably empower the nursing licensure board to issue regulations that deal with specific areas of nursing practice such as the administration of medications, resuscitation, or defibrillation. Thus, nurses should understand that the true extent of their authority in any given state is usually found in the regulations, rather than the broad, general language of the nurse practice act itself. In addition, most hospitals and skilled nursing facilities have policies and procedures for special tasks not covered by the particular state's nurse practice act or the regulations promulgated thereunder.

DISCIPLINARY ACTION AGAINST NURSES

A license to practice nursing is not a right but a privilege that can be suspended or revoked by the state if the licensee does not continue to meet the state's licensing standards. The typical grounds for suspending or revoking a nurse's license include: unprofessional, dishonorable, immoral, or illegal conduct (both on the job or off-duty); habitual intoxication or drug addiction; physical or mental incapacity; and incompetence, negligence, or malpractice. Obviously, some grounds for revocation are easier to prove than others, e.g., conviction of a criminal act, or clear-cut cases of drug addiction or mental instability. Revocation on grounds of incompetence or malpractice is much more difficult to prove, and many licensing boards are less likely to initiate revocations based on those grounds than they are to take action after a nurse has been held liable for malpractice in a court action.

Unprofessional conduct is defined in different ways in many states, but generally refers to unethical conduct, misconduct, or nursing contrary to standards of practice. Specific acts of unprofessional conduct have included unnecessary treatment, refusal to provide professional service because of a person's race, creed, color, or national origin, sexual misconduct involving a patient, abandonment of one or more patients, physically abusing a patient, using improper and profane language and treating a patient with flagrant discourtesy, failure to assess a patient's condition, failure to inform the attending physician of the life-threatening nature of a patient's cardiac instability, practicing without a current license, and assisting another to practice nursing without a license.

While allegations of unprofessional conduct appear frequently in the legal literature, the most common grounds for disciplinary action involve issues of drug and alcohol impairment. When disciplining a nurse who has abused drugs or alcohol while on the job, most state nursing boards recognize that they are dealing with chemically dependent, ill persons and encourage such nurses to seek appropriate medical and psychological help. However, concern for the personal interests of impaired nurses is subordinated to the overriding public concern for the safety and welfare of the patients they are treating.

Additional grounds for disciplinary action include fraud and deceit, outright criminal acts—often involving the use or sale of controlled narcotics—falsification of patients' records, and so forth. In all disciplinary proceedings notice is given to the nurse stating the charges, as well as the time and place of the hearing. Due process of law requires that an accused nurse be permitted to have legal counsel, produce witnesses, and to cross-examine witnesses, as well as the right to judicial review of any adverse decision or sanction imposed by the state board of nursing.

SCOPE OF NURSING PRACTICE

5-1   The fundamental issue underlying all scope-of-practice questions is whether a particular act or procedure carried out by a nurse is legally within or beyond the scope of his or her license to practice.* Since state laws vary with respect to what a nurse may or may not do, each case involving a scope-of-practice question must be viewed in light of the applicable local law.

As a general proposition, scope of nursing practice questions are resolved

☐   essentially the same way from state to state, based on common law principles

☐   differently from state to state, based on the governing local statutes

☐   differently from state to state, based on common law principles

---

5-2   In most instances, a nurse in State A   ☐ could   ☐ could not   be sure of his or her legal position on a scope-of-practice question arising in State B.

5-3   Scope-of-practice legal questions concern primarily the following area of nursing practice:

☐   the degree of care with which a nurse executes a nursing procedure

☐   the patient's right to be treated by a doctor instead of a nurse

☐   the nurse's legal authority to carry out a particular assigned procedure

---

*Nursing care rendered by a nurse who is *unlicensed* raises a different question entirely. Most state nurse practice acts make practicing without a license a crime, punishable by a fine and/or imprisonment. These laws generally exempt nursing care rendered by family members, neighbors, and domestic help. As already noted, care rendered by unlicensed nursing students is also exempt under state nurse practice acts. Here we are concerned only with the conduct of duly licensed nursing personnel.

5-1   *differently from state to state, based on the governing . . .*

5-2   *could not*

5-3   *the nurse's legal authority to carry out a particu-lar . . .*

5-4   Not only is there little uniformity among the states regarding the definition of nursing practice, but their statutes generally describe authorized nursing functions in broad, general areas with few specifics. Medical practice acts, on the other hand, are generally rather clear. By and large, they define the practice of medicine in terms of the physician's authority to diagnose, treat, and prescribe. Moreover, the physician not only may do these things himself or herself, but may direct the carrying out of a specific procedure by a nurse under his or her direct orders or supervision.

The problem with most state statutes defining the practice of nursing is that

☐   they are too vague with respect to what a nurse may or may not do

☐   they are too specific with respect to what a nurse may or may not do

☐   they are not as authoritative as medical practice acts

5-5

▪ Doctor D, licensed professional Nurse N, and licensed practical Nurse L are licensed to practice in State X. Without knowing the scope of nursing practice as outlined in the nurse practice act of State X, indicate whether the following statements are true or false.

True	*False*	
☐	☐	Doctor D can delegate to Nurse N or Nurse L the performance of a medical procedure under D's supervision without violating the state medical practice act.
☐	☐	Nurse N can legally delegate the performance of the same medical procedure to Nurse L without violating the state nurse practice act.
☐	☐	Nurse N and Nurse L are authorized to perform whatever medical procedures are reasonably called for in an emergency situation before a physician can be summoned.

5-4   *they are too vague with respect to what a nurse may or may not do*

5-5

	True	*False*
	☑	☐
	☐	☑
	☑	☐

> **NOTE:**   Under most state medical practice acts, physicians can delegate the carrying out of various medical procedures to nurses working under their direct supervision, and under these circumstances the nurses will not be legally responsible for practicing medicine in violation of state law. For example, in *Hoffson v. Orentreich et al.*, 543 N.Y.S. 2d 242 (N.Y. 1989), an office nurse employed by a dermatologist was not held to be practicing medicine when she incised cysts on a patient's face pursuant to previously given instructions for this procedure. On the other hand, without knowing what the state's nurse practice act says, it is impossible to determine whether a particular nursing function is delegable by a professional nurse to other nursing personnel. Some state laws expressly authorize RNs to delegate selected tasks in the implementation of the nursing regimen to LPNs, nurse's aides, and ancillary nursing personnel. Nonetheless, it is still the RN's responsibility to ensure the delegatee is adequately trained and sufficiently competent to undertake the task being delegated, since liability will result for any harm that comes to the patient if the RN is found negligent in selecting the nurse to carry out the delegated function.

5-6   Numerous areas of medical and nursing practice overlap, so the same act may be considered the practice of medicine when performed by a physician and the practice of nursing when performed by a nurse. It is these overlapping areas that create legal problems for nurses who have assumed expanded responsibilities in highly technical areas of patient care.

Select from the list below those areas of medical or nursing practice that are *most likely* to raise legal questions about the nurse's authority to perform them within the scope of his or her license.

- ☐   giving general anesthesia
- ☐   deciding that IV therapy should be initiated
- ☐   removing sutures
- ☐   giving vaccinations

5-6   ☑
      ☑
      ☐
      ☐

5-7 We are concerned here with legal problems arising from the delegation of specific medical tasks. What fundamental rule of liability applies to the conduct of nurses who are directed to carry out medical tasks assigned to them?

☐ The nurse will avoid liability for harm to the patient provided the order comes from a duly licensed physician.

☐ The nurse will be held liable for harm to the patient if the nurse undertakes the task without knowing how to execute it competently.

☐ The nurse will avoid liability for harm to the patient provided he or she is properly licensed as a professional nurse.

5-8 In and of itself, the carrying out of a procedure by a nurse that is described as a medical function in the state medical practice act is sufficient to hold the nurse liable for exceeding the scope of his or her license to practice nursing.

True	*False*
☐	☐

5-9 Unless specifically authorized by statute, nurses may not make medical diagnoses or initiate medical treatment on their own without running the risk of exceeding the scope of their license to practice. However, in medical emergencies in which a physician is not present and cannot be quickly summoned, nurses may initiate such procedures as they deem necessary, whether or not medical in nature, in order to save patients' lives.

The emergency treatment role noted above is *most closely* related to

☐ the standard of care rule

☐ the informed consent rule

☐ the Good Samaritan rule

5-7 *The nurse will be held liable for harm to the patient . . .*   **5-8** *False*   **5-9** *the Good Samaritan rule*

5-10

■ P, a semiconscious adult man with a foreign body in his throat, is admitted to the ER of Hospital H at 1:30 AM. No doctor is present and Nurse N directs an attendant to summon the on-call physician. Without waiting for the physician, however, Nurse N immediately attempts to manually extricate the foreign object, but without success. Noticing P's increasingly cyanotic condition, Nurse N performs a tracheotomy, which opens the air passage and keeps the patient alive until the physician finally arrives.

Under the described circumstances, Nurse N's conduct

☐   was perfectly proper and within the law

☐   extended well beyond the practice of nursing and would be grounds for revocation of N's license

☐   was sufficiently flagrant to warrant the bringing of a malpractice suit by Patient P

5-11   Using the preceding example assume that, notwithstanding Nurse N's actions, the patient died. In what respect, if any, would the legal consequences of Nurse N's conduct be different from that noted above?

☐   Nurse N probably would be charged with negligent homicide.

☐   Nurse N's license to practice nursing would be summarily revoked.

☐   The legal consequences would be the same.

5-12   An act or procedure normally viewed as a medical function may be viewed as within the scope of nursing practice

☐   if it is specifically authorized by the state's nurse practice act

☐   if the nurse is directed to carry out the act or procedure by a duly licensed physician

☐   if the act or procedure is carried out under emergency circumstances

---

5-10	*was perfectly proper and within the law*	5-11	*The legal consequences would be the same.*	5-12	☑
					☑
					☑

5-13 In the hospital, nursing home, and occupational health setting, numerous medical functions are delegated to nurses (usually nurse-specialists) by means of "standing orders." The object of these orders is to anticipate and deal with critical emergency situations and legitimize the nurse's execution of clearly prescribed medical functions before the physician arrives. The courts have long recognized the legal validity of this type of delegated authority.

■ Nurse N is a specialist in coronary care assigned to the coronary care unit of Hospital H. Standing orders for coronary patients in the CCU call for administering prescribed drugs and for administering precordial shock to terminate life-threatening arrhythmias. One evening, the alarm in the CCU indicates that Patient P's heart has gone into ventricular fibrillation. Without first contacting a physician, Nurse N attempts to stabilize P by injecting lidocaine intravenously, and when this doesn't succeed, Nurse N administers precordial shock. Despite these efforts, P dies.

True   *False*

☐   ☐   N's conduct constitutes the unauthorized practice of medicine.

☐   ☐   P's estate can hold Nurse N liable for having performed medical acts instead of first calling a physician.

☐   ☐   Both Hospital H and Nurse N acted completely within the law in the described circumstances.

☐   ☐   Excepting the emergency and the standing orders, N's actions clearly would be beyond the scope of nursing practice.

5-14 It may be stated as a general rule that when faced with a life-threatening situation a nurse

☐ should do everything possible to assist the patient short of performing acts that may be medical in nature

☐ should do whatever is reasonably necessary to save the patient's life

☐ should exert all efforts to locate a physician before giving indicated treatment to the patient

	5-13	*True*	*False*	5-14	☐
		☐	☑		☑
		☐	☑		☐
		☑	☐		
		☑	☐		

5-15 A nurse who initiates medical treatment without a physician's order or approved standing orders in a nonemergency situation, and who injures the patient in the process, runs
the risk of

    ☐ being sued for malpractice

    ☐ being disciplined by the state licensing authority

    ☐ being discharged by his or her employer

5-16 In which of the following instances does it appear that the nurse acted within the scope of
his or her legal authority?

    ☐ Patient A (while hospitalized) experiences symptoms that might be attributable to
either acute indigestion or a coronary occlusion. Nurse A makes a diagnosis of
acute indigestion and, based thereon, provides the customary nursing care for that
condition.

    ☐ Patient B is scheduled to be released from the hospital following the amputation of a
limb, but his depressed mental condition prompts Nurse B to probe for underlying
causes. Nurse B diagnoses his condition as a fear of being unable to obtain gainful
employment and, acting on her own, arranges for him to receive appropriate psychological counseling to cope with his depressive reaction.

    ☐ Patient C seeks aid from occupational health Nurse C for a painful puncture wound
received on the job. Nurse C diagnoses the injury as a superficial surface wound only,
treats it with antiseptic and a bandage, and sends the patient back to her job.

THE EXPANDED ROLE OF NURSES

If nursing is to flourish as a distinct professional endeavor, it is inevitable that nurses will continue to seek out and assume more important responsibilities for patient care, which is exactly what has been happening over the past three decades in the United States. The advent of the Medicare and Medicaid programs in the 1960s provided the initial impetus to the expanded role of nurses primarily because of the shortage of primary-care physicians existing at the inception of those programs. Access to health care became a political issue, and it was shown that, at minimal additional cost and educational preparation, nurses could provide primary health care services safely to selected populations. Also during this period, the first formal nurse practitioner (NP) programs were established. Additional impetus was given to this development by the fast-growing women's movement, which demanded not only more female autonomy in general, but specifically in the providing of prenatal, obstetrical, and postpartum care to women.

At the forefront of the advanced practice movement today are an array of specialist nurses—RNs whose formal education and clinical preparation extend beyond the basic requirements for licensure, resulting in either a specialized nursing certificate or a master's degree. Advanced nursing practice specialties include certified nurse-midwives (CNMs), certified registered nurse anesthetists (CRNAs), clinical nurse specialists (CNSs), and nurse practitioners (NPs). Within those categories are various subspecialties, including neonatal, pediatrics, psychiatric/mental health, family practice, school health, geriatrics, and so forth. Care provided by advanced practice nurses extends well beyond the parameters of traditional nursing practice, which has always been more dependent on physician supervision; a greater emphasis is placed on early nursing intervention and ongoing nurse management of patient health status.

CRNAs currently provide anesthesia for dental, surgical, and obstetrical procedures in about 35% of all hospitals in the country. CNMs provide the independent management of care of normal newborns and women, usually practicing within systems that call for medical consultation and collaborative management. Clinical nurse specialists are found primarily in institutional settings in which their ongoing experience with patients and families provides the content and directs their participation in various related activities such as clinical research, consultation, teaching, and so forth. Most NPs work in primary care settings such as physicians' offices, health maintenance organizations, and community or public health clinics, where they perform a wide range of professional nursing functions including obtaining medical histories, performing physical examinations, providing prenatal care and family planning services, and so on. NPs are also trained to provide certain functions traditionally performed by physicians including the diagnosis and management of common acute health problems such as minor injuries and infections, as well as common chronic diseases such as diabetes and hypertension.

Because advanced practice nurses have assumed higher levels of responsibility for patient care and safety, they are held to higher standards of care by the courts, and face correspondingly higher exposure to legal liability, as was discussed in Part 1 (frames 1-84 through 1-90). Most state nurse practice acts have been updated within the past 22 years to include some kind of legal authority for advanced nursing practice, but the statutory language varies considerably, from very broad mention of specialty practice to very specific definitions (and limitations) of scope of practice. Having the legal authority to prescribe drugs is deemed an essential component of advanced nursing practice; thus, it is significant that legislation giving prescriptive authority to advanced practice nurses currently exists in 43 states, with similar legislation pending in several other states.

The issue of independence continues to be a major problem both for NPs and physicians, and in those states where NPs have not been accorded statutory recognition, the medical profession has lobbied strongly to make sure their state legislatures do not allow expansion of nursing roles. For this reason, nurses who engage in advanced nursing practice in states that do not recognize the NP role run a substantial risk of being charged with practicing medicine without a license.

Sermchief v. *Gonzalez*

Independence was the issue for two nurse practitioners in Missouri, a state where the nurse practice act does not specifically authorize advanced nursing practice. In *Sermchief* v. *Gonzalez*, 660 S.W. 2d 683 (1983), two nurse specialists employed by a rural Missouri family planning clinic performed a variety of sophisticated diagnostic and treatment functions—including breast and pelvic exams, Pap smears and gonorrhea cultures, blood serology, inserting IUDs, fitting diaphragms, and prescribing and administering oral contraceptives—all done pursuant to written standing orders and protocols issued by five physicians working for the clinic. The orders, incidentally, were specifically directed to the two nurses in question and to no one else.

The state's medical licensing board (called the Board of Registration for the Healing Arts) threatened to initiate proceedings to punish the nurses for practicing medicine without a license. The board also took steps to revoke the licenses of the physicians for aiding and abetting the unauthorized practice of medicine. The nurses and the physicians countered with a suit seeking a declaratory judgment on the issue, and when the trial court ruled that the acts of the nurses did, in fact, constitute the unlawful practice of medicine, the case was appealed directly to the Missouri Supreme Court.

The court's task was to interpret the language of the Missouri Nurse Practice Act, which contained a definition of professional nursing practice that had been substantially broadened in 1975. Although the statute enumerated the wide variety of functions in which a professional nurse could engage, it did not specifically mention nurse specialists or nurse practitioners as such. One of the court's principal conclusions was that the legislature had revealed "a manifest desire to expand the scope of authorized nursing practices." An equally important conclusion was that the legislature's formulation of an open-ended definition of professional nursing eliminated the requirement that a physician directly supervise nursing functions. Specifically, the court ruled that the acts performed by the two nurses—pursuant to standing orders and treatment protocols—fell within the legislative standard as set forth in the Missouri statute. The court further recognized that the act of diagnosing is not solely within the province of physicians, and that nurses can make diagnostic judgments and institute treatment in accordance with such standing orders and protocols.

Sermchief has been hailed as a significant victory for professional nurses seeking greater recognition of their expanding roles as specialists. Nevertheless, it did not resolve all of the issues surrounding the authority to engage in specialized fields of nursing practice. Without a doubt, critical legal liability and scope-of-practice problems will continue to arise whenever a nurse assumes patient-care functions that (1) traditionally have been held to be within the province of physicians, (2) are not subject to standing orders, or (3) are not generally recognized as legitimate nursing functions by accredited professional organizations. On the other hand, the judicial trend in the United States is definitely toward recognizing the gradual expansion of nursing practice into specialty areas. Nurse specialists in states that have legitimized such practice by statute are not likely to suffer any unusual exposure to legal liability while so engaged.

5-17   The scope of a nurse's license to practice is defined principally by the state nurse practice act and accompanying regulations. Those nursing functions that are not specifically enumerated in the act or regulations are legally deemed to be excluded. The nurse who ignores these limitations does so at his or her peril, running the risk of disciplinary action, license revocation, criminal charges, and possible loss of malpractice insurance coverage. To the extent that the language of the nurse practice act (or its implementing regulations) is vague or nonspecific, a court may, in determining the scope of the nurse's authority, consider functions set forth in such sources as (1) nursing specialty organization guidelines, (2) institutional job descriptions and policies, and (3) educational curricula for various nurse-specialist certification programs.

■ Nurse N is a certified nurse specialist in medical-surgical nursing who is employed by Hospital H in State X. The state's nurse practice act recognizes this category of nurse specialist and specifically enumerates the permissible medical functions nurse specialists in medical-surgical nursing may perform. It makes no mention of such nurses acting as surgical first assistants. Hospital H has a long-standing policy permitting certified nurse specialists in medical-surgical nursing to act as first assistants at operations other than those classified as "major surgery." Nurse N acts as first assistant to Doctor D on a patient undergoing a cholecystectomy, and due to her negligence, the patient suffers a permanent disabling injury.

Since Nurse N was duly certified as a medical-surgical nursing specialist pursuant to the state nursing practice act, this fact situation   ☐ does   ☐ does not   present a scope-of-practice question.

5-18   Whether Nurse N could legally act as first assistant in this situation would depend primarily on

☐   Nurse N's professional qualifications and experience as a medical-surgical nursing specialist

☐   the language of the nurse practice act of State X

☐   the validity of Hospital H's policy permitting this practice

5-17 *does*	**5-18**	*the language of the nurse practice act of State X*

5-19   A malpractice suit brought by the patient in this case would undoubtedly focus *primary* attention on

     ☐   the alleged negligence of Nurse N and Doctor D

     ☐   the alleged violation of the state nurse practice act by Nurse N

     ☐   the alleged illegality of Hospital H's policy allowing persons like Nurse N to act as first assistants at surgery

---

5-20   In this case, what legal significance would attach to Hospital H's policy permitting the use of medical-surgical nursing specialists as first assistants?

     ☐   The policy established the standard of care for the type of surgery undertaken.

     ☐   The policy granted legitimacy to Nurse N's authority to act as first assistant at the surgery.

     ☐   The policy was of no legal significance, since it was in direct conflict with the state nurse practice act on the authority of medical-surgical nursing specialists to act as first assistants.

5-21   If Nurse N's negligence is found to be the sole or principal cause of the patient's injuries, which (if any) of the following would apply?

     ☐   Nurse N alone could be held liable in damages under the rule of personal liability.

     ☐   Doctor D alone could be held liable in damages for Nurse N's conduct under the borrowed servant doctrine.

     ☐   Nurse N, Doctor D, and Hospital H all could be held liable in damages under various legal liability doctrines.

     ☐   Hospital H alone could be held liable in damages, since it sanctioned N's use as a first assistant notwithstanding the language of the state nurse practice act.

5-19   *the alleged negligence of Nurse N and Doctor D*

5-20   ☐ ☐ ☑   *If you checked the 2d box, turn to Note A, p. 285.*

5-21   ☐ ☐ ☑ ☐

5-22 Because there is no statutory authority for N to act as a first assistant, what standard of care would apply to her conduct during the surgery?

☐ the standard of care of a surgeon acting as a first assistant

☐ the standard of care of a medical-surgical nursing specialist

☐ the standard of care of an RN experienced in OR procedures

5-23 If the court in this case were to find that Nurse N's activities did not fall within the scope of nursing practice under state law, what likely effect would this have on Nurse N personally and professionally?

☐ N's nursing license could be revoked for violating the state nurse practice act.

☐ N could face possible criminal charges for engaging in the unauthorized practice of medicine.

☐ N's malpractice insurance carrier more than likely would disclaim coverage for the injuries caused by N's negligence.

5-24 Proof of N's violation of the state nurse practice act would be sufficient to hold N liable to the patient in this case even if no injuries were suffered.

True	*False*
☐	☐

5-22 *the standard of care of a surgeon acting as a first assistant*

5-23 ☑ ☑ ☑

5-24 *False*

If you answered this wrong, turn to Note B, p. 285.

5-25   Indicate whether the following statements are true or false.

True	*False*	
☐	☐	Regulations promulgated pursuant to a state nurse practice act have the same legal effect as the act itself.
☐	☐	When a state nurse practice act is silent on the functions a nurse with specialist certification can perform, guidelines promulgated by professional organizations and accrediting bodies may be utilized to determine the scope of the nurse's authority to practice.
☐	☐	Scope-of-practice issues apply to LPNs and RNs.
☐	☐	Scope-of-practice questions are of greater importance to nurse practitioners than to nonspecialist RNs because of the greater risk of liability faced by nurses with specialty training in expanded nursing roles.
☐	☐	A scope-of-practice question in a malpractice suit is important from the standpoint of its relevance in determining the applicable standard of care.

5-25   *True*
           True
           True
           True
           True

The Disciplinary Proceeding Process

State nurse practice acts define, as well as limit, the practice of nursing and thereby determine not only what constitutes authorized nursing practice but what constitutes unauthorized practice or practice that exceeds the scope of the nurse's authority to practice. Grounds for disciplinary action are set forth in the nurse practice acts, and while the grounds differ somewhat from state to state, the general categories usually include fraud and deceit, criminal acts, professional incompetence, substance abuse, mental incompetence and unprofessional conduct. Set forth below are the steps typically applicable in the disciplinary proceeding process when a complaint is filed against a nurse for misconduct.

- **Sworn Complaint Filed.** The process begins with the filing of a sworn complaint with the state board of nursing by (1) an individual, (2) a health care agency, or (3) a professional organization.

- **Review of Complaint.** The state board of nursing conducts a hearing in which it reviews the allegations, obtains evidence, calls witnesses, and determines whether the nurse is guilty of misconduct.

- **Disciplinary Action.** If the board finds the nurse guilty of misconduct, it can take the following disciplinary action:

  - issue a reprimand
  - place the nurse on probation
  - Refuse to renew the nurse's license
  - suspend the nurse's license
  - revoke the nurse's license

- **Court Review.** If the nurse wants to challenge the board's decision or disciplinary action, he or she can file an appeal in court. Depending on the state, the court either (1) will examine the board's decision and decide whether the board's hearing was conducted properly, or (2) order a trial *de novo* at the appellate level. Finally, if either the nurse or the board wants to challenge the appeals court's ruling, they can appeal the ruling to a higher court.

NOTE: A final comment is necessary before concluding Part 5 on scope-of-practice issues. Without question, the knowledge and technical skill of physicians and nurses at the turn of the century were vastly different from the competencies expected of today's practitioners. Common nursing practices today include not only those functions that have long been held to be within the province of standard nursing practice (e.g., monitoring, observing, and assessing patient condition) but now also include such additional activities as conducting health education classes, nutrition counseling, initiating range-of-motion exercises, administering immunizations, ordering routine laboratory tests, and so forth.

Nursing is in a constant state of evolution, and we can anticipate that nursing's scope of practice will continue to evolve in response to social forces and trends, scientific advances, new interpretations by the courts, and curriculum changes in schools of nursing. Astute undergraduate and graduate nurses will strive to keep abreast of these evolutionary forces and prepare themselves for new modes of practice in the future, when nursing role expectations (and concomitant legal liabilities) undoubtedly will be far greater than they are today.

EXPLANATORY NOTES

Note A (from Frame 5-20)

There is no doubt that the hospital policy statement *appears* to legitimize Nurse N's authority to act as first assistant at surgery, which is obviously what it was intended to do. Nevertheless, when a state's nurse practice act (or its implementing regulations) *specifically* enumerates the permissible medical functions of a nursing specialist—as was the case in the given example—functions that are *not* listed are legally deemed to be outside the scope of practice. Thus, regardless of the hospital's attempt to legalize the use of medical-surgical nursing specialists as first assistants through its own policy statement, the language of the state's nurse practice act always takes precedence. Certainly, both the existence and thrust of the hospital policy statement would be a factor taken into consideration if disciplinary action were to be brought against Nurse N for violating the state nurse practice act.

Proceed to Frame 5-21.

Note B (from Frame 5-24)

You will recall from Part 1 that proof of harm or injury is one of the fundamental elements that must be proved in every case before a nurse can be held liable for malpractice. In the example in Frame 5-24, the patient suffered no injury, so whether Nurse N violated the state nurse practice act would be of no consequence on the issue of her liability for malpractice. However, even assuming that injury *was* sustained in this example, liability would result only if the patient could show a clear cause-and-effect relationship between the statutory violation and the harm or injury suffered. Returning to the original fact situation in frame 5-19, one could not say with certainty that the statutory violation was *in and of itself* the cause of harm to the patient. There is no clear connection or direct link between the injury suffered and the fact that Nurse N exceeded the scope of her nursing license. Thus, her violation of the statute would not be enough to hold her liable without proof of actual negligence.

Proceed to Frame 5-25.

POINTS TO REMEMBER

1. A scope-of-practice question is one that examines whether a particular act or procedure performed by a nurse is legally within the scope of his or her license to practice; it applies to LPNs and RNs.

2. State laws vary considerably in their delineation of what a nurse may or may not do.

3. Most state nurse practice acts describe authorized areas of nursing practice in broad, general terms; state medical practice acts, on the other hand, are generally more detailed and complete.

4. Medical practice acts commonly authorize physicians to delegate medical functions to RNs and LPNs, under the physician's supervision.

5. Unless authorized by statute, and with the exception of emergencies, nurses may not make medical diagnoses or initiate medical treatment.

6. Medical functions are often delegated to nurses in "standing orders," and this mode of delegation has long been sanctioned by the courts.

7. The nurse who exceeds the scope of his or her license may be disciplined by the state nurse licensure board and may also face criminal charges for practicing medicine without a license.

8. Most of the states have enacted laws authorizing nurses with specialty training and certification to engage in functions that would otherwise be deemed the practice of medicine.

9. A nurse's violation of the state nurse practice act will not, in itself, make the nurse liable in damages to a patient. The patient must always prove negligence as well as a causal connection between the negligence and the injuries suffered.

SELECTED REFERENCES—PART FIVE

The Expanded Role of Nurses

Stafford MJ and Appleyard J, "Clinical Nurse Specialists and Nurse Practitioners." In McKloskey JC and Grace HK, editors, *Current Issues in Nursing*, ed 4, Mosby–Year Book, Inc., St. Louis, 1994, Ch. 3.

Diers D, "Nurse-Midwives and Nurse Anesthetists: The Cutting Edge in Specialist Practice." In Aiken LH and Fagin CM, editors, *Charting Nursing's Future—Agenda for the 1990s,* J.B. Lippincott, Philadelphia, 1992.

Hamrick AB and Spross JA, *The Clinical Nurse Specialist in Theory and Practice*, W.B. Saunders, Philadelphia, 1989.

McGivern DO, *Nurses, Nurse-Practitioners, The Evolution of Primary Care*, Scott, Foresman & Co., Glenview, Ill., 1986, pp. 1-14.

Inglis AD and Kjervik DK, "Empowerment of Advanced Practice Nurses: Regulation Reform Needed to Increase Access to Care," *Law Med & Ethics* 21(2):193, 1993.

Pearson L, "1992-1993 Update: How Each State Stands on Legislative Issues Affecting Advanced Nursing Practice," *Nurs Pract* 18(1):23, 1993.

Safriet BJ, "Health Care Dollars and Regulatory Sense: The Role of Advanced Practice Nursing," *Yale J on Regulation* 9:417, 1992.

Hadley EH, "Nurses and Prescriptive Authority: A Legal and Economic Analysis," *Am J Law & Med* 15:245, 1989.

Hall JK, "How to Analyze Nurse Practitioner Licensure Laws," *Nurse Pract* 18(8):31, 1993.

Pearson LJ, "1991-1992 Update: How Each State Stands on Legislative Issues Affecting Advanced Nursing Practice," *Nurse Pract* 17(1):14, 1992.

National Council of State Boards of Nursing, Inc., "Advanced Nursing Practice Survey Results," *Issues* 12(2), 1991.

Elder RG and Bullough B, "Nurse Practitioners and Clinical Nurse Specialists: Are the Roles Merging?" *Clin Nurse Specialist* 4(2):78, 1990.

Forbes KE, Rafson J, Spross JA, and Kozlowski I, "The Clinical Nurse Specialist and Nurse Practitioner: Core Curriculum Survey Results," *Clin Nurse Specialist*, 4(2):63, 1990.

Tingle J, "Nurses and the Law: Responsible and Liable? . . . Extended Role," *Nurs Times* 86(25):42, 1990.

Wright JE, "Joining Forces for the Good of Our Clients," *Clin Nurse Specialist* 4(2):76, 1990.

Mechanic HF, "Redefining the Expanded Role," *Nurs Outlook* 36(6):280, 1988.

Sermchief v. *Gonzalez*, 660 S.W. 2d 683 (Mo. 1983)

Fraijo v. *Hartland Hospital*, 160 Cal. Rptr. 331 (Cal. 1979)

Disciplinary Action Against Nurses

Northrup CE, "Licensure Revocation." In Northrup CE and Kelly ME, editors, *Legal Issues in Nursing* C.V. Mosby, St. Louis, 1987, Ch. 25.

Fiesta J, "Why Nurses Lose Their Licenses—Part I," *Nurs Management* 24(10):12, 1993.

Fiesta J, "Why Nurses Lose Their Licenses—Part II," *Nurs Management* 24(11):14, 1993.

Fiesta J, "Why Nurses Lose Their Licenses—Part III," *Nurs Management* 24(12):16, 1993.

Fiesta J, "Safeguarding Your Nursing License," *Nurs Management* 21(8):20, 1990.

Annotation, 55 ALR 3d 1141, "Revocation of Nurse's License to Practice Profession."

Burns v. *Board of Nursing*, 495 N.W. 2d 698 (Iowa 1993)

Yeary v. *Board of Nurse Examiners*, 855 S.W. 2d 236 (Texas 1993)

Henley v. *Alabama Board of Nursing*, 607 So. 2d 256 (Ala. 1992)

Husher v. *Commissioner of Education*, 591 N.Y.S. 2d 99 (N.Y. 1992)

Heinecke v. *Department of Commerce, Division of Occupational and Professional Licensing*, 810 P. 2d 459 (Utah 1991)

Wallace v. *Veterans Administration*, 683 F. Supp. 758 (Kan. 1988)

Stevens v. *Blake*, 435 So. 2d 108 (Ala. 1983)

Derrick v. *Commonwealth of Pennsylvania*, 432 A. 2d 282 (Pa. 1981)

Tighe v. *State Board of Nurse Examiners*, 397 A. 2d 1261 (Pa. 1979)

Ullo v. *State Board of Nurse Examiners*, 398 A. 2d 764 (Pa. 1979)

Scope of Practice and Related Issues

Smith JA and Kelly ME, "Nurses Employed as Practitioners, Anesthetists, Midwives, Clinical Specialists." In Northrup CE and Kelly ME, editors, *Legal Issues in Nursing*, C.V. Mosby Co., St. Louis, 1987, pp. 363-378.

Hall R, "The Legal Scope of Nurse Practitioners under Nurse Practice and Medical Practice Acts." In *The New Health Professionals*, Aspen Systems, Rockville, Md., 1977.

Pearson L, "1992-1993 Update: How Each State Stands on Legislative Issues Affecting Advanced Nursing Practice," *Nurs Pract* 18(1):23, 1993.

Safriet BJ, "Health Care Dollars and Regulatory Sense: The Role of Advanced Practice Nursing," *Yale J on Regulation* 9:417, 1992.

Tingle J, "Nurses and the Law: Responsible and Liable? . . . Extended Role," *Nurs Times* 86(25):42, 1990.

Mechanic HF, "Redefining the Expanded Role," *Nurs Outlook* 36(6):280, 1988.

Barton CL, "The Scope of Nursing Practice," *Nebr Med J* 72(12):398, 1987.

George JE and Quattrone MS, "Safeguard Your License," *J Emerg Nurs* 13(6):369, 1987.

Wolff M, "Court Upholds Expanded Practice Roles for Nurses," *Law Med Health Care*, 12:26, 1984.

"Tennessee Board of Nursing Revokes Non-Certified Midwife's RN License," *Am J Nurs* 79:574, 1979.

Eccard WT, "A Revolution in White—New Approaches in Treating Nurses as Professionals," *Vanderbilt L Rev* 30:839, 1977.

Fein v. *Permanente Medical Group*, 695 P. 2d 665 (Cal. 1985)

Arkansas State Nurses Association v. *Arkansas State Medical Board*, 677 S.W. 2d 293 (Ark. 1984)

Carlsen v. *Javurek*, 526 F. 2d 202 (S. Dak. 1975)

Barber v. *Reinking*, 411 P. 2d 861 (Wash. 1966)

Magit v. *Board of Medical Examiners*, 366 P. 2d 816 (Cal. 1961)

Chalmers-Francis v. *Nelson*, 57 P. 2d 1312 (Cal. 1936)

Frank v. *South*, 194 S.W. 375 (Ky. 1917)

PROVING THE NURSE'S LIABILITY

Part 6

INTRODUCTORY NOTE

The procedural aspects of law, while of secondary concern to the nurse, cannot be ignored entirely. The injured patient who wishes to sue a nurse for malpractice faces a number of procedural obstacles, and although there may be a substantial *medical* basis for bringing the suit, the patient will not be successful unless he or she can overcome these *legal* procedural obstacles.

In Part 6 the basic elements of a lawsuit, the role of the Court and the jury, the question of burden of proof, and several of the more important legal doctrines that apply in the trial of malpractice cases in the United States will be discussed. Although the fundamental legal principles of malpractice law are the same both in Canada and the United States, there are many differences between the two countries in the way malpractice cases are prosecuted in the courts. For example, juries are customary in malpractice cases in U.S. courts but decidedly not customary in Canadian courts.

Because of these procedural differences, Part 6 is based solely on the law as it applies in U.S. courts. Many (if not most) of the principles discussed will be equally applicable in Canada and therefore of interest to the Canadian nurse.

WHO CAN SUE AND BE SUED

6-1   The complaining party in a malpractice suit is called the "plaintiff," and may or may not be the injured patient himself or herself since, under certain circumstances, the law permits such a suit to be brought by the injured person's spouse, parent, or appointed legal representative. As a *general rule*, however, the plaintiff in a malpractice suit is usually the injured patient.

Which of the following persons, under appropriate circumstances, might legally bring a malpractice suit against a nurse?

☐   the injured patient

☐   the patient's spouse

☐   the patient's legal guardian

☐   all of the above

6-2   The formal term used in referring to the complaining party in a malpractice suit is
☐   accuser   ☐   suitor   ☐   plaintiff

6-3   Under what circumstances might a malpractice suit be brought by someone other than the patient?

☐   if the patient is hospitalized

☐   if the patient is deceased

☐   if the patient is unable to afford a lawyer

6-1   *all of the above*   **6-2**   *plaintiff*   **6-3**   ☐   *If you checked the 1st or 3d*
                                                                              ☑   *box, see p. 303, Note A.*
                                                                              ☐

6-4   Does the law *require* that a malpractice suit be brought only by the injured patient?

                              Yes   *No*
                               ☐   ☐

6-5   The responding or answering party in a lawsuit is called the "defendant." Where the suit involves nursing malpractice, the defendant is usually the nurse alone although the plaintiff *may,* in some cases, have the right to sue the nurse's employer and the nurse.

■ Nurse N is employed by a private physician. In the course of her work she negligently injures a patient while taking a blood sample.

Who *could be* the defendant in a lawsuit brought by the patient?

☐   only Nurse N

☐   both Nurse N and her employer

☐   only Nurse N's employer

6-6   A single lawsuit may involve multiple plaintiffs and defendants, and more than one legal issue. For example, the plaintiff may sue a hospital and one of its nurses, alleging different types of negligence against each of the defendants.

Which of the following (if any) are true?

☐   There can be more than one defendant in a lawsuit involving a nurse's malpractice.

☐   A lawsuit against a hospital and a nurse may involve malpractice and ordinary negligence.

☐   There may be several plaintiffs in a lawsuit against a single defendant.

☐   None of the above.

6-4   *No*   6-5   *both Nurse N and her*   6-6   ☑
                            employer   ☑
                                                                   ☑
                                                                   ☐

> **NOTE:**   We now begin our discussion of the elements that a plaintiff must prove to win a malpractice suit against a nurse. Before doing so, it might be helpful to review the discussion in Frames 1-99 through 1-105 concerning the various "surrounding circumstances" that courts and juries consider in determining whether a nurse's conduct has been negligent.

ELEMENTS OF A MALPRACTICE SUIT

6-7   In every nursing malpractice suit, the following basic elements must be proved for the plaintiff to prevail in the litigation: (1) the defendant nurse owed a special duty of care to the plaintiff (the patient), the breach of which would foreseeably cause harm to the plaintiff, (2) the defendant nurse was required to meet a particular standard of care in carrying out the nursing act or function in question, and failed to do so, (3) such failure or breach of duty was the direct and proximate cause of the plaintiff's injury or harm, and (4) the plaintiff suffered compensable money damages as a result thereof.

The preceding list of basic elements does not refer to any particular class of nurses. What is the significance of this observation?

- ☐   Different principles of law apply to RNs, LPNs, and nursing students.

- ☐   The same principles of law apply whether the defendant is an RN, LPN, or nursing student.

- ☐   Some classes of nurses are immune from suit entirely.

6-8   One of the basic elements of every malpractice suit is that the defendant nurse owed the patient a special duty of care.

What would be the best way for a plaintiff to prove this duty?

- ☐   by proving the nurse's status as an RN or LPN

- ☐   by proving the existence of a nurse-patient relationship

- ☐   by proving the nurse's employment status at the time of the incident

---

6-7   *The same principles of law apply whether the defendant is an RN, LPN, or nursing student.*

6-8   *by proving the existence of a nurse-patient relationship*

6-9   Foreseeability of injury or harm to the patient is an integral aspect of the nurse's special duty of care to the patient. Thus, in the exercise of ordinary judgment and foresight, it should be apparent to the reasonably prudent nurse what would happen if that duty is not performed. Stated differently, if a particular type of harm or injury is foreseeable and preventable, the nurse owes the patient the special duty of making sure it does not happen.

Indicate whether the following statements are true or false.

True	*False*	
☐	☐	There can be no special duty of care to prevent harm or injury to a patient if that harm or injury is not reasonably foreseeable.
☐	☐	To say that the nurse owes a special duty of care to a patient implies that the duty may be different from the duty of care owed other patients.
☐	☐	The special duty of care owed a patient may require the nurse to refrain from carrying out even a direct medical order in certain treatment circumstances.
☐	☐	A duty of care that is not tied to the concept of foreseeability of harm cannot be the basis of a claim for malpractice.

NOTE: There are limitations to the doctrine of foreseeability. Neither a nurse nor a physician is a guarantor of a patient's safety; the law does not require it. The rules of common sense apply in this area. All the physician and nurse must do is to act reasonably and prudently to secure and maintain the patient's safety. What *is* and *is not* reasonable, in terms of the patient's safety, is always one of the key issues in a malpractice suit.

6-9	*True*
	True
	True
	True

6-10 Another basic element of every nursing malpractice suit is a claim that the nurse failed to meet the required standard of care in carrying out a specific nursing act or function. This issue is generally the most disputed in the entire case, since it relates to the fundamental question of negligence.

In a nursing malpractice suit, which of the following issues would be considered the most significant?

☐ the degree to which the defendant conformed or deviated from the applicable standard of care

☐ the nature and severity of the plaintiff's injuries

☐ the amount of damages claimed by the plaintiff

6-11 What do we mean when we say that a nurse failed to meet the required standard of care in a given situation?

☐ The nurse went beyond the scope of his or her license to practice.

☐ The nurse did not do what other reasonably prudent nurses would have done under the same or similar circumstances.

☐ The nurse did not strictly follow the doctor's orders or the hospital's policies and procedures.

6-10 ☑   6-11 ☐
      ☐   ☑
      ☐   ☐

PROVING THE NURSE'S BREACH OF THE STANDARD OF CARE

As we have just seen, the law says the nurse must do what other reasonably prudent nurses would have done under the same or similar circumstances. What *is* "reasonably prudent" nursing conduct, and how does the plaintiff prove the applicable standard of nursing care in an actual court case?

Breach of the standard of care may be—and usually is—proved in court in several ways. Primarily, it is accomplished by taking the testimony of expert witnesses. For example, if the case involves hospital treatment, a supervisory nurse may be called to testify as to the normal nursing procedure(s) in dealing with a given medical problem. Frequently, a physician will testify as to the required degree of nursing care.

Documentary evidence is also critical in proving a departure from the applicable standard of care; the patient's medical record is the principal form of documentation. Unfortunately, documentation is often scanty, and the defendant nurse, when called on to testify, cannot remember what was done or said on a specific occasion years earlier. Documentary evidence is not limited to the medical record alone, however. A particular standard of nursing practice may be ascertained by looking at, and introducing into evidence, the state's nurse practice act and regulations, other relevant state and federal statutes, the American Nurses Association's Standards of Practice, the Joint Commission on Accreditation of Healthcare Organizations' nursing care standards, institutional policies and procedures, nursing journal articles, and other written standards.

Remember, however, that all the described standards of practice are merely guidelines or evidence of what should be the applicable standard of care in a specific situation. Statutory standards, institutional standards, and accrediting body standards are minimal in nature; sometimes even if the nurse can show that one or more technical standards of nursing practice were met, a jury may find that the nurse did not act as a reasonably prudent nurse would have acted in the same or similar circumstances. Therefore, the testimony of experts with respect to the applicable standard of care is important in nursing malpractice cases.

6-12 The third important element in every malpractice suit is the necessity to prove that the nurse's breach of duty and departure from the required standard of care was the direct and proximate cause of the plaintiff's injury or harm. There must be a direct and clear chain of events leading from the wrongful act to the resultant harm; no intervening or chance causes must be capable of having produced the harm or injury. If a proximate causal connection cannot be shown, the plaintiff will lose the case.

■ Nurse N, in direct violation of Doctor D's orders that Patient P should not have any oral intake, gives P solid food before abdominal surgery. Because of postoperative complications, a second operation is undertaken 8 days later. P's condition continues to worsen and he suffers a permanently disabling injury. Not long afterward, P brings suit against Doctor D and Nurse N.

If P is to prevail in his suit against Nurse N, what must he prove?

☐ Nurse N's conduct was a direct violation of Doctor D's orders

☐ Nurse N's conduct was the direct cause of P's injury

☐ Nurse N's conduct went beyond the scope of her license as a nurse

---

6-13 It would be reasonable to say that the doctrine of proximate cause is most closely related to

☐ the contributory negligence doctrine

☐ the doctrine of *respondeat superior*

☐ the doctrine of foreseeability

6-14 If there is an intervening cause—one that the nurse could neither control nor anticipate—the nurse's conduct, even if negligent, cannot be said to be the *proximate* cause of the patient's injury. A surgeon's negligence would be a typical intervening cause; however, the patient's own negligent conduct will not absolve the nurse from liability where the nurse's negligent act or omissions put the patient in a position of danger in the first instance.

- Nurse N fails to strap dizzy, hypotensive, and semisedated Patient P to an x-ray table and when Nurse N leaves the room to find the x-ray technician Patient P falls off the table and breaks a limb.

Nurse N's conduct in this case probably would not be deemed to be the proximate cause of Patient P's injuries.

True	*False*
☐	☐

6-15

- Nurse N, assisting Doctor D in abdominal surgery, loses track of a sponge and gives Doctor D an erroneous sponge count. A week later, the patient dies of lobar pneumonia.

In a lawsuit brought against Doctor D and Nurse N alleging the wrongful death of the patient, what would be the most likely outcome?

☐ Both Doctor D and Nurse N more than likely would be held liable for their negligence in not getting an accurate sponge count.

☐ Neither Doctor D nor Nurse N would likely be held liable, because the patient's death could not be directly linked to the leaving of the sponge in her abdomen during the surgery.

☐ Nurse N more than likely would be held liable, because her failure to keep track of the sponges was the most probable cause of death.

NOTE: Proving causation is often difficult, and the courts have applied two somewhat different tests to establish injury causation. The more rigid test, adopted by the courts in some states, is called the "but-for" test. Under that test, the plaintiff must prove that the injury would not have occurred *but for* the defendant's conduct. Obviously, this test can be applied only when a single health professional was involved in the patient's care at the time of injury.

Rarely is a single individual in a hospital or skilled nursing facility the only person responsible for a particular harm or injury to a patient. Consequently, the courts in most states have resorted to what is known as the "substantial factor" test. Under that test, to hold a particular health professional liable, all that the plaintiff's attorney has to prove is that the conduct of the person in question was a *substantial factor* contributing to the patient's harm or injury. It need not be the exclusive causative agent.

Because of the complexities inherent in deciding proximate cause issues, expert testimony is almost always required. We will deal with the use of expert testimony shortly.

6-16 The fourth essential element of every nursing malpractice suit is proof of actual loss or damage that is proximately caused by the nurse's negligent conduct. Of course, there can be no recovery if there is no damage. Money damages are awarded to compensate for actual physical harm to the patient, and such harm must be shown before liability for compensation arises. Pain and suffering alone are not sufficient to prove damage. Other allowable items of compensatory damages include medical and hospital bills, loss of earnings and wage earning capacity, and loss of support, companionship, and comfort.

True	*False*	
☐	☐	A lawsuit seeking damages for medical injury must include a claim for pain and suffering.
☐	☐	The plaintiff's loss of possible future earnings, as opposed to loss of past earnings, is not a legitimate item of damages in a nursing malpractice suit.
☐	☐	Property damage alone is not a legitimate item of damages in a nursing malpractice suit.
☐	☐	The principal purpose of allowing damages in a nursing malpractice suit is to punish the defendant for his or her negligent conduct.

6-17

- A patient sues Nurse N, claiming that the nurse bullied her constantly while she was in the hospital and generally made her hospital stay an unpleasant and emotionally upsetting experience.

What *significant* element of a malpractice suit is missing in this case?

☐ no special duty of care shown

☐ no standard of care shown

☐ no compensable harm shown

6-16 *False* *If you marked the last response*   **6-17** ☐ *If you did not check the 3d*
      False *true, turn to p. 303, Note B.*   ☐ *response, turn to p. 304, Note*
      True   ☑ *C.*
      False

6-18   The following are the essential elements of every nursing malpractice suit:

A.   A special duty of care owed to the plaintiff by the defendant nurse

B.   The specific standard of care applicable to the nursing function in question

C.   The nurse's departure from the applicable standard of care (i.e., his or her negligence)

D.   Compensable harm or injury proximately resulting from the nurse's negligent conduct

The plaintiff's attorney's summation to the jury includes the statements quoted below. Referring to the items listed above, indicate which legal element shown there corresponds with each statement that follows.

☐   "As several witnesses have testified, it is standard nursing practice in this state to report all unusual symptoms and reactions of the patient to the treating physician."

☐   "Because of her depressed state of mind, the plaintiff unfortunately attempted to take her life and, in the process, suffered permanently disabling injuries."

☐   "The defendant was a registered nurse who was specifically assigned to care for the plaintiff while she was at the hospital."

☐   "The medical record clearly shows that the defendant made no mention to the treating physician of the plaintiff's strange behavior."

NOTE: Later in this part, we will discuss in some detail the subject of defenses to the allegations made by plaintiffs in malpractice suits. We shall first, however, address other matters pertaining to the litigation process.

6-18 B
        D
        A
        C

EXPLANATORY NOTES

Note A (from Frame 6-3)

As a rule, a malpractice suit would be brought by someone other than the injured patient only if the patient was no longer alive or had been declared legally incompetent. In that case, a court-appointed legal representative would be the complaining party. A patient can legally file a lawsuit when he or she is hospitalized even though the actual trial of the case might have to be delayed until the patient is out of the hospital.

A patient's inability to afford a lawyer would not be a legal basis for permitting someone else to bring the lawsuit in his or her behalf, assuming the financial issue is a valid argument in the first place. Actually, it is not, since most personal-injury lawyers do not require payment of legal fees in advance and will generally handle a malpractice case on a contingent-fee arrangement under which the plaintiff agrees to pay the lawyer an agreed percentage of the amount actually recovered, provided there is a recovery. Otherwise, the patient pays no legal fee whatsoever.

Proceed to Frame 6-4.

Note B (from Frame 6-16)

Although we have not mentioned it specifically, punishment is not the main purpose of tort litigation. Damages are supposed to be *compensatory*, not *punitive*. Nevertheless, when there is evidence of gross negligence, the plaintiff's attorney usually will ask for punitive damages. If the evidence shows that ordinary negligence has been compounded by the defendant's malice, recklessness, callousness, or deceit, the court may permit the issue of punitive damages to be submitted to the jury. The intention, of course, is to discourage a repetition of such actions.

Proceed to Frame 6-17.

EXPLANATORY NOTES

Note C (from Frame 6-17)

The really *significant* element missing from the given example is compensable harm or injury to the patient. From the standpoint of the law, displeasure, disgust, anger, and other similar subjective states of mind are not a sufficient basis for bringing a lawsuit. On *rare* occasions, in which a particularly unnerving experience due to a nurse's negligent conduct has resulted in psychic trauma to the patient, the courts have permitted a recovery, but only where the psychic trauma has produced fairly severe physiological effects. Generally speaking, however, a nurse will not be held liable unless his or her negligence is the direct cause of injury to the patient.

Note carefully, however, that bullying tactics on the part of a nurse and other similar behavior may be an important *psychological* mechanism leading to a later malpractice suit. This point is examined more thoroughly in Part 7 of this course.

Proceed to Frame 6-18.

POINTS TO REMEMBER

1. The complaining party in a malpractice suit is called the plaintiff. Usually the plaintiff is the injured patient although the law also permits other persons to bring such a suit.

2. The answering party in a malpractice suit is called the defendant. Usually the defendant is the nurse himself or herself, although in some instances the law permits the suit to be brought against the nurse's employer, as well as the nurse.

3. The basic elements of every nursing malpractice suit are claims that (1) the nurse owed the plaintiff a special duty of care, (2) the nurse was required to meet a specific standard of care in carrying out the nursing function in question, (3) the nurse's failure to meet the required standard of care proximately resulted in harm or injury to the plaintiff, and (4) call for money damages to compensate the plaintiff for the harm or injury sustained.

4. The most significant legal element in a nursing malpractice suit is whether the defendant nurse failed to meet the required standard of care. The degree to which the nurse meets the required standard of care or deviates from it is the basis of the fundamental question of negligence (or malpractice).

QUESTIONS OF FACT AND LAW

6-19 At the trial of a malpractice action some of the elements listed in Frame 6-18 are considered questions of fact and others are considered questions of law. The importance of the distinction is that questions of fact are *normally* left to the *jury* to decide, while questions of law are *always* left to the *Court* (the trial judge). Not all cases are tried before juries, since the parties may waive trial by jury in a civil proceeding. When there is no jury, the Court will decide the factual and the legal questions presented by the parties.

In the *usual* malpractice action, all questions of fact are resolved by   ☐   the Court
☐   the jury

6-20 The Court will decide all questions, both those of law and fact, when

☐   the attorneys for the parties agree to this process

☐   the complexity of the case requires that the judge act alone

☐   trial by jury is waived

6-21 Before a jury is permitted by the Court to hear any evidence on disputed questions of fact, the Court itself must decide that the defendant nurse owed the plaintiff a special duty of care. The finding of a nurse-patient relationship is usually the necessary determination, and if the Court so finds, the case will proceed on the remaining legal issues. However, if the Court determines that a nurse-patient relationship did *not* exist, it will immediately dismiss the plaintiff's case without further proceedings.

To the plaintiff, proving the existence of a nurse-patient relationship is

☐   important but not essential

☐   important and essential

☐   unimportant

when bringing a malpractice suit against a nurse.

6-19   *the jury*   **6-20**   *trial by jury is waived*   **6-21**   *important and essential*

6-22

■ General-duty Nurse N has a casual conversation about the merits of cosmetic surgery with the wife of a patient hospitalized for severe angina. Based on this conversation, the wife, who has been contemplating such surgery for a long time, decides to proceed with a face lift. The surgery turns out poorly and she later brings suit against both the plastic surgeon and Nurse N.

At the trial, the issue of Nurse N's legal relationship to the plaintiff would be

☐   a question of fact

☐   a question of law

to be decided by

☐   the judge

☐   the jury

6-23 The most important question of fact for the jury to decide in a nursing malpractice suit is whether the defendant nurse failed to conform to the required standard of care. In cases in which no jury is present, the Court decides this crucial issue of fact in addition to all questions of law.

If the jury in a malpractice case were to decide that the plaintiff failed to prove that the nurse deviated from the applicable standard of care, the jury would have decided

☐   a question of law

☐   a question of fact

which would

☐   for all practical purposes decide the case in the nurse's favor

☐   still leave many other equally important issues of law and fact to be resolved

<table>
<tr><td>**6-22** *a question of law*
the judge</td><td>**6-23** *a question of fact*
for all practical purposes decide the case in the nurse's favor</td></tr>
</table>

6-24 It was stated earlier that the standard of care *normally* is considered a question of fact for the jury to decide. There are circumstances, however, under which the jury is not permitted to decide this question. One example is when a statute prescribes the applicable standard of care. In this situation, the Court will so rule as a matter of law, leaving it to the jury to determine only whether the prescribed standard (the statute) was violated.

A state or provincial statute that prescribes a particular type of conduct on the part of a nurse is an example of ☐ a statutory standard of care ☐ statutory negligence

---

6-25

■ A practical nurse employed by a general hospital is sued by a former patient, who alleges in his complaint that the nurse negligently gave him an injection of morphine and that, in any event, the nurse was not legally authorized to give injections of narcotic drugs.

At the trial of this malpractice suit, which of the following would be questions of fact for the jury to decide and which would be questions of law for the Court to decide?

Fact	*Law*	
☐	☐	Did the nurse violate the state statute that relates to the administration of narcotic drugs by giving the injection in question?
☐	☐	Is the state statute regarding the licensure of practical nurses applicable in this case?
☐	☐	Did the nurse's actions give rise to a nurse-patient relationship?
☐	☐	Was the nurse negligent in the manner in which the plaintiff was given the injection of morphine?

6-24 *a statutory standard of care*

6-25	*Fact*	*Law*
	☑	☐
	☐	☑
	☐	☑
	☑	☐

LEGAL PRECEDENTS

6-26 Over the years, many court decisions have been handed down involving numerous types of nursing activities and functions. Once a common-law decision has established the standard of care for a particular activity or function, it is referred to by later courts in cases involving similar facts. Such decisions are called "legal precedents." They not only serve as guidelines to the courts in deciding future cases but establish authoritative guidelines for future conduct of nurses in carrying out specific nursing activities and functions.

Indicate *two* important effects of a court decision that lays down a specific rule of law (e.g., a standard of care) in a suit involving a particular nursing activity or function.

☐ The decision gives the Court added prestige and an opportunity to display its wisdom in a technical field of law.

☐ The decision becomes an authoritative guide to future nursing conduct on the part of nurses.

☐ The decision lends stability to the judicial process by serving as a guideline for deciding future similar cases.

☐ The decision automatically decides other malpractice suits involving nurses in that particular nursing activity or function.

6-27 Is a legal precedent in a malpractice case an example of statutory or common law?

Statutory law	*Common law*
☐	☐

NOTE: A related doctrine comes into play when a legal precedent is announced by a court. That doctrine is called *stare decisis* (*"Let the decision stand"*). The thrust of the doctrine is that prior decisions should be followed and settled points should not be disturbed when the same point or points are raised in subsequent litigation involving similar facts and issues. On the other hand, appellate courts are seldom reluctant to overturn legal precedents they believe are clearly erroneous or arrived at through faulty reasoning.

6-26 ☐
      ☑
      ☑
      ☐

6-27 *Common law*

If you selected the wrong answer, you should reread Frames 1-4 through 1-9.

JUDICIAL NOTICE

6-28   When a Court determines that a particular prior decision or a particular statute applies to the facts of the case at hand, it takes "judicial notice" thereof, which means that it officially recognizes the earlier court decision or the statute as controlling. Thus, the doctrine of *stare decisis* is implemented.

If in the course of a malpractice case the Court takes judicial notice of a prior court decision, what is the legal effect of this action?

☐   The case under consideration will be decided without regard to the earlier court case.

☐   The case under consideration will be decided exactly the same way as the earlier case.

☐   The case under consideration will be decided in accordance with the legal principles decided in the earlier case.

6-29

■   A patient files suit against a nurse for malpractice alleging negligence in the nurse's manner of carrying out a particular nursing function. The state in which the suit is brought has never had a similar case before its courts, and there is no state statute regulating the activity in question.

Under these facts, which of the following statements would be true?

☐   There is no legal standard of nursing care in this situation, so the Court has nothing it can judicially notice.

☐   The Court will judicially notice the lack of an existing legal standard of nursing care.

☐   The Court will take judicial notice of the novel facts presented and decide the case by itself.

6-28   ☐   6-29   ☑   *If you did not select the correct*
       ☐   ☐   *answer, turn to p. 317, Note A.*
       ☑   ☐

6-30 The decision in a case of this type will probably establish a judicial precedent with respect to the applicable standard of care for the nursing technique in question.

True	*False*
☐	☐

6-31 In which *two* of the following instances would a Court most likely take judicial notice of a standard of care already applicable to the case under consideration?

☐ when the case under consideration presents novel facts involving a gap in the existing rules of law regarding the standard of care

☐ when the case under consideration involves a nurse who has been sued in several prior malpractice cases

☐ when the case under consideration involves a nurse's violation of a statute that pre-scribes or prohibits a particular nursing function or responsibility

☐ when the case under consideration involves the same type of nursing function or responsibility adjudicated in an earlier court case in the same state

---

6-32 The way in which a Court officially rules that a particular statute or prior legal decision is controlling in a malpractice suit is to

☐ request briefs on the issue from each of the parties

☐ hear evidence on the issue before making a ruling

☐ take judicial notice thereof

6-30 *True*   **6-31** ☐
                                    ☐
                                    ☑
                                    ☑

6-32 *take judicial notice thereof*

POINTS TO REMEMBER

1. At a jury trial, questions of fact are normally left to the jury to decide, while questions of law are left to the Court. When there is no jury, the Court decides both the factual and the legal questions presented by the case.

2. A preliminary legal question is whether the defendant nurse owed the plaintiff any special duty of care. If the Court finds that a nurse-patient relationship existed between the parties, the case will proceed; otherwise, the Court will dismiss the suit without further proceedings.

3. While the standard of care is normally a fact question for the jury to decide, when a statute prescribes the governing standard of care, the Court will so rule as a matter of law, leaving it to the jury to determine only whether the statute was in fact violated.

4. Common-law court decisions in malpractice cases provide authoritative guidelines for the future conduct of nurses in carrying out the specific nursing functions that were the subject of these suits. They also serve as legal precedents in deciding future similar cases.

5. The doctrine of *stare decisis* provides that legal precedents should be followed and settled points not disturbed when the same or similar points are raised in subsequent litigation involving similar facts or issues.

6. The way a Court officially rules that a statute or a prior court decision is controlling in a malpractice suit is to take judicial notice thereof.

BURDEN OF PROOF

6-33 One of the most important rules of evidence applied in a malpractice suit is the rule that the plaintiff has the burden of proving that the defendant nurse was negligent. In other words, until the plaintiff can satisfactorily *prove* the defendant's negligence, he or she is legally presumed to be free from liability (i.e., not negligent). If the plaintiff cannot meet this burden of proof, he or she will lose the case.

When a malpractice suit is brought against a nurse, there is an initial presumption of law that the nurse

☐ was negligent

☐ was neither negligent nor free from negligence

☐ was free from negligence

6-34 This initial presumption of law has the following effect:

☐ It places a burden on the plaintiff to prove the nurse's negligence.

☐ It places a burden on the nurse to prove the absence of any negligence on his or her part.

☐ It places a burden on the Court to see that both parties to the suit introduce substantial evidence on the question of negligence.

6-35 Why does the burden-of-proof rule give the defendant nurse an initial courtroom advantage?

☐ the defendant nurse does not have to prepare a defense

☐ the defendant nurse is generally blameless and has the jury's sympathy

☐ the defendant nurse does not have to prove his or her freedom from negligence, while the plaintiff must affirmatively prove the nurse's negligence

6-33 *was free from negligence*	**6-34** *It places a burden on the plaintiff . . .*	**6-35** *the defendant nurse does not have to prove his or her freedom from negligence . . .*

6-36   Why is the rule relating to the plaintiff's burden of proof so important in a malpractice suit?

☐   it effectively relieves the defendant of all liability for his or her negligent conduct

☐   it assures the orderly presentation of evidence at the trial

☐   the plaintiff's inability to meet the burden of proof will result in the plaintiff's losing the case

6-37

■ Patient P sues Nurse N for an act of alleged malpractice while he was hospitalized. P claims N failed to take adequate precautions to see that he did not fall out of his bed following a subtotal gastrectomy. The undisputed evidence showed that P fell out of bed and severely injured his hip, although when he was discovered on the floor, the side rails of his bed were up (i.e., in proper position).

Based on the above facts alone, the standard of care in this case would be   ☐ a question of fact   ☐ a question of law

6-38   Would P's injury, sustained in the manner described above, be legal proof of N's negligence?

Yes   *No*
☐   ☐

6-39   Which two of the following items will P have to prove?

☐   N's professional background and experience

☐   existence of a nurse-patient relationship between N and himself

☐   N's failure to take adequate precautions

6-36 ☐	6-37 *a question of fact*	6-38 *No*	6-39 ☐
☐			☑
☑			☑

6-40 In order to sustain the burden of proof in a malpractice suit, the plaintiff must prove his or her case by a "preponderance of the evidence." The plaintiff must therefore introduce enough credible (believable) evidence to persuade the jury (or Court) that all the essential allegations of his or her complaint are *more probably true than not.* If the evidence is evenly balanced on both sides or favors the defendant more than the plaintiff, the latter has not sustained the burden of proof and will lose the case.

Which of the following ideas comes closest to describing what is meant by a preponderance of the evidence?

☐ evidence beyond all reasonable doubt

☐ evidence more likely true than not

☐ evidence convincing to more than half of the jurors

6-41 Three scales of justice are illustrated below. Symbolically, in which of the illustrations below has the plaintiff (P) failed to meet the burden of proof in his or her suit against the defendant (D)? (The blocks on each scale represent the relative weight of the evidence presented by each party.)

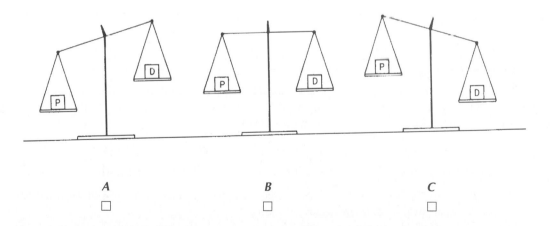

A	*B*	*C*
☐	☐	☐

6-40 *evidence more likely*   **6-41** *B and C*
true than not

6-42 To meet the burden of proof, the plaintiff must present convincing evidence in his or her favor on the following fundamental issues:

1. The existence of a special duty of care owed the plaintiff by the defendant nurse

2. The specific standard of care applicable to the nursing function involved in the case

3. The nurse's departure from the applicable standard of care

4. The nature and extent of damages suffered as a proximate result of the nurse's negligent conduct

The failure to sustain the burden of proof on any one of the first three issues ordinarily will result in the plaintiff's losing the case. The plaintiff must always prove he or she has suffered some damages, but even if the plaintiff cannot prove *all* the alleged damages, he or she may still win the case.

Which *two* of the following facts would be *essential* items for the plaintiff to prove in a malpractice case against a nurse?

☐ the accreditation status of the hospital in which the nurse was employed

☐ the existence of a nurse-patient relationship

☐ the nurse's age, place of schooling, and date of licensure

☐ the amount of the plaintiff's future anticipated loss of earnings as a result of the injury

☐ the act or omission that constituted negligent conduct on the part of the nurse

---

6-43 Assume that the plaintiff in a malpractice suit is able to prove the nurse's negligence without difficulty.

If the plaintiff claims a total of 20,000 dollars, comprised of 2,000 dollars for medical expenses, 1,000 dollars for wage loss, and 17,000 dollars for pain and suffering, but is able to prove only the first two items, what will be the result?

☐ The case will be dismissed for lack of proof of all claimed damages.

☐ The plaintiff will recover the full amount of the damages claimed.

☐ The plaintiff will recover all provable expenses plus an additional amount for pain and suffering, as determined by the jury.

6-42 ☐   6-43 ☐   *If you are uncertain about the*
     ☑   ☐   *correct answer, turn to p. 317,*
     ☐   ☑   *Note B.*
     ☐
     ☑

EXPLANATORY NOTES

Note A (from Frame 6-29)

When no prior court decision or statute applies to a particular nursing function, the concept of judicial notice does not come into play—at least not with respect to the standard of care applicable to that function. There are, of course, many other legal issues presented in a court case, and a Court may be required to judicially notice a variety of matters during the course of a trial so that time will not be wasted in having them proved repetitiously. For example, Courts are required to take judicial notice of the statutes and judicial decisions applicable within their respective jurisdictions. Courts are also required to take judicial notice of widely accepted scientific facts, mortality tables, and a multitude of other established facts. The doctrine of judicial notice is a legal extension of the rules of common sense and common knowledge, and is designed to expedite the proceedings of the trial.

Proceed to Frame 6-30.

Note B (from Frame 6-43)

Pain and suffering are considered a compensable item of damages in every malpractice suit in which liability of the defendant is established. As a matter of fact, damages awarded for pain and suffering generally comprise the major portion of a malpractice suit and the amount awarded is generally left to the jury to decide. In recent years, malpractice recoveries have kept pace with general inflationary trends and it is not uncommon for some awards to total several hundred thousand or even several million dollars where injuries have been devastating.

The plaintiff's suit will not be dismissed, therefore, merely because of an inability to precisely prove the value of his or her pain and suffering. On the other hand, no one can predict with any certainty what a jury will allow for this rather speculative element. In practice, when a jury award seems out of proportion to the injury sustained (as happens on occasion), the Court will set the verdict aside as excessive, in which event the case either may be retried or an appeal may be taken by the plaintiff.

Proceed to Frame 6-44.

POINTS TO REMEMBER

1. It is a fundamental rule of evidence in every malpractice suit that the plaintiff has the burden of proving the defendant's liability throughout the case. This burden of proof results from the basic legal proposition that the defendant is presumed to be free from liability until proved otherwise.

2. The plaintiff's inability to sustain the burden of proof on the question of the defendant's alleged negligence will cause the plaintiff to lose the case.

3. The plaintiff must prove his or her case by a preponderance of the evidence in order to win. A preponderance of the evidence is sufficient, believable evidence to persuade the jury (or Court) that the allegations of the complaint are more probably true than not.

4. In every nursing malpractice suit the plaintiff must prove (1) the existence of a special duty of care owed him or her by the nurse, (2) the particular standard of care applicable in the case, (3) that the nurse's failure to meet the standard of care (i.e., the nurse's negligence) proximately caused the plaintiff's injury, and (4) the nature and extent of damages sustained due to the nurse's negligence.

6-44 Another essential issue that the plaintiff must prove by a preponderance of the evidence is that he or she suffered some compensable harm or injury as a result of the defendant's conduct. Negligent conduct that does not cause any harm or injury reducible to monetary terms will not give rise to legal liability.

■ A month after she has been discharged from the hospital, Patient P is informed by her physician: "There was a mix-up one day while you were at the hospital. It seems that Nurse Simpson gave you the wrong medication, but we learned about it in time and your present condition shows that you suffered no harm."

P goes to a lawyer the following day to ask whether the above facts are sufficient to entitle her to bring suit against Nurse Simpson.

Which of the following responses by the lawyer expresses the legal position most accurately?

☐ "You have a good case because the doctor has already admitted that Nurse Simpson was negligent, and the doctor's admission is sufficient to hold the nurse liable for damages."

☐ "I would be happy to take your case since the nurse was clearly negligent, but unless we can prove you have sustained damages, there is no point in filing suit."

☐ "The fact that you know something went wrong while you were at the hospital is enough proof of legal harm, and we should have little difficulty in recovering a substantial amount by way of damages."

6-45 The preceding case *best* illustrates the following:

☐ Negligent conduct that does not cause any harm will not give rise to legal liability.

☐ The chance of winning a malpractice case is practically assured if one has a doctor as a witness.

☐ A nurse can be sued for negligence even though the patient may not have been aware of the nurse's negligence at the time.

6-44 *"I would be happy to take your case since the nurse was clearly negligent, but unless . . ."*

6-45 *Negligent conduct that does not cause any harm will not give rise to legal liability.*

6-46 The process of deciding whether the plaintiff has met the burden of proving the defendant's negligence (by a preponderance of the evidence) requires the jury to weigh the evidence presented by both sides. What counts is not the *number* of witnesses produced by a
given side but rather the *quality, relevance,* and *persuasive character* of the evidence. Members of the jury must evaluate all this evidence on the basis of their own general experience and knowledge of human affairs.

Which of the following statements is correct?

☐ It is generally recognized in malpractice litigation that the party who presents the
greatest number of expert witnesses is most likely to win the case.

☐ In a malpractice suit, it is for the Court to decide as a matter of law whether the plaintiff has sustained the burden of proof.

☐ In a malpractice suit, it is the express function of the jury to sift and weigh all the evidence presented and to decide whether the burden of proof has been met.

6-47 Since members of the jury must evaluate all the evidence presented in a malpractice case
on the basis of their individual experiences and knowledge of human affairs, it is reasonable to say that

☐ the outcome of a malpractice suit is impossible to forecast with any degree of certainty

☐ the outcome of a malpractice suit is nearly always predictable once all the evidence is
presented

☐ members of a jury almost always agree in their evaluation of the truthfulness of witnesses or the weight to be attached to their testimony

6-46 ☐
      ☐
      ☑

6-47 *the outcome of a malpractice suit is impossi-
ble to forecast with any
degree of certainty*

NOTE: As we have seen, under our system of justice the plaintiff has the burden of proving all the essential elements of his or her malpractice suit, and if the plaintiff cannot sustain that burden, he or she will lose. In other words, the defendant nurse can win merely by disputing the plaintiff's primary allegations and forcing the plaintiff to prove, for instance, that the nurse failed to meet the applicable standard of care or owed a particular duty of care to the plaintiff. This burden is never easy in a malpractice suit, which is one reason why most of these cases are won by the defendants, notwithstanding all the attention given by the media to plaintiffs' victories involving huge sums of money.

As we shall see in the discussion that follows, sometimes the defendant nurse can assert one or more affirmative legal defenses to the plaintiff's malpractice claim in addition to merely refuting the primary allegations made; when these defenses apply, they can be quite effective. An important point to note: when a defendant asserts one of these defenses in the course of a malpractice trial, he or she has the burden of proving that defense by a preponderance of the evidence—a reversal of roles with respect to who normally has the obligation or burden to establish proof.

CONTRIBUTORY NEGLIGENCE

6-48   One of the standard defenses in any malpractice action (as in any negligence action) is the defense of contributory negligence, which may be stated as follows: When a patient's failure to exercise reasonable care aggravates an injury initially caused by a nurse's negligence, the patient will *not* be permitted to recover damages in some U.S. states and Canadian provinces (i.e., the nurse will not be held liable under these circumstances).

In view of the rule of contributory negligence, a nurse who admits to an act of malpractice causing injury to a patient may avoid liability by showing that

☐   the patient was aware of the negligent conduct at the time it was committed

☐   the patient either caused or contributed to his or her own injury

☐   the patient anticipated the negligent conduct that occurred

6-48   *the patient either caused or contributed to his or her own injury*

6-49

■ Patient P is hospitalized for elective surgery. The day before the operation he sustains an injury to his foot caused by his own negligence in getting out of bed.

Why would the rule of contributory negligence not apply in this case?

☐ because the patient had not yet undergone surgery

☐ because the patient did not exercise reasonable care and was negligent

☐ because there was no negligence on the part of another person to which the patient's negligence could contribute

---

6-50 When the defense of contributory negligence is established and proved by the defendant, it normally constitutes a *complete defense* to the plaintiff's claim. In effect, the defendant will win the suit by proving that the injury received (or aggravated) was the plaintiff's own fault.

■ Patient P had been hospitalized for a leg fracture, requiring that her leg be placed in a cast. Nurse N gave P specific instructions about leaving the cast alone. Nevertheless, P pushed a traction weight down with her leg until the weight became useless, and also attempted to remove the cast with a table knife. When her leg became permanently disabled, P sued Nurse N for the resulting damages.

Based on the foregoing, which of the following would be the most likely result?

☐ P could recover full damages against Nurse N for failing to supervise her more closely.

☐ P could not recover any damages against Nurse N because P's conduct aggravated the fracture and subsequent disability.

☐ P could recover damages against Nurse N only for the additional disability she suffered while hospitalized.

6-49 *because there was no negligence on the part of another person to which the patient's negligence could contribute*

6-50 *P could not recover any damages against Nurse N . . .*

6-51 Failure of the patient to follow the doctor's or nurse's orders or instructions is the usual ground for raising the defense of contributory negligence. As long as patients are physically and mentally able to understand and follow such instructions, their failure to use reasonable care for their own safety will prevent them from recovering damages from the doctor or nurse in a malpractice action.

- P, a 45-year-old male machinist, suffered a cut while at work. Occupational health Nurse N sutured the wound and advised P he would need a tetanus antitoxin shot. Because her own supply of the antitoxin was exhausted, N (in accordance with standing orders) instructed P to get a tetanus shot from his personal physician immediately. P went home instead, and did not contact his physician. Several days later, P developed tetanus and died.

Should P's estate prevail in its claim for damages against Nurse N, and for what reason?

☐   Should not—because P's failure to follow N's instructions was the primary factor leading to his death

☐   Should—because P had a right to expect Nurse N to follow up on her instructions and make sure that P got his tetanus shot

☐   Should not—because P's death was completely unrelated to Nurse N's conduct

---

6-52 Why would the defense of contributory negligence not apply to a person who was unconscious when the treatment was rendered?

☐   the law allows no defense to a claim brought by a person who was unconscious while undergoing treatment

☐   an unconscious person cannot contribute to his or her own injuries

☐   the law presumes medical or nursing negligence where an unconscious person suffers injury

---

6-51   *Should not—because P's failure to follow N's instructions was . . .*   6-52   ☐ ☑ ☐

COMPARATIVE NEGLIGENCE VERSUS CONTRIBUTORY NEGLIGENCE

As previously discussed, when the rule of contributory negligence comes into play, the injured plaintiff's claim is defeated in its entirety. Because of the obvious inequities that have resulted from this harsh rule, the defense of contributory negligence has been greatly limited, and in some states entirely nullified, by what is known as the doctrine of comparative negligence. Comparative negligence operates on the theory that even if an individual (e.g., the patient) has been careless in some slight manner, he or she should not be prevented from recovering some of the damages incurred from the party mainly responsible for the harm (e.g., the treating nurse).

Under this doctrine, when a plaintiff brings a tort suit seeking to recover damages for the allegedly negligent acts of the defendant, the degree of negligence of both plaintiff and defendant are compared, and the damages awarded to the plaintiff, if any, are apportioned according to the relative degree of negligence found. For example, if a plaintiff were to suffer injuries of 20,000 dollars as a direct result of a defendant nurse's negligence, and the jury were to find the plaintiff 20% negligent and the nurse 80% negligent, the nurse would be required to pay only 16,000 dollars to the patient. In a state that adheres to the contributory negligence rule, however, the plaintiff would recover nothing from the nurse.

Because the doctrine of comparative negligence seeks to achieve fairness and equity, it has been adopted by the courts in a growing number of states.

ASSUMPTION OF RISK

6-53 A second legal defense to a malpractice suit is the doctrine of assumption of risk. Simply stated, this doctrine says that when a patient understands all the risks of unpreventable adverse results of treatment and knowingly consents thereto, he or she cannot prevail in a later malpractice claim alleging that an adverse result he or she was informed of was attributable to negligence.

- P, a diabetic, is warned in advance of surgery that her condition is susceptible to unavoidable infection. She authorizes the surgeon to proceed, and when postoperative infection occurs, her leg must be amputated.

Did P assume the risk of surgery in this case?

Yes	No
☐	☐

6-54 If P decides to sue the surgeon, what, if anything can she legally recover in the way of damages?

☐ nothing at all

☐ only her actual out-of-pocket expenses

☐ all losses suffered, including her pain and suffering

6-55 Patients do not assume the risks of treatment unless

☐ they do not want the doctor to refuse their case

☐ they fear they may not recover from the illness

☐ they know what the risks are

6-53 *Yes*	**6-54** *Nothing at all*	**6-55** *they know what the risks are*

6-56 The doctrine of assumption of risk is closely related to the doctrine of informed consent. Just as with informed consent, a patient who has been informed of possible adverse results of treatment never assumes the risks of *negligent* treatment.

- Patient P is told by his doctor that radiation therapy is the preferred mode of treatment for his condition. In describing the therapy, the doctor tells P about the possibility of radiation burns, but P nevertheless decides to proceed. Through an error in calibration, P receives an overdose of radiation and is severely burned.

P ☐ would be ☐ would not be within his rights to bring a malpractice claim against the doctor because

    ☐ he did not assume the risk of being burned

    ☐ he assumed the risk of being burned

    ☐ he did not assume the risk of negligent use of the equipment

---

6-57 A patient may assume the risks of treatment if he or she chooses to proceed in spite of being warned *against* being treated.

- P comes to Doctor D's office without an appointment to have her ears irrigated to remove excessive wax. Since the doctor is not there, P asks Nurse N to perform the procedure. N tells P he is not qualified to perform the irrigation procedure but, at P's insistence, he reluctantly agrees to perform the procedure. In the process N causes P's eardrum to be ruptured.

P's later malpractice claim against Nurse N will probably

    ☐ succeed, because N carried out the procedure negligently

    ☐ fail, because P knew N was not qualified to perform the procedure and willingly assumed the risk of possible injury

    ☐ fail, because there was no nurse-patient relationship in effect

---

6-56   *would be*   6-57   ☐
        he did not assume the   ☑
        risk of negligent use of   ☐
        the equipment

EMERGENCY

6-58   As noted earlier in this course, the law takes the surrounding circumstances into consideration whenever a malpractice claim is brought against a doctor or nurse. Thus, treatment given in a life or death emergency may provide a complete defense to a suit claiming negligence in treatment if it can be shown that the urgent circumstances required a relaxed standard of care.

■ A patient choking on a bone is brought to the emergency room. ER Nurse N attempts to remove the bone but is unsuccessful. Noticing the patient's cyanotic condition, Nurse N performs a tracheotomy and breathing is restored, but in the process, she injures the patient's vocal chords.

Yes	*No*	
☐	☐	Is this the type of emergency that would appear to provide a good defense to a malpractice suit against Nurse N?
☐	☐	Was Nurse N justified in performing the tracheotomy under the circumstances described?
☐	☐	Would Nurse N have been justified in performing the tracheotomy if a doctor was available in 15 minutes?
☐	☐	Has Nurse N run the risk of losing her license for performing the tracheotomy in the described circumstances?

6-59   The legal defense of emergency will be effective in a nursing malpractice suit only when the defendant nurse can prove that

☐   there were insufficient nurses on duty to assist when the emergency arose

☐   the treatment in question was a matter of life or death

☐   the emergency circumstances were brought about by the patient's own willful conduct

6-58	*Yes*	*No*	**6-59**	*the treatment in ques-*
	☑	☐		*tion was a matter of life*
	☑	☐		*or death*
	☑	☐		
	☐	☑		

NOTE: We have just reviewed the three most significant legal defenses available to a defendant in a malpractice suit. In addition to these defenses based on the merits of the case, there are certain *procedural defenses* that might also come into play. The first of these is the defense of statute of limitations. Every lawsuit seeking money damages must be brought within a specified period after the incident giving rise to the cause of action occurred. The period is always prescribed by statute and is thus commonly referred to as the "statute of limitations." Since the statutory periods within which malpractice claims must be brought vary from state to state, they are not detailed here. The nurse's legal defense counsel will know when (and how) to invoke the defense of statute of limitations when it is applicable.

Another procedural defense relates to the doctrine of governmental immunity, as noted earlier in this course. Pursuant to special federal statutes, nurses who are employed by the Department of Defense, Department of Veterans Affairs, National Aeronautics and Space Administration, and United States Public Health Service all enjoy immunity from suit for any acts of malpractice that occur while on duty. In addition, Congress passed the Federal Employees Liability Reform and Tort Compensation Act in 1988 (P.L. 100-694), which made it absolutely clear that the Federal Tort Claims Act was to be the *exclusive* remedy against the United States for suits based on the allegedly tortious acts of its employees while acting within the scope of their employment.

The fellow-servant doctrine is yet another procedural defense that might be asserted by an occupational health nurse who is sued by a co-worker seeking to recover damages from the nurse for aggravation of an on-the-job injury normally covered only by workers' compensation. As mentioned above, the nurse's lawyer will know when and how to invoke any of these legal defenses once the lawsuit has been instituted.

We return now to the trial process itself, covering briefly those areas of trial practice that are of relevance to nurses who may be sued.

POINTS TO REMEMBER

1. Unless the plaintiff has sustained some compensable harm, the defendant cannot be held liable in a malpractice suit.

2. Weighing the evidence in a malpractice case is the function of the jury, which must decide whether the plaintiff has met the burden of proof on all essential factual issues.

3. Some jurisdictions permit a defendant to assert the legal defense of contributory negligence if it can be shown that the plaintiff's own failure to exercise reasonable care contributed to or aggravated an injury caused by a nurse's negligence. When this defense is applicable, it is a complete bar to any recovery of damages by the plaintiff.

4. A growing number of jurisdictions have adopted the comparative negligence rule, under which damages are awarded to the plaintiff in proportion to the relative degree of negligence of both plaintiff and defendant, as determined by the jury.

5. When a patient is fully informed of all the risks of unpreventable adverse results of treatment and accepts them, legally he or she assumes those risks and cannot later prevail in a malpractice suit seeking to recover damages arising out of a risk he or she assumed.

6. A patient never assumes the risk of negligent treatment, even when the patient is informed of and has agreed to assume specified risks of unpreventable adverse results.

7. When treatment is given in a life or death emergency, the law relaxes the normal standard of care, and the plaintiff will not be allowed to recover damages for injuries arising out of those emergency circumstances, unless even that relaxed standard has not been met.

DIRECTED VERDICTS

6-60   As noted earlier, questions of fact ordinarily are left to the jury to decide, but on rare occasions a Court may "direct a verdict" in favor of the plaintiff or the defendant. When this occurs, the case is removed from consideration by the jury and is decided solely by the Court.

The Court is legally *required* to direct a verdict in favor of one party or the other when *both* of the following occur: (1) There is no substantial dispute in the evidence as to what events took place, and (2) the conclusion of whether the nurse was negligent is so clear and obvious that reasonable minds could not arrive at a different conclusion.

Consider the following case:

- Patient P sues Nurse N for malpractice. In her suit P claims only that Nurse N gave her an oral medication that caused her to suffer an allergic reaction. N admits these allegations but claims he was in no way negligent.

Which of the following best explains why the Court would be inclined to direct a verdict in N's favor in this case?

- ☐ Courts tend to be more inclined to believe the defendant than the plaintiff in a malpractice suit involving an adverse reaction to medication.

- ☐ The facts are not in dispute, and since N is legally presumed to be free from negligence, the Court must rule in N's favor in the absence of proof of specific negligent conduct.

- ☐ Many people react adversely to medications and the Court, aware of this fact, will rule in N's favor to avoid unnecessary speculation on the part of the jury about what caused P's reaction.

NOTE: In actual practice a directed verdict for the plaintiff is extremely rare in a malpractice case; occasionally, though, a Court will direct a verdict in favor of a defendant where the plaintiff's evidence is so weak as to warrant the dismissal of the case.

6-60   *The facts are not in dispute, and since N is legally presumed to be free from negligence, the Court must rule in N's favor in the absence of proof of specific negligent conduct.*

NEED FOR EXPERT TESTIMONY

6-61 In a nursing malpractice case the key question of whether the nurse acted with reasonable care ordinarily is a matter that requires the opinions of *expert witnesses*. Expert witnesses are necessary because members of the jury are lay persons and cannot be expected to know what nursing skills or procedures should have been followed in the case at hand. Accordingly, the plaintiff must introduce the testimony of one or more experts to prove the applicable standard of care and thereby help the jury decide what a reasonable nurse would have done in the given situation.

Why is the question of whether a nurse acted in a reasonable manner usually not left to the jury to decide?

☐ members of a typical jury are incapable of judging fairly what is reasonable conduct on the part of others

☐ members of a typical jury often are confused when confronted with novel fact situations, particularly those that relate to the acts of medical personnel

☐ members of a typical jury are lay persons and therefore do not have an adequate basis for arriving at a judgment with regard to the professional conduct of a nurse

---

6-62 The expert witness is someone who qualifies as an expert by demonstrating that he or she has expert knowledge of the particular subject area of the lawsuit and advanced professional training, extensive practical experience, or a combination of the two.

Which two of the following persons would logically qualify as experts in a nursing malpractice case arising out of the administration of a general anesthetic?

☐ an intensive care nurse specialist

☐ an anesthesiologist

☐ a hospital clinical pharmacist

☐ a nurse specialist in anesthesiology

6-61 *members of a typical jury are lay persons and therefore do not have an adequate basis for arriving at a judgment . . .*

6-62 *an anesthesiologist*

a nurse specialist in anesthesiology

6-63

■ A malpractice suit is filed against a pediatrician's office nurse for leaving an unconscious child in the pediatrician's office unattended.

Which of the following would probably qualify as an expert witness in a case of this type?

☐   a pediatric nurse-specialist

☐   an experienced office nurse

☐   a pediatrician

☐   all of the above

6-64   Since the jury ordinarily is not permitted to decide the issue of a nurse's alleged negligence without some expert testimony concerning the applicable standard of care, if no expert testimony on this issue is introduced by the plaintiff, the Court must direct a verdict in favor of the defendant nurse.

■ Patient P sues Nurse N for negligence in administering x-ray therapy that resulted in scalp burns. At the trial P seeks to prove N's negligence by introducing evidence of his injuries and of the good working condition of the x-ray machine that was used. N defends by claiming that P was fully informed of the potential risks involved and consented to the proposed course of treatment. N further claims that in any event there was no evidence to show she acted without reasonable care in giving the x-ray therapy.

The Court directs a verdict in N's favor. Which of the following reasons explains why?

☐   N more than adequately proved she acted with reasonable care

☐   P failed to prove by expert testimony that N's conduct did not constitute reasonable care

☐   N's conduct could not be held negligent where the patient was fully informed of the risks involved

---

6-63   *all of the above*   **6-64**   ☐   *If you checked the last box,*
                                              ☑   *turn to p. 339, Note A.*
                                              ☐

6-65   Expert testimony is not required where the alleged negligence involves something so common or ordinary that even a lay person would know that the injury could result only from negligent conduct. This determination is made by the Court.

Indicate in each of the following cases whether an expert witness would be needed by the plaintiff (P) to prove Nurse N's alleged negligence.

Expert needed	No expert needed	
☐	☐	P claims N negligently placed on his body an excessively hot heating pad, resulting in a severe burn.
☐	☐	P claims N erroneously gave her medication that was intended for another patient.
☐	☐	P claims N improperly administered an anesthetic agent.
☐	☐	P claims N failed to raise the side rails of his bed, permitting him to fall.

6-66   Which of the following best expresses the rule regarding the need for expert testimony?

☐ Expert testimony is always required in a malpractice suit, and a plaintiff who fails to introduce such testimony will lose his or her case.

☐ The jury is permitted to decide, on the basis of all the evidence submitted, whether expert testimony is needed in order for the plaintiff to win his or her case.

☐ Whether expert testimony is needed will depend on the facts of each case, with the Court deciding whether the jury will be permitted to decide the issue of negligence without expert testimony.

6-65	Expert needed	No expert needed	**6-66**	*Whether expert testimony is needed will depend on the facts of each case . . .*
	☐	☑		
	☐	☑		
	☑	☐		
	☐	☑		

THE MALPRACTICE LITIGATION PROCESS

All nurses should have at least a basic understanding of the process by which malpractice claims are handled in our legal system. There are three principal stages of the process: the pretrial stage, the trial stage, and the posttrial or appeals stage. Each is discussed briefly below.

Pretrial Stage. Litigation doesn't begin until the aggrieved party files a formal complaint with the appropriate court and the complaint is then personally served on the defendant(s)—usually by a sheriff's deputy or a special process-server—accompanied by a summons. The summons notifies the defendant of the date by which a formal answer to the complaint must be filed. The filing of the complaint begins the official discovery period, that is, the period before trial during which the parties are given an opportunity to discover from each other what evidence exists to substantiate their respective positions, claims, and defenses. The principal discovery devices include (1) *interrogatories*, which are written questions directed to the opposing side, (2) *depositions*, which are out-of-court examinations under oath of the parties or their experts (to be used at trial to impeach the testimony of the person if it is different than that given at the deposition), (3) *requests to produce documents* such as medical records, hospital policy and procedure manuals, and correspondence, and (4) *requests for an independent medical examination of the plaintiff*. A variety of procedural rules govern the discovery process. Thus, a party may object to discovery requests on the grounds that they are unduly burdensome, seek confidential or privileged information (e.g., the minutes of official peer review panels, whose deliberations are typically protected by statute), or are part of the attorney's work product. In general, however, the scope of discovery is quite liberal and courts tend to permit the parties to discover all relevant evidence that would be deemed admissible at trial.

Trial Stage. In a typical malpractice case, the discovery period may last as long as 2 years, during which period the parties may make efforts to settle the case before trial. If such informal efforts are not successful, the trial judge assigned to the case will hold a pretrial hearing to review the facts, narrow the legal issues, and make one final effort to settle the case without trial. If these attempts are still unsuccessful, the trial will begin. First, the jury is selected, and the lawyers for each side make opening statements outlining their respective positions and the facts they intend to prove (or disprove). As we have discussed, the plaintiff has the burden of proof, which means that the plaintiff must introduce credible evidence of each element of the claim and has the burden of proving each element by a preponderance of the evidence so introduced. Once the plaintiff has concluded its presentation of evidence, the defendant usually asks the court to direct a verdict in his or her favor on the ground that the plaintiff has failed to sustain the legal burden of proof. More often than not, the court reserves judgment on this request until the evidence for both sides has been heard.

At this point in the trial, the burden shifts to the defendant to dispute or disprove the plaintiff's evidence, or raise one or more affirmative defenses—such as contributory negligence or assumption of risk. Cross-examination of the plaintiff's witnesses by the defendant's lawyer is the process by which the testimony of plaintiff's witnesses is refuted or discredited. At the conclusion of the plaintiff's case, the defense elicits testimony from its witnesses, which is followed by cross-examination of these witnesses by plaintiff's counsel. Often, the plaintiff's attorney will request the court to direct a verdict in its favor at this point.

Throughout the trial, the judge's job is to monitor the testimony, decide evidentiary questions, and rule on legal questions raised by the attorneys for the parties. Thus, at the conclusion of all the evidence, the court will rule on the motions for directed verdicts made by either or both parties, and if these are denied, the case will go to the jury. The court instructs the jury on the law involved and what the jury's responsibilities are in applying the law to the facts introduced into evidence in order to arrive at a fair and just verdict. The jury decides whether negligence has occurred and what damages should be awarded, and its verdict is announced in open court. Needless to say, if the parties have waived their right to a jury trial, the trial judge alone will decide the case.

Posttrial Stage. A party who believes that the final decision of the court or jury is in error may appeal the decision to a higher court. Grounds for reversal by an appellate court usually relate to the improper admission or exclusion of evidence at trial, particularly evidence that is substantially prejudicial to one or another of the parties. The appellate court reviews the trial record and written briefs and hears oral arguments of the attorneys. Once the appeal is decided, an opinion is prepared explaining the reasons for the decision. If the court decides that significant error has in fact been made at the trial level it may reverse the verdict and remand the case for a new trial. On rare occasions, a party who feels aggrieved with an appellate court's decision may appeal the case to a still higher court. Appellate courts have their own body of procedural rules, and it goes without saying that the costs of appeals can be significant, both in direct legal fees and the costs of producing the required printed briefs for the appellate court.

Assuming damages have been awarded to the plaintiff, the final stage of the litigation is the process for collecting those damages, called the execution of judgment. Where responsible malpractice insurers are involved, this rarely presents a problem. Where financially solvent defendants (such as insurers) are not involved, however, it may take a successful plaintiff years to recover some—let alone all— of the damages awarded in the case, and may require considerable additional legal expense and emotional trauma. The table that follows summarizes the steps previously described.

The Basic Procedural Steps in a Malpractice Suit

Pretrial Stage

Summons and Complaint	Answer or Counterclaim	Discovery Proceedings	Pretrial Hearing	Settlement Negotiations
The complaining party files a complaint that, together with summons, is served on the defendant. This event begins the case.	Defendant files an answer within a stated period and may also file a counterclaim to plaintiff's charges.	Information-gathering stage for both parties. Interrogatories and depositions, plus review of documents and other evidence takes place.	This is an informal review of the facts by attorneys for both sides before the trial judge to narrow the issues.	Attorneys for the parties attempt to resolve the case through settlement negotiations before the trial begins.

Trial Stage

Opening Statements	Plaintiff's Case	Cross-Examination	Defendant's Case	Cross-Examination
Attorneys for both sides present to the jury their positions and what facts they intend to prove.	Direct testimony of plaintiff's witnesses (including expert witnesses) is presented in court.	Defendant's attorney asks questions of the plaintiff's witnesses to weaken the effect of their testimony.	Direct testimony of defendant's witnesses (including expert witnesses) is presented.	Plaintiff's attorney asks questions of the defendant's witnesses to refute or weaken points made by them.

Closing Statements	Jury Instructions	Jury Deliberations		
Attorneys for both sides summarize the facts and evidence for the jury.	The judge instructs the jury on the law involved and its duty to apply the law to the facts in the case.	The jury reviews the evidence in the case and arrives at a verdict, which is announced in open court.		

Posttrial Stage

Appeal	Further Appeal	Execution of Judgment
The aggrieved party may appeal the case to a higher court if that party believes the judge made erroneous rulings or didn't give proper instructions to the jury.	Either party may appeal the initial appeals court decision to the next higher appeals court if the party believes the first appeals court was in error in its decision.	The legal process begins for collecting the damages awarded in the initial jury trial, or as subsequently modified by an appellate court.

THE DOCTRINE OF *RES IPSA LOQUITUR*

6-67   As noted earlier, in the usual nursing malpractice suit the plaintiff has the burden of proving the defendant's negligence by a preponderance of the evidence. Sometimes, however, the plaintiff cannot possibly meet this burden due to unusual circumstances surrounding the injury; in these instances the legal doctrine known as *res ipsa loquitur* ("the thing speaks for itself") comes into play. When the doctrine is applicable in a given case, the usual rule regarding burden of proof is modified and the jury is permitted to find the defendant negligent without any expert testimony on the part of the plaintiff.

Under ordinary circumstances the jury in a malpractice suit is permitted to find the defendant liable for malpractice only on

- ☐ the defendant's admission of negligent conduct
- ☐ the testimony of expert witnesses
- ☐ specific instructions from the trial judge

6-68   Which of the following statements accurately describes the procedural advantage that results when the doctrine of *res ipsa loquitur* comes into play?

- ☐ Plaintiff does not have to introduce expert testimony to prove the defendant's negligence.
- ☐ Defendant does not have to introduce evidence proving his or her freedom from negligence.
- ☐ Evidence of the defendant's negligence can be ignored entirely.

6-67   *the testimony of expert witnesses*

6-68   *plaintiff does not have to introduce expert testimony to prove the defendant's negligence.*

6-69 The special circumstances that will permit the doctrine of *res ipsa loquitur* to be applied in a nursing malpractice suit are:

1. The injury must be of a type that does not ordinarily occur unless someone has been negligent.

2. The conduct that caused the injury must have been under the exclusive control of the nurse.

3. The patient must not have contributed to his or her own injury.

Consider the following illustrative case:

■ The parents of a 1-year-old infant bring a malpractice suit against Nurse N, claiming damages for burns sustained by the infant while under N's care. The plaintiffs are able to prove that N placed a heat lamp near the infant's crib and that when the infant was next observed, she had been severely burned by the heat lamp that had fallen into her crib. Plaintiffs seek to invoke *res ipsa loquitur*.

Yes *No*

☐ ☐ Was the injury one that ordinarily would not occur unless someone was negligent?

☐ ☐ Was the cause of the injury within the exclusive control of the defendant nurse?

☐ ☐ Did the patient contribute to her own injury?

☐ ☐ Should the doctrine reasonably apply in this case?

6-70 Keeping in mind the first requirement of *res ipsa loquitur*—that the injury must be of a type that ordinarily does not occur unless someone has been negligent—in which of the following situations might the doctrine reasonably be applied?

☐ fracture of an anesthetized patient's arm during surgery for removal of his gall bladder

☐ injury resulting from leaving a foreign object in the patient's body during surgery

☐ injury to a patient resulting from a fall out of bed

☐ injury to a patient resulting from administration of the wrong drug or wrong dosage form of a drug

6-69   Yes   No   6-70   ☑   *If you are in doubt about any of*
        ☑   ☐   ☑   *these answers, turn to p. 339,*
        ☑   ☐   ☐   *Note B.*
        ☐   ☑   ☐
        ☑   ☐

EXPLANATORY NOTES

Note A (from Frame 6-64)

The final item raised an entirely new issue, and perhaps your unfamiliarity with the subject of consent to treatment caused you to select the wrong answer. You must always bear in mind that the general rule regarding burden of proof requires the plaintiff to prove the applicable standard of care by one or more expert witnesses. Thus, a Court is *required* to direct a verdict when no such expert testimony is introduced. In the given example P did not introduce any expert testimony, and the Court had no choice but to direct a verdict in N's favor on that ground alone.

However, of what concern is P's consent to the x-ray therapy? Would that in itself be a sufficient basis for denying P a recovery? The answer is no, at least not without more facts than given in the example. A patient's consent to treatment may prevent a later claim by the patient that he or she was given unauthorized treatment (the technical tort known as battery), but it would *not* absolve a nurse of any *negligence* while giving such treatment.

Proceed to Frame 6-65.

Note B (from Frame 6-70)

The doctrine of *res ipsa loquitur* has been applied in many different types of cases, but only where the injury was produced in such a manner as to leave little doubt that someone was negligent. The doctrine is widely applied in cases involving foreign objects left in a patient's body during surgery. It has also been applied in cases of burns or other injuries suffered by a patient while under anesthesia or otherwise unconscious, infections caused by unsterile instruments, and injuries from defective diathermy apparatus or other electrical equipment. In the cited examples, only the first two are clearly within the category of unusual types of injuries that normally do not occur unless *someone* is negligent. The remaining examples might or might not be due to negligence but, in any event, are not considered the sort of occurrences that raise an *inference* of negligence; they might involve contributory negligence on the part of the patient or might occur even if no one was negligent.

Proceed to Frame 6-71.

6-71   The doctrine of *res ipsa loquitur* does not become operative automatically. The plaintiff generally urges the Court to permit the doctrine to apply in the case. If the Court decides that the doctrine should be applied, it will instruct the jury that the circumstances under which the injury occurred raise a presumption or inference of the defendant's negligence. The presumption is rebuttable, however, which means that it may be contradicted or disproved. Thus, when *res ipsa loquitur* is applied under a given fact situation, the burden shifts to the defendant to prove that he or she was *not* negligent.

When we say that the doctrine of *res ipsa loquitur* permits an *inference* of negligence on the part of the nurse, what do we mean?

☐   The nurse is considered liable whether or not he or she can show proof of due care.

☐   The circumstances under which the injury occurred are considered evidence of the nurse's negligence, which the nurse must disprove.

☐   The nurse's negligence is a purely legal question to be decided by the Court.

NOTE: You should be aware that the doctrine of *res ipsa loquitur* is not recognized in all jurisdictions. Moreover, this area of law is rapidly undergoing transition, and hence only the broad outlines of the doctrine will be touched on in this course. However, because the doctrine has such far-reaching consequences to a nurse when it is applied, you should be at least familiar with the fundamental legal concept involved.

6-71   *The circumstances under which the injury occurred are considered evidence of the nurse's negligence, which the nurse must disprove.*

POINTS TO REMEMBER

1. When the evidence is not in dispute and reasonable minds could not arrive at a different conclusion, the Court is required to direct a verdict (as a matter of law) in favor of the prevailing party.

2. The plaintiff ordinarily is required to introduce the testimony of expert witnesses to prove the standard of care and whether the defendant nurse conformed to that standard of care. Expert testimony is required because a jury of lay persons cannot be expected to know from their own experience what a reasonable nurse would do in a given situation.

3. When the plaintiff presents no expert testimony in a case requiring such testimony, the Court must direct a verdict for the defendant.

4. Expert testimony is not required to prove negligent conduct involving something within the knowledge or experience of most lay persons. The Court decides whether expert testimony is required in any given case.

5. The doctrine of *res ipsa loquitur* emerges when a plaintiff sustains injury under circumstances that make it difficult or impossible to prove *how* the injury was sustained or *who* was legally responsible.

6. The Court decides whether the doctrine of *res ipsa loquitur* will apply in any given fact situation. When *res ipsa loquitur* is applied, the jury is permitted to infer that the defendant nurse was negligent without the need for any expert testimony.

    Res ipsa loquitur can apply only when the following elements are present:

    a. The injury is of a type that ordinarily does not occur unless someone has been negligent.

    b. The conduct causing the injury is under the exclusive control of the defendant.

    c. The patient did not contribute to his or her own injury.

SELECTED REFERENCES—PART SIX

Elements of a Malpractice Claim

Nurse's Handbook of Law & Ethics, Springhouse Corporation, Springhouse, Pa., 1992, p. 202.
Kelly ME, "Professional Negligence Overview." In *Legal Issues in Nursing* (Northrop CE and Kelly ME, eds.), The C.V. Mosby Company, St. Louis, 1987, Ch. 4.
Louisell D and Williams H, *Medical Malpractice*, Matthew Bender & Co., New York, 1983, §§ 8.04-8.07.
Hemelt M and Mackert M, *Dynamics of Law in Nursing and Health Care*, Reston Publishing Co., Reston, Va., 1978, pp. 13-18.
Restatement (second) TORTS, § 281

Proximate Causation

Prosser W, *Handbook of the Law of Torts*, ed 4, West Publishing, St. Paul, 1971, §§ 236-237.
Annotation, 13 ALR 2d 11, "Proximate Cause in Malpractice Cases."
Dent v. *Perkins*, 629 So. 2d 1354 (La. 1993)
Flores v. *Cyborski*, 629 N.E. 2d 74 (Ill. 1993)
Porter v. *Lima Memorial Hospital*, 995 F. 2d 629 (Ohio 1993)
Vincent By Staton v. *Fairbanks Memorial Hospital*, 862 P. 2d 847 (Alaska 1993)
Godeaux v. *Rayne Branch Hospital*, 606 So. 2d 948 (La. 1992)
Pitre v. *Opelousas General Hospital*, 530 So. 2d 1175 (La. 1988)

Questions of Fact and Law

75 *Am Jur 2d*, TRIAL, § 714
Annotation, 71 ALR 2d 332, "Anxiety as to Future Disease, Condition, or Death Therefrom, as Element of Damages in Personal Injury Action."
Dooley v. *Skodnek*, 529 N.Y.S. 2d 569 (N.Y. 1988)
Wilsman v. *Sloniewicz*, 526 N.E. 2d 645 (Ill. 1988)
St. Petersburg v. *Austin*, 335 So. 2d 486 (Fla. 1978)
Hamilton v. *Hardy*, 549 P. 2d 1099 (Colo. 1976)
Capella v. *Baumgartner*, 494 F. 2d 36 (Fla. 1974)
Ferrara v. *Galluchio*, 152 N.E. 2d 249 (N.Y. 1958)
Leonard v. *Watsonville Community Hospital*, 305 P. 2d 36 (Cal. 1956)

Legal Precedents and *Stare Decisis*

20 *Am Jur 2d*, COURTS, § 183
Wise G, "The Doctrine of *Stare Decisis*," *Wayne L. Rev* 21:1043, 1975.
Stewart v. *Volkswagen of America, Inc.*, 584 N.Y.S. 2d 886 (N.Y. 1992)
Maislin Industries, U.S., Inc. v. *Primary Steel, Inc.*, 110 S. Ct. 2759 (1990)
San Antonio v. *Gonzales*, 737 S.W. 2d 78 (Texas 1987)
Exxon Corp. v. *Butler*, 585 S.W. 2d 881 (Texas 1979)
Adkins v. *St. Francis Hospital*, 143 S.E. 2d 154 (W.Va. 1965)

Judicial Notice

75 *Am Jur 2d*, TRIAL, § 717
29 *Am Jur 2d*, EVIDENCE, §§ 24-154
Stone v. *Sisters of Charity*, 469 P. 2d 229 (Wash. 1970)
Daiker v. *Martin*, 91 N.W. 2d 747 (Iowa 1958)
Agnew v. *City of Los Angeles*, 218 P. 2d 66 (Cal. 1950)

Burden of Proof

29 *Am Jur 2d*, EVIDENCE, §§ 155-180

Louisell D and Williams H, *Medical Malpractice*, Matthew Bender & Co., New York, 1983, § 14.03.

Gordon v. *Bossier*, 594 So. 2d 1332 (La. 1991)

Bacon v. *Mercy Hospital of Fort Scott, Kan.*, 756 P. 2d 416 (Kan. 1988)

Ogletree v. *Willis-Kinghton Memorial Hospital, Inc.*, 530 So. 2d 1175 (La. 1988)

Guilbeau v. *St. Paul Fire & Marine Ins. Co.*, 325 So. 2d 395 (La. 1976)

Pederson v. *Dumouchel*, 431 P. 2d 973 (Wash. 1967)

Beaudoin v. *Watertown Memorial Hospital*, 145 N.W. 2d 166 (Wis. 1966)

Contributory Negligence as a Defense

Creighton H, *Law Every Nurse Should Know*, W.B. Saunders Company, Philadelphia, 1986, pp. 107-8.

Cazalas MW, *Nursing and the Law*, Aspen Systems Corporation, Germantown, Md., 1978, p. 27.

Prosser W, *Handbook of the Law of Torts*, ed 4, West Publishing, St. Paul, 1971, p. 417.

Comment, "Contributory Negligence in Medical Malpractice," *Cleveland St. L Rev.* 21:58, 1972.

Annotation, 100 ALR 3d 723, "Medical Malpractice: Patient's Failure to Return, as Directed, For Examination or Treatment as Contributory Negligence."

McGill v. *French*, 424 S.E. 2d 108 (N.C. 1993)

Hoffson v. *Orentreich et al.*, 543 N.Y.S. 2d 242 (N.Y. 1989)

Fabianke v. *Weaver, by and through Weaver*, 527 So. 2d 1253 (Ala. 1988)

Mikkelsen v. *Haslam*, 764 P. 2d 1384 (Utah 1988)

Ostrowski v. *Azzara*, 545 A. 2d 148 (N.J. 1988)

Haynes v. *Hoffman*, 296 S.E. 2d 216 (Ga. 1982)

Moon v. *United States*, 512 F. Supp. 140 (Nev. 1981)

Comparative Negligence Rule

Prosser W, *Handbook of the Law of Torts*, ed 4, West Publishing, St. Paul, 1971, pp. 436-7.

Dent v. *Perkins*, 629 So. 2d 1354 (La. 1993)

Oxford v. *Upson County Hospital*, 438 S.E. 2d 171 (Ga. 1993)

St. Paul Medical Center v. *Cecil*, 842 S.W. 2d 809 (Texas 1992)

Carreker v. *Harper*, 396 S.E. 2d 587 (Ga. 1990)

Cowan v. *Doering*, 545 A.2d 159 (N.J. 1988)

Ostrowski v. *Azzara*, 545 A. 2d 148 (N.J. 1988)

Brazil v. *United States*, 484 F. Supp. 986 (Ala. 1979)

Assumption of Risk as a Defense

Annotation, 50 ALR 2d 1043, "Contributory Negligence or Assumption of Risk as Defense in Action Against Physician or Surgeon for Malpractice."

Smith v. *Hospital Authority*, 287 S.E. 2d 99 (Ga. 1981)

Olsen v. *Molzen*, 558 S.W. 2d 429 (Tenn. 1977)

Charrin v. *Methodist Hospital*, 432 S.W. 2d 572 (Texas 1968)

Du Blanc v. *Southern Baptist Hospital*, 207 So. 2d 868 (La. 1968)

Tunkl v. *Regents of the University of California*, 383 P. 2d 441 (Cal. 1963)

Directed Verdicts

Cazalas MW, *Nursing and the Law*, Aspen Systems Corporation, Germantown, Md., 1978. p. 10.

75 *Am Jur 2d*, TRIAL, §§ 857, 907.

Annotation, 82 ALR 3d 974, "Propriety of Direction of Verdict in Favor of Fewer than All Defendants at Close of Plaintiff's Case."

Savold v. *Johnson*, 443 N.W. 2d 656 (S.Dak. 1989)

Mantz v. *Continental Western Insurance Co.*, 422 N.W. 2d 797 (Neb. 1988)

Bryan v. *Luverne Community Hospital*, 217 N.W. 2d 745 (Minn. 1974)

Larson v. *Harris*, 231 N.E. 2d 421 (Ill. 1967)

Roberts v. *Gale*, 139 S.E. 2d 272 (W.Va. 1965)

Ahola v. *Sincock*, 94 N.W. 2d 566 (Wis. 1959)

Thomas v. *Merriam*, 337 P. 2d 604 (Mont. 1959)

Leonard v. *Watsonville Community Hospital*, 305 P. 2d 36 (Cal. 1956)

Seneris v. *Haas*, 291 P. 2d 915 (Cal. 1955)

Need for Expert Testimony

Fiesta J, "The Nurse's Role as Expert Witness," *Nurs Management* 22(3):28, 1991.

Sweeny P, "Proving Nursing Negligence," *Trial* 27:34, 1991.

Beyer EW and Popp P, "Nursing Standard of Care in Medical Malpractice Litigation: The Role of the Nurse Expert Witness," *J Health & Hosp*, Dec. 1990, 363.

Bahr v. *Harper-Grace Hospitals*, 497 N.W. 2d 526 (Mich. 1993)

Elias v. *Suran*, 616 N.E. 2d 134 (Mass. 1993)

Landes v. *Women's Christian Association*, 504 N.W. 2d 139 (Iowa 1993)

Vogler v. *Dominguez*, 624 N.E. 2d 56 (Ind. 1993)

Minster v. *Pohl*, 426 S.E. 2d 204 (Ga. 1992)

St. Paul Medical Center v. *Cecil*, 842 S.W. 2d 809 (Texas 1992)

Bacon v. *Mercy Hospital of Fort Scott, Kan.*, 756 P. 2d 416 (Kan. 1988)

Bell v. *Maricopa Medical Center*, 755 P. 2d 1180 (Ariz. 1988)

Guzzi v. *New Britain General Hospital*, 547 A. 2d 944 (Conn. 1988)

St. Francis Regional Medical Center v. *Hale*, 752 P. 2d 129 (Kan. 1988)

Doctrine of *Res Ipsa Loquitur*

Louisell D and Williams H, *Medical Malpractice*, Matthew Bender & Co., New York, 1983, § 14.08.

Prosser W, *Handbook of the Law of Torts*, ed 4, West Publishing, St. Paul, 1971, p. 39.

Annotation, 9 ALR 3d 1315, "Res Ipsa Loquitur in Actions Against Hospital for Injury to Patient."

Annotation, 67 ALR 4th, "Applicability of Res Ipsa Loquitur in Case of Multiple Medical Defendants— Modern Status."

Vogler v. *Dominguez*, 624 N.E. 2d 56 (Ind. 1993)

Lecander v. *Billmeyer*, 492 N.W. 2d 167 (Wis. 1992)

Scribner v. *Hillcrest Medical Center*, 866 P. 2d 437 (Okla. 1992)

Cangelosi v. *Our Lady of Lake Regional Medical Center*, 564 So. 2d 654 (La. 1989)

Barkei By Barkei v. *Delnor Hospital*, 531 N.E. 2d 413 (Ill. 1988)

Calvin v. *Jewish Hospital of St. Louis*, 746 S.W. 2d 457 (Mo. 1988)

Jones v. *Levy*, 520 So. 2d 602 (La. 1988)

Morgan v. *Children's Hospital*, 480 N.E. 2d 464 (Ohio 1985)

Parks v. *Perry*, 314 S.E. 2d 287 (N.C. 1984)

PART SEVEN

PRINCIPLES OF MALPRACTICE CLAIMS PREVENTION

Part 7

INTRODUCTORY NOTE

If malpractice claims arose *solely* because of errors in nursing practice, there would be no need for a separate part of this course dealing with
the subject of malpractice claims prevention. To *prevent* malpractice claims,
nurses would simply render the best possible nursing care to their patients
as consistently as possible. The fact is that malpractice suits also arise from
several other causes, including sociological and psychological causes.

Teaching you about the various sociological and psychological
causes of malpractice suits will be the function and aim of Part 7 of this
course. This information will offer insights into the fundamental bases of
patient dissatisfaction and ways to reduce the causes of such dissatisfaction and the lawsuits generated thereby.

MALPRACTICE CLAIMS PREVENTION

7-1   Every nurse involved in direct patient care should regard malpractice claims prevention as an integral part of daily nursing responsibilities for two fundamental reasons: (1) All affirmative measures taken to minimize the occurrence of malpractice claims will minimize the nurse's exposure to personal liability, and (2) such measures will necessarily result in higher-quality patient care.

The subject of malpractice claims prevention is something the nurse should want to know

☐   in order to provide the best possible care to patients

☐   in order to ensure the successful defense of potential malpractice claims

☐   in order to avoid potential licensure problems arising out of malpractice claims

---

7-2   The concept of malpractice claims prevention implies that the nurse

☐   can take affirmative steps to prevent malpractice claims from arising

☐   can avoid personal liability for his or her negligent conduct

☐   can limit the specific types of malpractice claims brought against him or her

---

7-3   Is the following statement true or false?

There is no direct relationship between improved patient care and the subject of malpractice claims prevention.

True	*False*
☐	☐

| **7-1** *in order to provide the best possible care to patients* | **7-2** *can take affirmative steps to prevent malpractice claims from arising* | **7-3** *False* |

7-4   Nurses should want to prevent malpractice claims if for no other reason than to avoid the psychological disadvantages that generally accompany such claims. A malpractice suit represents an attack on the professional judgment and integrity of the nurse, and no matter how competent he or she is, the nurse who is challenged in this manner is bound to suffer anxiety and nervous tension while the case is in process.

Which of the following statements *best* expresses the foregoing?

☐   Malpractice claims are psychologically disturbing to the nurse primarily because he or she may have to pay damages to the injured party.

☐   Although malpractice claims often create psychological disadvantages for nurses who are professionally incompetent, they rarely affect competent nurses in this manner.

☐   Because their professional reputations are at stake when they are sued for malpractice, all nurses experience the psychological tensions that customarily accompany such suits.

7-5   What would be the *best* way for nurses to avoid the psychological disadvantages that accompany malpractice claims?

☐   They should become proficient in the workings of the legal system.

☐   They should do what they can to prevent such claims from arising.

☐   They should learn the psychological techniques for reducing stress.

NOTE: Malpractice claims and suits against nurses have increased considerably within the recent past, and all indications are that they will continue to grow in frequency in the future. Essential to any program of malpractice claims prevention is a basic understanding of the general and specific factors that influence *all* malpractice claims. Some of these factors are directly related to the quality of physical care given, while others represent sociological or psychological influences. All these factors will be discussed in the material that follows.

7-4   ☐
      ☐
      ☑

7-5   *They should do what they can to prevent such claims from arising.*

THE CAUSES OF MALPRACTICE SUITS

7-6   One of the important sociological reasons why malpractice suits are becoming more frequent is the public's growing interest in medicine and awareness of medical facts. Discussions of medical topics appear daily in family magazines. Television programs dealing with medical subjects likewise have educated the public in many areas of medical practice. One of the unfortunate side effects of all this has been the tendency to underrate the dangers and overrate the benefits of medical care, leading to expectations that may not be fulfilled.

Which of the following *best* explains the sociological basis for the increasing number of malpractice suits?

☐   Malpractice suits are on the increase as a direct result of the effects on the public of magazine articles and television programs dealing with medical subjects.

☐   Malpractice suits have become more numerous because of the public's increasing familiarity with medical subjects and the erroneous expectations they often acquire from the mass media with regard to medical cures.

☐   Malpractice suits have increased as the public has become more conscious of lowered standards of medical care and the increased likelihood of negative medical outcomes.

7-7   The public's attitude toward health professionals has changed considerably within recent years. As the public has become more sophisticated, its attitude has shifted from one of great respect and near reverence for those engaged in the healing arts to a more realistic view that doctors and nurses are fallible human beings who can and should be held legally responsible for their negligent conduct.

All other things being equal, the physician or nurse in practice today faces a threat of being sued for malpractice that

☐   is probably no greater than

☐   is probably greater than

☐   is probably smaller than

the threat of being sued faced by the physician or nurse practicing 20 years ago.

7-6   ☐
           ☑   **7-7**   *is probably greater than*
           ☐

7-8   Answer yes or no to the following questions.

Yes	No	
☐	☐	Is the increase in malpractice suits due principally to changes in social attitudes?
☐	☐	Could the fact that more lawyers now specialize in handling malpractice cases be a sociological factor behind the growing number of malpractice suits?
☐	☐	As the public becomes more aware of the fact that physicians and nurses generally maintain malpractice insurance coverage, is it reasonable to conclude that the public will become less reluctant to sue a physician or nurse for malpractice?

7-9   Notwithstanding the sociological factors behind malpractice suits that have just been mentioned, *there can be no malpractice suit without some unfavorable medical result.* In Part 3 we saw examples of different types of negligent nursing conduct. When harm results from such conduct, the event invariably focuses the injured patient's thinking on a malpractice claim.

As a basic cause of malpractice suits, unfavorable medical results are

☐   more significant than

☐   no different than

☐   less significant than

the various sociological causes for malpractice suits.

7-8	Yes	No	7-9	*more significant than*
	☐	☑		
	☑	☐		
	☑	☐		

7-10 Without evidence that a nurse's negligence resulted in some harm or injury to the patient, there can be no malpractice claim.

	True	*False*
	☐	☐

7-11 When we refer to an unfavorable medical result as the basis of a malpractice suit, what do we mean?

☐ The patient and nurse have had one or more serious arguments, leading to a breakdown in their relationship.

☐ The nurse's conduct has resulted in some objective physical harm to the patient.

☐ The patient's condition has steadily worsened, notwithstanding proper care and treatment by the patient's physician and attending nurse.

7-10 *True*

If you checked the wrong answer, turn to p. 355, Note A.

7-11 ☐
        ☑
        ☐

POINTS TO REMEMBER

1. Malpractice claims prevention should be an integral part of the nurse's daily patient care responsibilities, because the same steps taken to avoid malpractice claims are those that result in better patient care.

2. When a nurse is sued for alleged malpractice, the psychological disadvantages generally outweigh any possible financial loss.

3. Malpractice suits are attributable to medical, sociological, and psychological causes, each of which plays an important part in the patient's ultimate decision to sue.

4. A major sociological cause of malpractice suits is the public's tendency to overrate the curative power of medicine and to underrate the dangers and limitations of medical treatment. This tendency has been greatly fostered by the mass media.

5. As a result of greater public awareness of medicine and medical facts (including its awareness of malpractice claims insurance), there is far less hesitancy today about suing a physician or nurse for malpractice.

6. Sociological factors have combined with other causes of malpractice suits to bring about a decided increase in the number of such suits within recent years.

7-12 One point should be made perfectly clear: Not *every* unfavorable medical result is preventable, nor is *every* such result automatically the basis of legal liability. The law does not expect the nurse to be a guarantor against harm to the patient. It merely requires that the nurse exercise the degree of care other reasonably prudent nurses would exercise under similar circumstances in caring for their patients.

■ Patient P enters the hospital for elective surgery, which proves to be uneventful. Postoperatively, he suffers an infection that extends his hospital stay an additional 3 weeks. He consults a competent lawyer for advice about the chances of success in a lawsuit against the medical personnel involved in his case while at the hospital.

What is the lawyer most likely to tell him?

☐ "Postoperative infection is an untoward medical event that may or may not be due to negligence. Under these facts you do not appear to have the basis for a lawsuit, but I'll investigate the circumstances more carefully."

☐ "Even if we cannot prove the postoperative infection was due to someone's negligence, the hospital and medical staff can and should be sued, because you suffered the infection while under their care."

☐ "Postoperative infection is always attributable to someone's negligence, and there is no doubt you can recover damages for the harm suffered in this case."

7-13 Which of the following unfavorable medical results, *in and of itself*, would reasonably be the basis of legal liability, and which of them would not?

Basis for liability	No basis for liability	
☐	☐	The patient was given 6 ounces of paraldehyde instead of 6 drams due to a nurse's failure to check the physician's questionable handwriting.
☐	☐	The patient died from cardiac arrest during a cesarean delivery.
☐	☐	The patient suffered injury to his ulnar nerve while undergoing abdominal surgery.
☐	☐	The patient suffered burns from a heat lamp placed too close to her bed.

7-12 ☑   7-13 *Basis* *No Basis*   *If you missed more than one of*
      ☐   ☑   ☐   *these questions, turn to p. 355,*
      ☐   ☐   ☑   *Note B.*
                     ☑   ☐
                     ☑   ☐

EXPLANATORY NOTES

Note A (From Frame 7-10)

Negligent conduct, in and of itself, does not establish legal liability on the part of the nurse. As pointed out in Part 6, the courts do not recognize tort claims where there has been no injury to the plaintiff, no matter how emotionally upset the plaintiff may be. To illustrate, a patient enters the hospital for surgery and the operation proves to be entirely uneventful. He later learns that the nurse anesthetist was unlicensed to practice in the state in question and immediately files suit against her for damages. Unless he can prove the nurse anesthetist's conduct was in some way harmful to him, he cannot possibly prevail. As a matter of fact, the Court will most likely direct a verdict in the nurse's favor. The same result would occur if the unlicensed nurse had been negligent but no harm resulted from the negligence.

To repeat: Negligent conduct that creates no harm does not give rise to legal liability.

Proceed to Frame 7-11.

Note B (from Frame 7-13)

Of all the unfavorable medical events listed, only the cardiac arrest during childbirth cannot reasonably be attributable to someone's negligence. Were we given more facts, even *that* incident might be the basis of liability against someone (e.g., the anesthetist). However, all the remaining events are explainable *only* as the product of negligent conduct on someone's part, and each could be the basis of liability against the responsible party.

Proceed to Frame 7-14.

7-14 The basis of every malpractice suit must be some unfavorable medical result in the treatment process, but not every unfavorable medical result affords a basis for a malpractice suit.

True	*False*
☐	☐

7-15 From the standpoint of physical care of the patient, nurses can do many things to lessen the possibility of malpractice suits. Select from the following list those things a nurse can and should do that might reasonably prevent a later malpractice suit.

☐ accurately record and report all significant facts relating to the patient's condition

☐ never question a physician's instructions

☐ determine whether a patient's needs can be safely carried out by another nurse

☐ administer medications prepared by other nurses

☐ anticipate which patients might suffer injuries from falls

☐ diagnose the patient's ailment in the physician's absence

☐ clarify instructions whenever he or she is in doubt

7-16 Nursing is the core of the many activities that center on the hospitalized patient. In view of the frequency of nurse-patient contacts in the hospital setting, hospital nurses should be constantly aware of the malpractice claims potential of any improperly executed nursing functions. From the viewpoint of malpractice claims prevention, nothing is more effective than scrupulous attention to the requirements of good nursing practice.

Hospital nurses are more likely to be sued for acts of malpractice than other categories of health personnel because

☐ most hospitals do not carry large amounts of malpractice insurance

☐ hospital nurses have more patient contacts than other health personnel

☐ hospital nurses tend to make more professional errors than do other health personnel

---

7-17 Which category of nurses should pay the *most* attention to the requirements of good nursing practice?

☐ hospital nurses

☐ private-duty nurses

☐ occupational health nurses

☐ public health nurses

☐ school nurses

☐ office nurses

☐ home health nurses

7-16 *hospital nurses have more patient contacts than other health personnel*

7-17 ☐ *none of the boxes should have*
☐ *been checked. The question*
☐ *was purposely designed to*
☐ *emphasize the fact that all*
☐ *nurses should pay attention to*
☐ *the requirements of good nurs-*
☐ *ing practice, no matter where*
or for whom they work.

> **NOTE:**   Thus far we have examined some of the sociological and direct medical causes of malpractice suits. We now turn to a less obvious but extremely important cause of many malpractice suits: the patient's *psychological* dissatisfaction with the nursing care received.

7-18   A malpractice suit against a nurse often is merely the final stage of a deteriorating nurse-patient relationship. Whether the patient will resort to this dramatic way of showing dissatisfaction with the nurse will depend on a number of interpersonal factors, the most important of which are the patient's personality and the nurse's personality, particularly the way these two interacted during key treatment situations.

In analyzing the causes of malpractice claims, it is not often realized that interpersonal factors

☐   play a relatively minor role as causes of such claims

☐   are the principal causes of such claims

☐   are extremely important causes of such claims

7-19   a malpractice claim is always founded on some unfavorable medical result, but whether a particular result will trigger a suit against a nurse will depend in large part on

☐   the patient's prior attitude toward the nurse

☐   the patient's prior experience in courtroom cases

☐   the patient's knowledge of medicine and law

7-18   *are extremely important causes of such claims*

7-19   *the patient's prior attitude toward the nurse*

7-20   The tone and character of the nurse-patient relationship are determined by the daily interaction of the patient's personality and the nurse's personality.

Which of the following would be evidence of a poor nurse-patient relationship?

☐   The nurse and the patient's physician continually argue over the patient's nursing
needs in the patient's presence.

☐   The nurse and the patient neither like nor respect each other.

☐   The nurse and the supervisor disagree on how the patient should be treated.

7-21   If malpractice claims are founded in part on the interaction of the patient's and the nurse's
personalities, then the role played by the nurse's personality in precipitating malpractice
claims can be described as

☐   essentially neutral and, at most, secondary

☐   critical and more significant than all other factors

☐   decidedly influential but secondary to direct medical factors

---

7-22

True   *False*

☐   ☐   It is fair to state that a nursing malpractice claim will result whenever
there is an unfavorable event in the treatment process causing harm or
injury to the patient.

☐   ☐   It is fair to state that a nursing malpractice claim will result whenever
there is a breakdown in the nurse-patient relationship.

7-20 ☐   **7-21** ☐   **7-22** *True*   *False*
☑   ☐   ☐   ☑   *If you checked the wrong*
☐   ☑   ☐   ☑   *answer to either statement, turn*
to p. 372, Note A.

POINTS TO REMEMBER

1. A malpractice suit cannot be successfully pursued unless there has been some unexpected or unfavorable medical result directly related to a nurse's negligence.

2. Since the law does not require the nurse to be a guarantor against harm to the patient, not every unfavorable medical result will necessarily be grounds for a malpractice suit. Malpractice is said to exist only if the occurrence was preventable in the exercise of reasonable care by the nurse.

3. From the viewpoint of malpractice claims prevention, nothing is more effective than giving the highest-quality nursing care in accordance with recognized practices and procedures.

4. Psychological and interpersonal factors play an extremely important role as determinants of malpractice suits. More often than not a patient's decision to sue, although triggered by some adverse medical result, is one way the patient can obtain revenge for what he or she considers unsatisfactory treatment (in the psychological sense) on the part of the nurse.

5. Since malpractice claims are founded in part on the daily interaction between the nurse and patient, the nurse's personality plays a significant role in the fostering or prevention of malpractice claims.

6. Because the psychological component can greatly influence whether a patient sues a nurse, all nurses should become familiar with the principles of patient psychology.

7-23   Careful study has shown that most nursing malpractice suits can be traced to patients' general dissatisfaction with the way they received care from the nurses they eventually sued. In order to understand the root causes of patient dissatisfaction and how to prevent it, a nurse must learn the fundamental principles of patient psychology.

Which of the following statements *best* summarizes the previous paragraph?

☐   The nurse should understand that patient dissatisfaction frequently leads to malpractice claims against nurses.

☐   A nurse's knowledge of patient psychology can uncover many of the causes of patient dissatisfaction and possibly prevent later malpractice claims.

☐   A knowledge of patient psychology is important to the nurse in carrying out everyday nursing responsibilities, but it is not likely to prevent malpractice claims from arising.

7-24   It may be stated as a fundamental rule that the less personal the relationship, the more likely the patient will think of suing for damages if something eventually goes wrong in the treatment process. Most patients want to be regarded as individuals and not as impersonal objects of medical treatment.

Which type of nurse is *most likely* to be sued for an act of malpractice, following some untoward medical event?

☐   the nurse who is generally efficient but always impersonal

☐   the nurse who is both efficient and friendly

☐   the nurse who is generally careless but always helpful

7-23   ☐
       ☑
       ☐

7-24   *the nurse who is generally efficient but always impersonal*

7-25   Quality nursing care is more than just caring *for* the patient; it is caring *about* him or her as well. Although it may seem too obvious to state, all patients want to be treated with dignity and respect. Considerably more attention should be given to the interpersonal and emotional aspects of patient care, and the nurse should never forget that patients' emotional and psychological needs are as important as their physical comfort and safety.

Which of the following statements best summarizes the foregoing?

☐   Quality nursing care is concerned solely with patients' physical needs and safety.

☐   Nurses tend to place too much emphasis on ways of satisfying their patients' emotional needs.

☐   Nurses who pay attention to their patients' emotional needs thereby give recognition to an important aspect of patient care.

7-26   Three nursing students are discussing ways to prevent malpractice claims.

Nurse A: "The surest way to prevent malpractice claims is to be careful in meeting the patient's physical requirements."

Nurse B: "The surest way to prevent malpractice claims is to satisfy the patient's emotional needs."

Nurse C: "The surest way to prevent malpractice claims is to recognize the patient's emotional and physical needs and to treat both in a competent manner."

Which of these nursing students is most nearly correct?

Nurse A	*Nurse B*	*Nurse C*
☐	☐	☐

7-25   *Nurses who pay attention to their patients' emotional needs thereby give recognition to an important aspect of patient care.*

7-26   *Nurse C*

PSYCHOLOGICAL ASPECTS OF PATIENT CARE

7-27   A basic understanding of the psychological aspects of patient behavior is important to the nurse not only from the standpoint of malpractice claims prevention but from the standpoint of stimulating and encouraging the patient's participation in the treatment process, thereby hastening his or her recovery.

Name two principal benefits for the nurse with a knowledge of patient psychology:

☐   prevention of malpractice claims

☐   greater psychological satisfaction

☐   greater respect by the medical staff

☐   improved patient care

☐   enhanced opportunity for career advancement

7-28   The current emphasis on patient-centered treatment is based on the philosophy that the nurse should interact with the patient as a human being, instead of simply doing things for (or *to*) the patient in a stereotyped fashion. The patient is encouraged to understand and participate in his or her care, thereby assuming a degree of responsibility for the outcome of that care. With the focus on the patient rather than the task, the interaction between nurse and patient becomes more personal, less businesslike, and more satisfying to patient and nurse alike.

What does the patient-centered approach emphasize?

☐   prompt completion of the nursing task by enlisting the patient's help

☐   more nursing commands and less discussion with the patient, to prevent patient anxiety

☐   greater understanding by the patient concerning the treatment to be undertaken and how he or she can effectively participate therein

7-27   *prevention of malprac-*   7-28   ☐
       tice claims   ☐
       improved patient care   ☑

7-29   An underlying assumption of the patient-centered approach to nursing is that

☐   the patient wants to and should be encouraged to participate in his or her care

☐   the patient's cooperation is relatively insignificant in the treatment process

☐   the patient's participation in the treatment process tends to interfere with necessary nursing functions

---

7-30   From the point of view of malpractice claims prevention, the key to the success of the patient-centered approach is

☐   the ability to enlist the patient's help in performing necessary nursing functions

☐   the development of a more wholesome therapeutic interaction between patient and nurse

☐   the opportunity given the nurse to experience more satisfying emotional relationships with patients

---

7-31   Since most patients react strongly to threats (real or implied) to their individuality, maturity, and adulthood, any procedure that requires them to be submissive is bound to give rise to feelings of helplessness, anxiety, and (to differing degrees) antagonism. On the other hand, when the patient is adequately informed of the procedure and encouraged to participate in it, feelings of helplessness diminish, and the patient becomes a more willing and cooperative partner in the therapeutic relationship.

■ A nurse informs a youthful maternity patient expecting her first child that standard hospital procedures require all maternity patients to get a predelivery enema.

What would be the best way for the nurse to cope with the patient's apparent apprehensiveness?

☐   Assure her that the procedure is a routine one, generally safe, and in any event *necessary* in accordance with hospital policy.

☐   Say as little as possible to her since the more she is told, the more her anxiety is likely to increase.

☐   Give her a chance to express her reaction to the procedure and then explain how her conscious cooperation in relaxation and retention of the enema will have more effective results.

7-29 ☑	**7-30**	*the development of*	**7-31** ☐	*If you selected the*
☐		*a more wholesome*	☐	*wrong answer, turn to*
☐		*therapeutic interac-*	☑	*p. 372, Note B.*
		tion between pa-		
		tient and nurse		

7-32 The nurse's ability to develop effective interpersonal relationships with patients requires a conscious effort. The nurse's words and actions must convey genuine interest and warmth so that the patient gets a feeling of real caring. Insincere mouthings, intended merely to give the impression of the nurse's interest, can prove to be more harmful than no conversation at all.

Nurse A begins her conversation with a patient as follows:

"I'm supposed to tell you about the barium enema you are scheduled for today."

Nurse B begins his conversation with a patient as follows:

"Good morning, Mr. Smith. I see that you're scheduled to undergo a barium enema, which is a simple diagnostic procedure. I'll be happy to tell you whatever you want to know about it."

What does nurse A's introductory statement immediately reveal?

- ☐ She is genuinely concerned about keeping the patient posted on the treatment he is to undergo.
- ☐ She is making a routine explanatory statement that conveys neither warmth nor personal interest.
- ☐ She shows a sincere personal interest in the patient and his welfare.

7-33 What psychological effect is generally associated with addressing a patient by name, as Nurse B did in the example above?

- ☐ The patient's personal identity is recognized, and he feels that he has been treated with respect.
- ☐ The patient generally feels his personal privacy has been invaded.
- ☐ The patient generally does not care one way or another.

7-32 *She is making a routine explanatory statement that conveys neither warmth nor personal interest.*

7-33 *The patient's personal identity is recognized, and he feels that he has been treated with respect.*

POINTS TO REMEMBER

1. Most malpractice suits are traceable to the patient's psychological dissatisfaction with some aspects of the nursing care received.

2. The less personal the nurse-patient relationship, the greater the likelihood that the patient will think of suing the nurse should something go wrong in the treatment process.

3. All patients want to be treated with dignity and respect, and the intelligent nurse will always give appropriate recognition to patients' emotional and physical needs.

4. Understanding patients' attitudes and behavior will not only prevent malpractice suits but will stimulate patients' participation in their treatments.

5. By definition, patient-centered treatment focuses on the patient rather than the task, and this personal approach is calculated to be more beneficial to patient and nurse alike.

6. Patients should be encouraged to participate in their care to the greatest extent practicable, thereby assuring a more wholesome therapeutic relationship between patient and nurse.

7. Nurses should consciously try to develop effective interpersonal relationships with their patients and should demonstrate by their words and actions that they not only care for but about their patients.

7-34   Hostility is a very common reaction to something that is viewed as a threat, and the hospital atmosphere has a tendency to heighten the anxiety and insecurity of many patients, making them extremely uncooperative and difficult to care for. Understanding the causes of hostility and helping the hostile patient to identify what he or she perceives as a threat will not only bring about a better therapeutic relationship but will greatly reduce the malpractice threat to the nurse that the hostile patient always presents.

Hostility in the hospital setting is

☐   something virtually all patients exhibit

☐   a trait exhibited by relatively few patients

☐   a rather common type of behavior

7-35

■ Patient P is scheduled to undergo surgery for amputation of her left leg. She is worried about the loss of this important organ, as well as her future chances of employment, and shows her concern by being hostile to all who attend her. One day she tells Nurse N, "You're a miserable nurse. Nothing you do is right."

What is the best way for Nurse N to react to this hostile patient?

☐   He should react no differently than in any other similar situation. If he feels anger or hostility toward the patient, he should tell her so.

☐   He should help the patient identify the cause of her hostility and patiently explore with her ways of dealing with the stressful situation.

☐   He should defend himself against the attack on him and make it clear to the patient that her behavior is disrupting the hospital routine.

7-34   *a rather common type of behavior*

7-35   *He should help the patient identify the cause of her hostility and patiently explore with her ways of dealing with the stressful situation.*

> **NOTE:**   Nurses who react to hostility by defending their own actions are not much help to patients and may even aggravate an already hostile attitude. Experienced nurses will always direct their responses to the patients' problems and assure them (in a sincere way) that they care and want to help. Under no circumstances should nurses take advantage of the situation by venting their *own* feelings of hostility, either toward difficult patients or other patients.

THE SUIT-PRONE PATIENT

7-36   There is one type of patient who is more likely than any other to bring suit alleging malpractice when something goes wrong in the treatment process. This individual is often referred to as the "suit-prone" patient. Because this person's psychological makeup breeds resentment and dissatisfaction in *all* phases of life, he or she poses a serious malpractice threat to all health personnel involved in his or her treatment. Nurses should learn to recognize the symptoms of suit-prone patients and make appropriate allowance for their emotional needs.

What can the nurse do, if anything, to cope with the suit-prone patient?

☐   The nurse should avoid dealing with this patient as much as possible.

☐   The nurse might possibly protect herself or himself against suit by a suit-prone patient by paying special attention to this patient's psychological needs.

☐   There is little or nothing a nurse can do to cope with a person who is suit-prone.

> **NOTE:**   Before proceeding with the discussion of the suit-prone patient, it should be made clear that *not every patient is suit-prone, nor should all patients be regarded as potential litigants.* The fact is, patients who are suit-prone are probably in the minority, but they can create serious problems for conscientious nurses and, for that reason, should be dealt with carefully. The key to prevention, as noted above, is to learn how to spot suit-prone patients in the first place, and then deal with them appropriately.

7-36   ☐
        ☑
        ☐

7-37 The concept of suit-prone means that this type of person frequently chooses to express dissatisfaction or resentment by seeking revenge in a lawsuit against the person who is the object of this dissatisfaction.

Which of the following would *best* describe patients who are suit-prone?

☐ They have an intimate knowledge of the law and are familiar with courtroom procedures.

☐ They have a genuine appreciation of the law and legal proceedings.

☐ Their preferred method of dealing with persons who antagonize them is to file lawsuits against them.

7-38 What is the threat to nurses posed by suit-prone patients?

☐ Their conduct tends to be overtly violent, which raises the constant threat of physical harm to a nurse.

☐ Their need to blame others whenever things do not go as expected may encourage them to sue a nurse for malpractice.

☐ Their behavior invariably is disruptive of the nurse's normal routine.

7-39 The attitudes of suit-prone patients reflect a basic immaturity that is revealed in *all* aspects of their lives. They are generally insecure persons who express their insecurity by being hostile and uncooperative. Perhaps the thing that characterizes them best is their need to shift blame to other persons as a way of coping with their own inadequacies.

Which of the following personality traits would a suit-prone patient generally *not* possess?

☐ a well-defined sense of personal responsibility

☐ dependency and a generally insecure nature

☐ immaturity and avoidance of responsibility

7-37	*Their preferred method of dealing with persons who antagonize them is to file lawsuits against them.*	7-38	☐ ☑ ☐	7-39	*a well-defined sense of personal responsibility*

7-40 Which of the following statements *most accurately* reflects the attitude of the suit-prone patient toward physicians and nurses?

☐ "I don't like medical people to begin with, and I'll get even with any one of them who treats me in a high-handed way."

☐ "Most doctors and nurses are competent, but even the best of them are bound to make mistakes occasionally, so I make the usual allowances for their failings."

☐ "Suing a doctor or nurse is no different than suing anyone else, and if it becomes necessary, that's just what I'll do."

7-41 Suit-prone patients, by their very nature, are likely to be uncooperative patients. They frequently fail to state their complaints accurately and are less likely to follow a prescribed therapeutic regimen. They react to their feelings of inferiority and insecurity by being difficult and negative in their dealings with medical personnel.

Which of the following traits would indicate to the nurse that a patient is probably suit-prone? (Select two.)

☐ The patient is argumentative and generally disagreeable.

☐ The patient is understanding and cooperative.

☐ The patient is a fault-finder and critic.

☐ The patient is a lawyer or the spouse of a lawyer.

7-40 ☑
☐
☐

7-41 ☑
☐
☑
☐

7-42 Studies have shown that the institutional structure of the typical hospital has a tendency to stimulate even greater dissatisfaction and resentment on the part of suit-prone patients than they normally display. The patients' enforced passivity, coupled with the invasion of their bodily privacy and control over their own actions, intensifies their feelings of inferiority, insecurity, and frustration.

Which of the following reactions might be expected to occur as a consequence of a patient's hospitalization? (Select two.)

☐ The patient is actively involved in most phases of his or her medical care.

☐ The patient generally receives more attention and hence is inclined to be more agreeable.

☐ The patient is required to be obedient, cooperative, and uncomplaining, all of which tends to make him or her more frustrated.

☐ The patient's enforced passivity tends to heighten his or her sensitivity and emotional reaction to any real or fancied slights by doctors or nurses.

7-43 It is well established that a suit-prone patient will sue for malpractice whenever he or she suffers some compensable harm or injury at the hands of a physician or nurse.

True   *False*

☐   ☐

7-42 ☐
        ☐
        ☑
        ☑

7-43 *False*
      If you checked True, turn
to p. 372, Note C.

EXPLANATORY NOTES

Note A (from Frame 7-22)

Both of these statements are false. Even if some unfavorable medical event occurs, a patient may or may not decide to sue the offending nurse, depending on a variety of factors. One of the most important of these factors is the way the patient believes he or she has been treated—emotionally and physically—before the incident in question. Looking at the other side of the coin, no matter how poorly patients believe they have been treated (both emotionally and physically), they cannot successfully bring malpractice suits unless they can prove some compensable harm. The important psychological bases for malpractice suits are discussed in the following frames.

Proceed to Frame 7-23.

Note B (from Frame 7-31)

Most studies have revealed that the most successful relationship between patient and nurse occurs when there is mutual planning and consent. It can be disastrous for the nurse to assume an authoritarian role and place the patient in a position of a recipient of care he or she may neither understand nor want. The failure to communicate with the patient generally results in *greater* anxiety on the part of the patient, not the reverse. All in all, it seems reasonably well established that encouragement of the patient's participation in matters such as administration of the predelivery enema has produced more effective results than when the patient was assigned a more passive role.

Proceed to Frame 7-32.

Note C (from Frame 7-43)

Generally speaking, suit-prone patients will *not* sue for malpractice unless they have been badly treated—in the emotional sense—before the act of malpractice. Recognizing suit-prone patients, therefore, and making proper allowance for their emotional needs in an intelligent manner can effectively eliminate one of the principal causes of malpractice suits. Dealing with persons who have unusual emotional needs calls for patience and genuine understanding on the part of the nurse. It is a challenge to which all nurses should rise, knowing that success will make their chosen career a much more satisfying one from every point of view.

Proceed to Frame 7-44.

POINTS TO REMEMBER

1. Since hostility is a common reaction of many patients to the various threats posed by the hospital atmosphere, the nurse should try to help the hostile patient identify the source of his or her hostility and then come to grips with the stress-producing situation.

2. Nurses should never permit their own feelings of hostility to override their primary responsibility to their patients. Their responses should always be therapeutically oriented.

3. Some patients are particularly suit-prone as a result of built-in personality defects that are typified by dissatisfaction and resentment in all phases of their lives. Since suit-prone patients pose the greatest malpractice threat to practicing nurses, nurses should learn to recognize their symptoms and make appropriate allowances for their emotional needs.

4. Suit-prone patients tend to be immature, dependent, uncooperative, and frequently hostile. Their hallmark is their inability to be self-critical, and they invariably shift blame to other persons as a way of coping with their own inadequacies.

5. Treating a suit-prone person is hazardous under the best of circumstances, so the nurse must be especially alert to the problems this type of patient presents in order to avoid a later malpractice claim.

> **NOTE:** How should you cope with suit-prone patients? First and foremost, you should make a conscious effort to *know* these patients, not simply as ill persons, but as human beings. This means cheering them up when they are obviously depressed or fearful, showing interest and sympathy in their pain and suffering, and expressing appreciation when they are cooperative. A genuine atmosphere of *attentiveness, patience,* and *understanding* will foster the respect and confidence necessary to help bring about these patients' ultimate recoveries.

7-44   In what way can a nurse be sensitive to a patient's latent or expressed fears?

☐   by trying not to discuss matters that are likely to enhance those fears

☐   by being sympathetic and attentive

☐   by letting him talk but not getting overly involved

7-45   If a patient is already suit-prone, any evidence that the nurse's sympathy and concern on his or her behalf are a pretense will probably

☐   reinforce the patient's belief that most nurses are basically false

☐   not affect the patient at all

☐   reinforce the patient's suit-prone nature

7-44   *by being sympathetic and attentive*

7-45   *reinforce the patient's suit-prone nature*

7-46 Any adverse nursing incident is sufficient for the suit-prone patient to conclude that malpractice has occurred. At that point, however, the patient's decision to sue the nurse may depend not so much on the adverse medical event itself but on how well the patient believes he or she has been dealt with by the nurse in the psychological sense—that is, the degree of understanding, sympathy, and respect the patient has received from the nurse *before* the time of the incident.

In which of the following cases would the otherwise suit-prone patient probably *not* sue the nurse?

☐ A. The nurse (acting on the doctor's orders) tells the patient he must get up and walk for 15 minutes. The patient tells the nurse he feels faint, nauseated, and slightly dizzy. The nurse insists he must walk anyway, and while so doing he falls and injures himself.

☐ B. The nurse is summoned to the patient's bedside, and when he arrives the patient asks several vague questions and engages him in general small talk. Although the nurse is busy, he chats amiably with the patient and then leaves. Later that day the nurse negligently injures the patient while giving an injection.

☐ C. The nurse is about to give the patient the second dose of a medicine when the patient reminds her that the first dose reacted very badly. "Never mind," says the nurse, "according to the chart you're supposed to get the second dose now, and I'm here to see that you get it." The second dose results in a more severe reaction than the first.

7-47 It is poor nursing practice to make special adjustments in a patient's care simply because the patient is known to be suit prone.

True   *False*

☐   ☐

7-46   *A*   *B*   *C*   **7-47**   *False*
          ☐   ☑   ☐   *If you checked True,*
                                        turn to p. 382, Note A.

7-48

- Mrs. P is 38-years-old, a widow, and an active career woman. She has no children and only distant relatives. During her hospitalization for removal of an ovarian cyst, she exhibits all the traits and symptoms of the suit-prone patient (anger, resentment, dissatisfaction, uncooperativeness, and so forth), and all the floor nurses are aware of these traits. Mrs. P. shows extreme concern for her physical health, and whenever a nurse is near she regularly complains of numerous vague symptoms. The three nurses who have been caring for her react to these complaints as follows:

Nurse A shows signs of annoyance and remarks, "Now, now, Mrs. P. It isn't as bad as all that. You are just upset about your operation, but you have nothing to worry about."

Nurse B listens carefully to Mrs. P's complaints and then remarks, "Don't worry, Mrs. P, I'm sure there's nothing seriously wrong, but I will make a note on your chart and tell Doctor D when he comes to see you."

Nurse C regards Mrs. P's complaints as exaggerated and (acting on her own) administers a sedative to keep Mrs. P from bothering the nursing staff.

Which nurse reacted to Mrs. P in the professional manner calculated to help the patient the most, as well as minimize the risk of a later malpractice suit?

Nurse A	*Nurse B*	*Nurse C*
☐	☐	☐

7-49   The fundamental reason why a nurse should be attentive, patient, and understanding in caring for patients is to forestall the possibility of later malpractice suits.

True	*False*
☐	☐

7-48   *A   B   C*
       ☐   ☑   ☐   7-49   *False*

7-50   Nursing psychiatric patients calls for the utmost in patience, judgment, and intelligence on the part of the nurse since the basic personality disturbances of mentally ill persons are greatly heightened in the hospital atmosphere. With respect to this class of patient, therefore, special attention is necessary to prevent the possibility of a later malpractice claim.

The significant threat to the nurse that psychiatric patients present is

☐   they are more likely to complain about a nurse's services to the physician or nurse-supervisor

☐   they will go out of their way to make the nurse's life miserable

☐   they are more likely to sue a nurse for malpractice if something goes wrong in their treatment

---

7-51   Since the suit-prone patient is one who (by definition) has unusual emotional needs, it follows that a mentally ill patient

☐   can be treated with considerably less attention to his or her emotional needs

☐   is probably not suit-prone at all

☐   is probably the most suit-prone patient of all

7-52   The nurses who are least likely to be sued by their patients, even though they may commit acts of malpractice, are

☐   the nurses who are most familiar with malpractice litigation procedures

☐   the nurses who are sensitive to all their patients' physical and emotional needs

☐   the nurses who keep up with the latest techniques in nursing practice through post-graduate courses

---

7-50   ☐
       ☐
       ☑

7-51   *is probably the most suit-prone patient of all*

7-52   *the nurses who are sensitive to all their patients' physical and emotional needs*

TIPS FOR RECOGNIZING THE SUIT-PRONE PATIENT

The suit-prone patient is one who exhibits many if not most of the personality traits and behaviors shown below. As the text has pointed out, treating these individuals is hazardous at best, so the intelligent nurse will be especially alert to the problems they present. Here are the traits and behaviors to look for in the suit-prone patient:

- The patient tends to be excessively critical of all aspects of the nursing care provided.

- The patient tends to be openly hostile to nurses and other hospital personnel.

- The patient tends to be immature and unjustifiably dependent on nurses for virtually all aspects of his or her nursing care.

- The patient refuses to accept responsibility for any aspect of his or her medical care, preferring to shift blame to the doctors and nurses who are providing such treatment.

- The patient is generally uncooperative and often fails to follow the designed plan of care.

- The patient projects his or her fear, insecurity, and anxiety onto nurses and other treating personnel, overreacting to any perceived slight in an exaggerated manner.

- Learn to recognize the personality traits and behaviors of suit-prone patients and make appropriate allowances for their emotional needs.

> **NOTE:** In the material that follows, we discuss briefly the problems associated with suit-prone nurses. Before doing so, however, it should be made clear that *most nurses do not fall within that category*; it should not be inferred simply because the topic is discussed.

THE SUIT-PRONE NURSE

7-53   Some nurses have great technical competence but nevertheless find it difficult to establish warm relationships with others. They may show their uneasiness with close interpersonal contacts by being authoritarian, aloof, or so busy with the mechanics of nursing care that they have little time for meaningful human interaction. It should be recognized that such personality patterns in nurses may be important causes of later malpractice suits.

From the human relations standpoint, the success of the nurse-patient relationship requires the nurse to develop which of the following abilities?

☐   the ability to interact favorably with patients on a personal level

☐   the ability to accomplish all his or her nursing tasks with the greatest degree of proficiency

☐   the ability to successfully manage patients by appropriate directions, orders, and discipline

---

7-54

- Nurse N has a fine record as a nurse who can initiate and carry out the most complex nursing procedures with technical perfection. Psychologically she is rigid and does not relate well to other persons. Although she gives the impression of one who "knows it all," she is extremely sensitive to criticism and reacts to criticism either by becoming verbally offensive or by stalking out of the room to show her displeasure.

What does nurse N have in common, if anything, with the patient who is suit-prone?

☐   She has nothing in common with a suit-prone patient.

☐   She has an insecure personality.

☐   She has the tendency to shift blame to others.

☐   She is probably just as suit-prone as a suit-prone patient.

7-53   *the ability to interact favorably with patients on a personal level*

7-54   ☐   *If you did not check the last box, turn to p. 382, Note B.*
          ☑
          ☑
          ☑

7-55 From the standpoint of her malpractice liability, under what circumstances would Nurse N be in *greatest* jeopardy?

☐ when she is working under close supervision

☐ when she is caring for a suit-prone patient

☐ when she is carrying out standing orders

7-56 What two steps should Nurse N take to minimize her malpractice liability potential

☐ She should learn the fundamentals of patient psychology and put them into practice as much as possible.

☐ She should devote more time to recognition and understanding of her own personality problems and make appropriate adjustments to enable her to relate more effectively to her patients.

☐ She should try to become more technically proficient in order to reduce the likelihood of errors.

☐ She should regard all patients as potential malpractice litigants and deal with them accordingly.

7-57 All other things being equal, a nurse who has a reputation for being tough and inflexible and for going "by the book" is

☐ more likely

☐ less likely

☐ neither more nor less likely

to be sued for malpractice than a nurse who is more flexible and agreeable.

7-55 *when she is caring for a suit-prone patient*	**7-56** ☑ ☑ ☐ ☐	**7-57** *more likely*

HALLMARKS OF THE SUIT-PRONE NURSE

The suit-prone nurse is one who shares many of the personality traits and behaviors of the suit-prone patient. These negative personality traits and behaviors may be important causes of later malpractice claims against these individuals. The suit-prone nurse is one who:

- has difficulty in establishing close and warm relationships with others.

- has an insecure personality and a tendency to shift blame to others when something goes wrong in the treatment process.

- has a tendency to be authoritarian, aloof, and more preoccupied with the mechanics of nursing care than in establishing meaningful human interactions with patients.

- tends to be insensitive to the patient's complaints or fails to take them seriously.

- fails to identify and meet the patient's underlying emotional and psychological needs.

- refuses to recognize the limits of his or her nursing skills and personal competency.

- inappropriately delegates responsibilities to colleagues or subordinates in order to avoid closer personal contact with patients.

Nurses who exhibit the previous characteristics would be well advised to recognize their limitations or deficiencies and make positive efforts to change their attitudes and behavior toward patients.

EXPLANATORY NOTES

Note A (from Frame 7-47)

The point that has been stressed throughout this discussion of psychological factors is that special attention *must* be paid to the patient who is suit-prone. In fact, it is one of the few things a nurse can do to prevent a later malpractice suit by such a person. Paying special attention to suit-prone patients means being aware of the way they react to illness, their attitude toward doctors and nurses, and their hidden fears and antagonisms. It means cheering them up when they are obviously depressed or fearful, showing interest and sympathy in their pain and suffering, and expressing appreciation for their efforts to cooperate in the recommended course of treatment. The worst mistake a nurse can make is to be insensitive to the suit-prone patient's unusual psychological needs. Indifference to the patient only adds fuel to a preexisting feeling of resentment, setting the stage for a later lawsuit.

Proceed to Frame 7-48.

Note B (from Frame 7-54)

It may seem far-fetched to refer to a nurse as suit-prone, but the fact is that some nurses (certainly not the majority) are just that. Suit-prone nurses cannot admit to themselves their own limitations of training and experience and, when confronted by dissatisfied patients, generally respond to the situation by neglecting the patient (rejection) or dismissing the complaints as trivial (ridicule). In an attempt to bolster their own faltering egos, suit-prone nurses refuse to accept responsibility for whatever may have gone wrong and tend to react to the situation by losing emotional control. Being more preoccupied with their own images, they tend to regard the patients as symbols of their own failure and punish them by total indifference to their emotional needs. In so doing, they completely distort the nurse-patient relationship and become prime targets for a patient's later desire for revenge. Thus, the nurses are just as suit-prone as suit-prone patients even though they are the ones who are sued rather than the ones who initiate the suit.

Proceed to Frame 7-55.

POINTS TO REMEMBER

1. To cope with suit-prone patients the nurse should make a genuine effort to know and understand them as individuals. The nurse should be attentive, patient, and understanding.

2. The more rigid and impersonal a nurse is, the more likely that he or she will be sued by a suit-prone patient.

3. Whether a suit-prone patient will sue the nurse, even after an adverse nursing incident, will depend on how well the patient believes he or she was treated by the nurse (in the psychological sense) before the incident.

4. Since the suit-prone patient is one who is dependent, insecure, and socially immature, persons who are mentally ill and have intensified emotional problems are probably the most suit-prone of all patients.

5. Nurses who cannot take criticism and who do not relate well to other persons are sure targets for the suit-prone patient. Accordingly, they should make a sincere effort to learn more about their own personality limitations and make necessary adjustments therein to prevent unwanted malpractice suits.

RISK MANAGEMENT IN THE HOSPITAL

Throughout this discussion emphasis has been placed on the things the individual nurse can do to prevent malpractice suits. There are a number of other measures, however, that can and should be taken in the hospital setting that concern not just the individual practitioner but the hospital as a whole. Taken collectively, these measures form part of the hospital's *risk management plan*, designed to identify the risks of potential accidents and injuries to patients (and staff as well) and thereby to improve the quality of patient care.

A well-functioning hospital risk management program will include at the very least the following:

1. Some form of in-house complaint mechanism by which patients and/or their family members can make management aware of inadequacies in treatment (by doctors as well as nurses), demeanor of personnel, potentially harmful practices, billing problems, and so forth. Many hospitals now employ patient advocates or ombudsmen on a full-time basis to work directly with patients and their families in resolving reported grievances promptly, both to increase patient satisfaction and to forestall possible later litigation.

2. The continuous collection and evaluation of data concerning specific patient grievances and negative health care outcomes in general. In most cases, these data are collected in the form of incident reports filed by staff members—frequently nursing personnel—as the grievances and outcomes are brought to their attention. A good incident-reporting program will alert both medical and administrative staff to those areas that need improvement, and is thus closely tied to item 3.

3. Mechanisms to evaluate the quality of medical care throughout the institution including medical audit, nursing audit, utilization review, and tissue committees. This process includes the formulation and implementation of corrective actions designed to reduce all potential causes of injuries to patients, whether or not they give rise to malpractice claims.

4. Special education programs for hospital medical, nursing, and technical personnel designed to anticipate and prevent all potential causes of medical injury, as well as programs dealing with the legal aspects of patient care and ways of improving rapport with patients.

A good hospital risk management program will also include a number of other elements and areas of responsibility to ensure the safety of patients, whether in the emergency room, the surgical suite, the recovery room, the corridors, or anywhere else in the hospital. Usually, a hospital will establish a special risk management committee, composed of representatives from each of the hospital's major departments and chaired by someone with expertise in the field of risk management who normally acts as coordinator and basic strategist for implementing corrective measures.

The importance of a formal hospital risk management program cannot be overemphasized, especially in an era when malpractice suits against all providers of health care are on the increase. Nurses who are employed in the hospital setting will make it their business to become familiar with the hospital's incident-reporting system and other risk management procedures. Of course, they will also make it their business to understand the importance of malpractice insurance protection, a subject covered more fully in Part 8.

SELECTED REFERENCES—PART SEVEN

Malpractice Claims Prevention

Barker SM, et al. "Quality Improvement in Action: A Falls Prevention and Management Program," *Mount Sinai J Med* 60(5):387, 1993.

Moore GM, "Surviving a Malpractice Lawsuit: One Nurse's Story," *Nursing '93* 23(10):55, 1993.

Mandell M, "Practical Ways to Survive a Lawsuit," *Nursing '92* 22(8):56, 1992.

Clark MD, "Toward Safer Nursing Practice," *Nurs Management* 22(3):88, 1991.

Kraus N, "Malpractice Litigation: A Painful Lesson in Professional Responsibility," *J Nurs-Midwifery* 35(3):166, 1990.

Kuhlman C, "Surviving a Malpractice Suit: Personal Experience and General Information," *J Nurs-Midwifery* 35(3):166, 1990.

Lacombe DC, "Avoiding a Malpractice Nightmare," *Nursing '90* 20(6):42, 1990.

Varga K, "How to Protect Yourself Against Malpractice," *Imprint* 36(5):33, 1989.

Bernzweig E, "How a Communication Breakdown Can Get You Sued," *RN* 48(12):47, 1985.

Knight M, "Our Safety Net Keeps Patients from Falling," *RN* 48(12):9, 1985.

Guariello D, "Can You Be Sued Without Cause?" *RN* 47(2):19, 1984.

Press I, "The Predisposition to File Claims: The Patient's Perspective," *Law, Med & Health Care* 12:54, 1984.

Psychological Aspects of Patient Care

Sundeen SJ, Stuart GW, and Rankin EAD, *Nurse-Client Interaction, Implementing the Nursing Process*, The C.V. Mosby Company, St. Louis, 1989.

Bernstein L and Bernstein RS, *Interviewing: A Guide for Health Professionals*, Appleton-Century-Crofts, New York, 1986.

Cormier LS, Cormier WH, and Weisser RJ, *Interviewing and Helping Skills for Health Professionals*, Wadsworth Health Sciences, Div., Monterey, Calif., 1986.

Louisell D and Williams H, *Medical Malpractice*, Matthew Bender & Co., New York, 1983, §§ 5.08-5.09.

Gerard B, Boniface W, and Love B, *Interpersonal Skills for Health Professionals*, Reston Publishing, Reston, Va., 1980.

Jessop AL, *Nurse-Patient Communication: A Skills Approach*, Microtraining Associates, North Amherst, Mass., 1979.

Larson PJ, "Patients' Satisfaction with Nurses' Caring During Hospitalization," *West J Nurs Res* 15(6):690, 1993.

Huggins KN, Gandy WM, and Kohut CD, "Emergency Department Patients' Perception of Nurse Caring Behaviors," *Heart & Lung* 22(4):356, 1993.

Messner RL, "What Patients Really Want from Their Nurses," *Am J Nurs* 93(8):38, 1993.

"Bossy Nurses Get Bad Results," *Diabetes Care* 16(5):714, 1993.

McKinney S, "The Nurse Who Listened," *Nursing '92* 22(5):71, 1992.

Podarsky DL and Sexton D, "Nurses' Reactions to Difficult Patients," *Image* 29(1):16, 1988.

Kivi D, "Did He Say It Was OK to Use His First Name?" *RN* 48 (4):13, 1985.

Kasch C, "Interpersonal Competence and Communication in the Delivery of Nursing Care," *Advanced Nurs Sci* 6(2):71, 1984.

Armstrong D, "The Fabrication of Nurse-Patient Relationships," *Soc Sci Med* 17(8):457, 1983.

Bernzweig E, "Soothing Patient Psyche May Prevent Lawsuit," *Mod Hosp* 112(2):83, 1969.

Suit-Prone Patients

"We Couldn't Come to Terms with Hank—Until He Signed a Contract," *Nursing '92* 22(1):50, 1992.

Bernzweig E, "How to Spot the Suit-Prone Patient," *RN* 48(6):63, 1985.

Miller A, "Nurse-Patient Dependency—Is It Iatrogenic?" *J Advanced Nurs* 10(1):63, 1985.

Barash D, "Defusing the Violent Patient—Before He Explodes," *RN* 47(3):34, 1984.

Brink P, "The Patient as Victim," *Am J Nurs* 84(7):964, 1984.

Gannon D, "On Being a Patient: Hate, Love and Nurses," *Med J Austr* 140(8):486, 1984.

Groves J, "Taking Care of the Hateful Patient," *N Engl J Med* 299:366, 1978.

Fox v. *Smith*, 594 So. 2d 695 (Miss. 1992)

Kakligian v. *Henry Ford Hospital*, 210 N.W. 2d 463 (Mich. 1973)

The Suit-Prone Nurse

"Nurses Fail to Listen to Patient's Complaints," *Regan Rep Nurs L* 34(5):1, 1993.

"Five Steps to Defusing Emotional Outbursts by Nurses," *Nursing '92* 22(2):32, 1992.

Bernzweig E, "When the Nurse Is Her Own Worst Enemy," *RN* 48(7):53, 1985.

Hardin S, "Nonverbal Communication of Patients and High and Low Empathy Nurses," *J Psychosoc Nurs Ment Health Serv* 21(1):14, 1983.

Schuster P, "Preparing the Patient for a Barium Enema: A Comparison of Nurse and Patient Opinions," *J Advanced Nurs* 7(6):523, 1982.

Duldt B, "Anger: An Occupational Hazard for Nurses," *Nurs Outlook* 29(9):510, 1981.

Harmon v. *Patel*, 617 N.E. 2d 183 (Ill. 1993)

Arnold v. *Haggin Memorial Hospital*, 415 S.W. 2d 844 (Ky. 1967)

Duling v. *Blufield Sanitarium, Inc.*, 148 S.E. 2d 754 (W.Va. 1967)

Medical and Nursing Liability Risk Management

Koch MW and Fairly TM, "Quality Management in Risk Management and Safety," Ch. 7 in *Integrated Quality Management*, Mosby, St. Louis, 1993.

Cohn SD, "Risk Prevention and Management," Ch. 1 in *Malpractice and Liability in Clinical Obstetrical Nursing*, Aspen Publishers, Inc., Rockville, Md., 1990.

Orlifoff JE and Vanagunas AM, *Malpractice Prevention and Liability Control for Hospitals*, American Hospital Publishing, Inc., Chicago, 1988.

American College of Surgeons, *Patient Safety Manual*, ed 2, Chicago, 1985.

Richards EP and Rathbun KC, *Medical Risk Management*, Aspen Systems Corp., Rockville, Md., 1983.

"Filling Out an Incident Report," *Nursing '92* 22(10):17, 1992.

Porter A, "Assuring Quality Through Staff Nurse Performance," *Nurs Clin N Am* 23(9):649, 1988.

Bowyer EA, "Risk Management." In *Legal Issues in Nursing*, Northrop CE and Kelly ME, editors. The C.V. Mosby Co., St. Louis, 1987, pp. 427-440.

Blake P, "Incident Investigation: A Complete Guide," *Nurs Management* 15(11):36, 1984.

Fife DD et al., "A Risk/Falls Program: Code Orange for Success," *Nurs Management* 15(11):50, 1984.

Joseph VD et al., "Incident Reporting: The Cornerstone of Risk Management," *Nurs Management* 15(12):22, 1984.

Press I, "The Predisposition to File Claims: The Patient's Perspective," *Law, Med & Health Care* 12:54, 1984.

Kay Laboratories v. *District Court*, 653 P. 2d 721 (Colo. 1982)

PART EIGHT

MISCELLANEOUS LEGAL MATTERS

Part 8

INTRODUCTORY NOTE

The prime objective of this programmed course is to teach nursing students and graduate nurses about their legal liability for malpractice. There are a number of other legal problem areas, however, that do not pertain to nursing malpractice *per se* but nevertheless directly relate to the daily activities of nurses. Awareness of these problem areas is of particular importance to the nursing student, whose familiarity with the underlying issues and how to cope with them is generally minimal.

The material presented in Part 8 is intended to bridge this information gap in a nonprogrammed format so that it can be a quick-reference source of help when dealing with these nonmalpractice issues. The inherent limitations of both time and space do not permit discussion of still other legal problems that affect the nurse's patient care activities, so nurses who are faced with specific legal problems should not hesitate to contact the hospital's legal counsel or the legal counsel for their state or local nursing association.

MEDICAL RECORDS AND DOCUMENTATION

In Part 3 of this course it was pointed out that one of the nurse's fundamental legal responsibilities is the duty to keep accurate records of the patient's physical and mental condition. The necessity for maintenance of accurate and complete medical records should be evident to all who work in the field of medicine. Such records are an integral and vital adjunct in patient care, providing the connecting links in the chain that extends from the patient's initial treatment for a medical complaint to his or her discharge from treatment after receiving the maximum benefits of care.

Medical records that are kept in a careful manner not only assist in the treatment of the patient—their primary and fundamental purpose—but incidentally can aid materially in the defense of any claim, should a malpractice suit later be instituted. To be of any real value in serving either purpose, all entries in medical records should be clear and legible.

Bearing in mind that medical records may one day be subpoenaed for use in litigation, physicians and nurses must guard against inserting gratuitous or defamatory statements in the patient's chart that might later prove embarrassing in court. Thus, the prudent nurse will avoid the temptation to include in the chart remarks concerning (1) the patient's personality traits or idiosyncracies (unless such remarks are relevant to the patient's treatment), (2) personal views to the effect that the patient is a malingerer or potential litigant, (3) gratuitous admissions of legal liability with respect to untoward medical or nursing events, or (4) otherwise inappropriate comments or observations that simply do not belong in a medical record. One physician, for example, wrote in an elderly patient's chart under "prognosis" the letters PBBB. After the patient died, the family—which had been unhappy with her treatment all along—sued and subpoenaed the patient's chart. When the family's lawyer was told that PBBB stood for "pine box by bedside," the hospital's insurer promptly settled the case out of court for a substantial sum.

Contents

The patient's medical record (or chart) is a written account of his or her illness and course of treatment by all members of the health care team during the patient's stay in the hospital, or by the physician in private practice providing treatment on an outpatient basis. Generally speaking, the medical record has two distinct parts. The first, usually prepared on the patient's admission, merely details the information necessary to identify the patient and to indicate the primary reason for his or her admission. The second part of the record is both dynamic and historic in that it details the clinical history of the patient's course of treatment. The information in this part of the patient's medical record is commonly prescribed by state licensing authorities, supplemented by the hospital's own rules and regulations. Normally it includes the patient's physical history, admitting diagnosis, follow-up diagnoses, temperature chart, therapy and medications prescribed, consultations ordered and the results thereof, x-ray and lab reports, doctor's progress notes, operative procedures performed, nurse's progress notes, signed consent forms (or refusals to execute such forms, properly documented), and similar medical-nursing data.

The failure to record essential information occasionally can have catastrophic consequences. In *Scribner* v. *Hillcrest Medical Center*, 866 P. 2d 437 (Okla. 1994), the facts showed that

Ronda Scribner was placed in Bed B of a semiprivate room following an uncomplicated hysterectomy. The following day, the patient in Bed A was moved to another location, but the hospital staff failed to note the move in its records. Later that morning, an orderly seeking the "Bed A patient" came to the room and informed Ms. Scribner of his intention to take her to the ultrasound laboratory for testing. Despite her repeated protests that she had just come from surgery, was told not to move without direction, and knew of no scheduled test, the orderly persisted without checking the patient's identity with the nursing staff, who had already treated the Bed A patient in her new room. Scribner was placed in a wheelchair and taken in excruciating pain to the laboratory where—only after her continued remonstrations—the laboratory personnel determined Scribner's true identity. Even then, however, the laboratory technicians failed to notify the patient's attending nurses of the error that had been made, nor was any notation made in the patient's chart. Shortly after her discharge from the hospital, Ms. Scribner suffered an incisional dehiscence and hernia, necessitating further surgery. A malpractice suit was filed against the hospital and the jury awarded Scribner 100,000 dollars in actual (compensatory) damages and *10 million dollars* in punitive damages based on the callous indifference of hospital employees, the lackadaisical attitude toward patient identification procedures, and the described reckless and wanton disregard of the patient's rights. Although the punitive damages were later reduced to 5 million dollars, it was a sobering lesson for the defendant hospital and its nursing personnel. Apart from showing some simple humanity towards a patient in obvious emotional and physical distress, prompt and accurate record keeping could have prevented the entire incident and the patient's resulting injuries from occurring.

Alteration of Records

The nurse's charts and notes are an important guide for the physician in diagnosing and prescribing for the patient; hence, they should always be legible, concise, and accurate. Where errors in the chart are noted, they should be corrected promptly and initialed appropriately. Under no circumstances should erroneous records—i.e., those containing inadvertently incorrect information—be removed from the overall record and new pages substituted. Both for ethical and legal reasons the error(s) simply should be noted, corrected, and initialed.

The matter of correcting chart errors raises a related question. In many hospitals there is a mistaken notion that nurses are duty bound to place on the patient's chart *anything the treating physician directs them to place on the chart*, as though it were a direct medical order not subject to challenge. Nothing could be further from the truth. Nurses who accede to the demands of a physician to cover up the true facts of an unusual clinical episode by deliberately not mentioning it in the patient's chart are begging for trouble. Not only will their conduct subject them to possible loss of their licenses, but in flagrant circumstances they may even subject themselves to criminal action, leading to a fine or jail sentence.

Perhaps even worse than altering one's own nursing notes is to tolerate an alteration of those notes by a physician whose sole purpose is to cover up his or her own negligence, which is exactly what happened in *Henry by Henry* v. *St John's Hospital*, 512 N.E. 2d 1044 (Ill. 1987). In that case, the physician, a first-year resident on her first rotation in obstetrics, amended the nursing notes to reflect the administration of a lesser dosage of marcaine to the patient in labor than the patient's physician had actually ordered. When this came out at the trial, the jury rendered a verdict of 10 million dollars for the resultant injuries to the newborn infant, which was upheld on appeal. As pointed out previously, nursing notes should be corrected if the nurse is convinced that an error or omission has occurred and that a correction is appropriate. However, the correction should be made *by the nurse and the nurse alone.*

Hospitalized patients have a legal right to assume not only that adequate health care will be provided, but also that all records relating to that health care will be accurate and truthful. Under no circumstances should the nurse place a doctor's order to falsify or alter a patient's record or delete pertinent information therefrom above a legal and ethical responsibility to record all clinical information truthfully. Also, the nurse should never permit the alteration of nursing notes by a physician seeking to avoid legal liability. When faced with such situations, the prudent nurse should respectfully decline to become an accessory to the doctor's bidding; if pressured further, the nurse should report the circumstances to the appropriate hospital authority without delay.

Countersigning

It has become increasingly common in teaching hospitals, and other hospitals as well, to require that all entries made in patient's charts by licensed practical nurses and nursing students be countersigned by a clinical instructor or other nurse acting in a supervisory capacity. While this practice may be justifiable from the hospital's point of view, it is fraught with legal risks for the nurse who routinely is required to countersign such records.

It should be clearly understood that to countersign a patient's chart is more than to simply add one's signature to a statement made by someone else. The countersigner is actually attesting to the authenticity of the observations and statements made by the original signer. From a legal standpoint, the countersigner is presumed to have personal knowledge of the information contained in the particular record, as though he or she had personally performed the procedure, given the particular medication, or made the specific observation recorded. Later, in a court case, the nurse who has countersigned statements made in the patient's chart can be held jointly liable with the original signer for any negligence traceable to the information so recorded.

The legal lesson is clear. The nurse who is required by hospital policy to countersign on a routine basis documents or information in the patient's chart should protect himself or herself in one of two ways: (1) by personally verifying the information being recorded, or (2) by noting in the record that his or her signature is included in accordance with hospital policy, and is not based on personal knowledge of the information in question.

Confidential Nature of Medical Information

A confidential communication is one that contains information given by one person to another under circumstances of trust and confidence with the understanding that such information must not be disclosed. Clearly, information about a patient—gathered by examination, observation, conversation, or treatment—is the type of confidential information the law has always protected. Thus, both nurses and physicians are legally and morally obligated to keep secret any information about a patient's illness or treatment that is obtained in the normal course of their professional duties. Indeed, the observance of confidentiality is one of the fundamental tenets of the Code for Professional Nurses adopted by the American Nurses Association.

Disclosure of Medical Information

The information contained in the patient's medical record customarily is used for a number of purposes. Those persons involved in the direct care of the patient obviously have a legitimate interest in seeing the chart; hence, there is no breach of confidentiality when the records are made available for this purpose. Medical and nursing personnel may also have occasion to see a patient's chart for the purpose of research, data gathering, or continuing education needs, and here again there is no breach of confidentiality so long as the records are used as intended.

In general, however, if information from a patient's chart is disclosed without the patient's express consent, or without a court order or express statutory authority, the hospital—as well as those who actually made the disclosure—may be held liable in damages should the patient be able to prove invasion of privacy or perhaps defamation of character. Most state statutes expressly require disclosure of medical record information where criminal matters are involved (e.g., attempted suicide, unlawful dispensing of narcotic drugs by a doctor or nurse, evidence of rape or other criminal abuse).

The patient may waive the right to have his or her medical information remain confidential either by actions or words. For example, by bringing a lawsuit in which he or she claims personal-injury damages, an individual thereby waives the right to confidentiality of his or her medical records, since the record will be the principal determinant of the patient's entitlement to damages. Waivers of this sort apply equally to workers' compensation cases and to actions brought against accident and health insurers for benefits due under disability policies. Of course, patients commonly give written consent to the disclosure of medical information to health care insurers, government agencies, prospective employers, and the like. The release of such information under these circumstances poses no question of breach of confidentiality.

Use of Medical Records in Court

Medical records often play an important part in the outcome of legal proceedings such as personal-injury actions, wrongful-death actions, will contests, workers' compensation cases, and so forth. They generally play an important role in determining mental competency in both civil and criminal proceedings. Clearly, in a malpractice action brought against a nurse, the nature and quality of the patient's chart may well prove to be a nurse's main avenue of defense, since it is there that systematic, organized notes reveal how well the nurse observed and reacted to the patient's symptoms.

Why is the medical record so important in a court case? Primarily because it is a contemporaneous record of events—a systematic description of the patient's problems and reactions and responses to treatment, and the judgments made by doctors and nurses concerning the patient's condition and progress. Nurses are with the patient more than any other health care provider and, thus, their documentation may provide the court in a medical or nursing malpractice case with valuable evidence of the patient's condition and the treatment that was provided. Often, nurses' notes are the only evidence to indicate whether the standard of care has been met. Further, since good nursing notes represent the recording of what the nurse has observed and heard first-hand, they can be of great value in determining the patient's state of mind or mental capacity—an issue that assumes great importance in informed consent cases, will contests, and so forth. They can also be of great importance in documenting the patient's lack of obedience to doctor's orders, which may give rise to the defense of contributory negligence.

While statements inserted in the patient's chart are not made under oath and are not self-authenticating, they are given credence by the courts precisely because they represent information and observations recorded at the time the events occurred. The law presumes that record entries of this nature kept in accordance with standard hospital procedures and not in anticipation of any particular legal proceeding are true statements, although this presumption is a rebuttable one. When a nurse is called as a witness in a legal action involving medical treatment in one way or another, he or she is permitted to refresh his or her recollection of the facts and circumstances of the particular case by reference to the patient's medical record. Statements contained in the medical record are not, in themselves, admitted into evidence; but rather, the testimony of the witness concerning the particular event—as reinforced by the medical record—becomes the direct evidence given under oath.

It should be apparent that failure to maintain well-documented medical records may cause great difficulty for nurses who later must defend their actions in malpractice cases. Since it is impossible to anticipate if or when they may have to defend their actions in court, prudent nurses will take pains to maintain medical records that include all matters of significance, favoring the inclusion of more rather than less detail. The attempt to convince a jury that something was or was not done on behalf of the patient several years earlier is more likely to be believed if it is substantiated in the patient's chart.

Some nurses make it a practice to keep a personal record or diary of unusual events that occur in the course of treatment. This can prove extremely helpful in recalling the details of these events should a malpractice case later result. All in all, keeping a diary of this sort is not a bad idea. It is a practice that could prove a boon to the nurse who may become involved in such litigation.

INVASION OF PRIVACY

Although the U.S. Constitution doesn't explicitly sanction a right to privacy, the Supreme Court in a number of landmark cases has recognized the distinct right of every person to withhold his or her person, personality, and property from unwarranted public scrutiny. In addition, 10 states have written some type of privacy provision into their constitutions, and all states have recognized the right to privacy either through statutes or common law decisions. This right of privacy includes the freedom to live one's life without having one's name, photograph, or private affairs made public against one's will. The legal concept of the patient's right of privacy—now an integral part of the Patient's Bill of Rights published by the American Hospital Association—is one with which every nurse should become familiar, since even a negligent violation thereof can have serious legal consequences.

All members of the health care team are duty bound to treat patients with decency, respect, and the greatest degree of privacy possible. At the very least, the patient should be seen, examined, and handled only by those persons directly involved in his or her care and treatment. Unnecessary exposure of the patient' body or unwarranted discussion of his or her case with third parties will give rise to a legal cause of action for invasion of privacy, with appropriate damages assessed against the offending party. The nurse must always be alert to any witting or unwitting violation of the patient's right of privacy.

On a practical level, patients who are moved through hospital corridors or into examining or treatment rooms always should be covered and not exposed unnecessarily to other hospital personnel, patients, or visitors. The careful nurse likewise will guard against such exposure in wards and shared rooms. We have already discussed the matter of the confidential nature of the information in the patient's chart. It bears repeating at this point that the nurse has both an ethical and a legal duty not to reveal confidential and personal information about the patient to unauthorized parties.

The publication of the patient's picture in a newspaper or magazine or showing it on videotape without his or her consent is also an invasion of privacy, and the person who permits such invasion is answerable in damages to the offended party. In an early New York case, *Griffin v. Medical Society of the State of New York*, 11 N.Y.S. 2d 109 (1939), plastic surgeons who had taken photographs of the patient before a rhinoplasty published four of the photos in the society's journal without obtaining the patient's permission and were held liable in damages for invasion of privacy. More recently, a California jury awarded 274,000 dollars in emotional distress damages to a patient whose name, photograph, and medical records were included without permission in a public relations brochure distributed by the hospital (*Banks* v. *Charter Hospital of Long Beach*, as reported in *Medical Malpractice Verdicts, Settlements & Experts*, 8[10]:19 [1992]).

Another type of invasion of privacy is the deliberate announcement of publication of information that, although not defamatory in nature, compromises the ordinary decencies to which all private persons are entitled. Thus, publishing or permitting to be published information about a patient's medical condition without the patient's permission is not just a breach of confidentiality but a basis for holding the offending health personnel liable in an invasion of privacy lawsuit. For example, in *Doe v. Roe*, 345 N.Y.S. 2d 560 (N.Y. 1973), a psychoanalyst was charged with violating the patient's right to privacy by writing a book in which the patient's entire case history was outlined, with only the feeblest attempt made to conceal her identity. In addition to compensatory damages, the court granted a permanent injunction against further sale of the book.

The right of privacy rule is relaxed somewhat where the individual in question is considered a "public figure" whose activities (whether hospitalized or not) are considered to be of legitimate interest to the public. Even so, the prudent nurse will follow hospital rules and regulations with respect to allowing reporters, photographers, television crews, or others to enter the patient's room to interview, photograph, or videotape the patient without his or her consent.

There are certain clear-cut exceptions to the right of privacy, one of which—the public-figure situation—we have already mentioned. Other exceptions include the duty to report communicable diseases, child-abuse cases, gunshot wounds, and other such matters to the appropriate law enforcement authorities. There can be no penalty for regarding privacy rights for doing what the law requires in these instances.

In conclusion, when entering a hospital, a patient places the integrity of his or her person and reputation in the hands of all health care personnel who attend him or her; personnel must always be aware of their legal and ethical responsibility to preserve and protect the patient's right to privacy.

REPORTING CHILD ABUSE

Throughout the 1960s and early 1970s public attention began to focus more intently on the problem of the physically abused or neglected child in U.S. society, a problem that previously had been considered of only minor significance. We know today that the number of reported cases of child abuse has not only increased markedly in the past 2 decades, but that most abused children are young and literally "battered babies." A major study in Denver, for example, indicated that 33.7% of the children abused were under 1 year of age, 56% were under 3 years, and 68% were under 5 years. Even though physicians had been aware of the problem for years, most failed to report their clinical findings of child abuse to the police or other appropriate authorities either out of fear of incurring civil or criminal liability or because they felt that such reporting would amount to meddling.

Eventually the problem attracted national attention, and following congressional hearings in 1973, the Child Abuse Prevention and Treatment Act of 1973 was enacted into law. This statute requires the states to meet certain federal standards in order to qualify for federal grant assistance in setting up state child abuse-prevention programs. One of the federal requirements was the mandatory reporting of abuse and neglect of minor children to the appropriate state and local authorities—usually the local welfare agency, department of social and rehabilitation services, or law enforcement agency. Following enactment of the federal statute, all of the states passed child abuse laws. Under these laws, failure of the nurse to report child abuse may lead to criminal and civil liability. In addition, failure to report a case of child abuse may make the physician or nurse liable for civil damages in a malpractice case.

Clearly, the success of any child abuse-prevention program depends on the early reporting of suspect child abuse or neglect cases. As noted previously, there was a time when physicians and nurses had good reason to avoid alerting the authorities, since the child's parents could bring suit claiming both an invasion of their privacy and defamation of their character. With passage of the Child Abuse Prevention and Treatment Act of 1973, however, state statutes almost uniformly granted protection (immunity) from suit to persons reporting suspected child abuse cases in good faith. Many of these statutes specifically mention nurses as being within the protection of the good-faith reporting requirements.

The various state laws differ in their definitions of abuse and neglect, as well as with respect to who is considered a child or minor in the eyes of the law. They also differ in their requirements about who must report suspected child abuse and to whom the reports must be made. A few states actually impose a penalty on certain categories of persons for failing to report suspected child abuse. In general, however, the laws call for the reporting of all cases in which a child has sustained serious physical injury inflicted by other than accidental means by either a parent or other person responsible for the child's welfare. Sexual abuse is included within the reporting requirements of a number of the states. Finally, as is discussed more fully in the material immediately following, Congress amended the Child Abuse Prevention and Treatment Act in 1984 to assure greater protection of the rights of severely handicapped newborns.

Nurses should become familiar with the child abuse-reporting requirements for their own states, including the procedures established within their own hospitals for making such reports. It goes without saying that the nurse who handles pediatric emergencies should be especially alert to the possibility of child abuse when confronted with unusual traumatic injuries to children—dislocations, head injuries, unusual burns, and so on—that are not readily explainable or seem to occur with greater than normal frequency. The conscientious nurse should look at the statutory reporting requirement as an opportunity to save the life or preserve the health of a defenseless child, not as a disagreeable bureaucratic waste of time.

HANDICAPPED NEWBORNS AND THE "BABY DOE" REGULATIONS

Closely related to the problem of child abuse is the enormously complex legal, ethical, social, and philosophical problem arising out of decisions by parents and doctors to withhold medical treatment from seriously handicapped newborns with life-threatening conditions. In 1982, under the Reagan Administration, the federal government attempted to intervene in this decision-making process in order to prevent such withholding of treatment, but its efforts were stymied at every turn.

What prompted the Administration's unprecedented intrusion into this area of social concern—a crusade it espoused with almost religious fervor—was the widely publicized case of "Baby Doe," an infant born in April of 1982 with Down's syndrome and a detached esophagus. The parents, in conjunction with the doctors, decided not to attempt correction of the infant's intestinal blockage with surgery, but the hospital sought court intervention to protect the rights of the infant. While the matter was being challenged in court, the baby died of starvation, but the public hue and cry at what had occurred did not end with the baby's death.

It was in the aftermath of this case that the Administration, acting through the Department of Health and Human Resources (HHS), attempted to invoke the sanctions of section 504 of the Rehabilitation Act of 1973 (the Rehabilitation Act) on behalf of handicapped newborns and it did so by hastily promulgating regulations—commonly referred to as the "Baby Doe Regulations"—that authorized HHS to investigate cases of alleged medical discrimination against "otherwise qualified" handicapped infants in federally funded hospitals. Under the regulations, any person working in such a hospital "having knowledge that a handicapped infant is being discriminatorily denied food or customary medical care" was directed to call a Handicapped Infant Hotline number in Washington, D.C., to report the circumstances. The regulations made it very clear that the withholding of treatment from infants with life-threatening but treatable conditions was a federal offense.

The Baby Doe regulations were immediately challenged in court and were struck down as arbitrary and capricious (*American Academy of Pediatrics* v. *Heckler*, 561 F. Supp. 395 [D.C. 1983]). HHS reacted to the court's ruling by proposing a new set of regulations dealing with discrimination against handicapped newborns in federally funded facilities. While comments were being received on the newly proposed regulations, a second "Baby Doe" case came to light in October, 1983, and it received extraordinary press and television coverage. This case involved a female infant (Baby Jane Doe) born with spina bifida and hydrocephalus in a New York hospital, and again the parents chose not to proceed with surgery to mitigate these life-threatening conditions.

A Vermont lawyer who was a right-to-life activist filed suit in the New York court to contest the denial of surgery and request his appointment as the infant's guardian. After extensive litigation, the New York Court of Appeals affirmed dismissal of the lawyer's suit on the basis that he lacked legal standing to bring the action (*Weber* v. *Stony Brook Hospital*, 469 N.Y.S. 2d 63 [N.Y. 1983]). The next day, HHS, acting on an anonymous report from the hospital that section 504 of the Rehabilitation Act was not being complied with, requested the hospital records on Baby Jane Doe to investigate the allegation further. When the hospital declined to release the records, the federal government sued to obtain them, but the government's suit was dismissed on the basis that, since there was no evidence of any discrimination under section 504, the federal government had no right to the records (*U.S.* v. *University Hospital of SUNY at Stony Brook*, 575 F. Supp. 607 [N.Y. 1983]). The government appealed, but the lower court's decision was sustained, and in its decision, the Second Circuit Court of Appeals held that although Baby Jane Doe was a "handicapped individual," section 504 of the Rehabilitation Act simply did not apply to her (*U.S.* v. *University Hospital of SUNY at Stony Brook*, 729 F. 2d 144 [2nd Cir. 1984]).

Meanwhile, HHS had issued its new regulations—also predicated on hospital compliance with section 504 of the Rehabilitation Act—and this time the regulations were not only successfully challenged, but were invalidated by the court (*American Hospital Association* v. *Heckler*, 585 F. Supp. 541 [N.Y. 1984]). The Justice Department appealed the case all the way up to the U.S. Supreme Court, which in 1986 upheld the lower court decisions invalidating the "Baby Doe" regulations (*Bowen* v. *American Hospital Association*, 106 S. Ct. 2101 [1986]). This decision effectively stalled the government's efforts to intrude directly in the decision-making processes where parents and medical personnel have to decide whether or not to withhold treatment from severely handicapped infants.

Recognizing the ineffectiveness of utilizing the Rehabilitation Act as the appropriate legislative mechanism for coercing doctors and hospitals to treat even the most severely handicapped newborns, Congress passed the Child Abuse Amendments of 1984, which directed the states, as a condition of receiving federal child abuse funds, to consider the withholding of medically indicated treatment from handicapped infants as medical neglect, and directing investigations into such matters by the states. It is far from clear how future cases involving handicapped newborns will be resolved, but all nurses, particularly those who work in neonatal units, should be aware of the potential liability that may exist for nontreatment of handicapped newborns under pertinent federal and state child abuse statutes and regulations. When faced with an actual situation in which the doctors and parents have chosen to withhold treatment, the prudent nurse in the neonatal unit should not hesitate to seek the immediate advice of the hospital's legal counsel as to the proper course of action.

REPORTING OF ELDER AND SPOUSE ABUSE

At the time of writing, the nation is transfixed by the virtually nonstop television and print media coverage of the O.J. Simpson double-murder trial in Los Angeles. Whether O.J. Simpson did in fact murder his ex-wife and a male companion on the scene is still undetermined, but the fact that a national sports hero battered and terrorized his wife over a span of years and ultimately may have murdered her has, at long last, focused national attention on the burgeoning problem of domestic violence and spousal abuse. Criminal justice statistics consistently show that about 95% of domestic violence victims are women, many of whom suffer from lack of self-esteem and behave passively, making it easier for their spouses to abuse them repeatedly without fear of retaliation. While spousal abuse generally takes the form of physical violence, elderly abuse is often accompanied by psychological abuse, threats, denial of essential human needs (such as withholding of food), financial exploitation, and general medical neglect. Several research studies have revealed that abuse of persons over 65 years of age occurs almost as often as abuse of children.

To address the problems of elder and spouse abuse, nearly all the states have enacted laws establishing intervention mechanisms to protect these victims of domestic violence. Most of these laws authorize the issuance of civil injunctions or restraining orders against the abuser. The abuser who disobeys the restraining order can be held in criminal contempt and may be punished by being fined, imprisoned, or both. Some statutes also authorize (and pay for) the temporary removal of the victim from the residence where the abuse has occurred.

All nurses should become familiar with the pertinent reporting laws of their own states, as well as the public agencies assigned primary responsibility for dealing with elder and spouse abuse. Nurses who customarily work in the home setting (e.g., community health nurses, visiting nurses, and home-care nurses) should be particularly alert to the signs and symptoms of abuse within the family. As with child abuse, trained nurses should have little difficulty recognizing the obvious physical symptoms of bruises, welts, sprains, and fractures, but they should also be perceptive of less obvious symptoms of psychogenic origin, such as gastrointestinal disorders, choking sensations, acute back pain, or constant headaches.

Few victims of abuse by family members will readily admit their plight to an outsider because of fear of reprisal by the family member-abuser. Thus, the conscientious nurse must act with courage in these matters, making the necessary inquiries and showing the degree of compassion and support for which these difficult situations always call. As in the case of child abuse-reporting statutes, a nurse's official report of elder or spouse abuse is a privileged communication and will not subject him or her to any legal action by the family member or spouse reported to the authorities as the abuser.

PATIENTS' RIGHTS, INCLUDING THE RIGHT OF SELF-DETERMINATION

Within recent years, much has been written about the concept of patients' rights in the health care field. These basic rights focus on human dignity, privacy, confidentiality, informed consent, and refusal of treatment. (We discussed the latter two at length in Part 4 of this course and cover invasion of privacy and confidentiality in this part.) The patients' rights movement evolved from significant changes in attitudes regarding health care in the 1960s and gained momentum with the advent and growth of the consumer movement in general. The 1973 *Report of the Secretary's Commission on Medical Malpractice* (U.S. Department of Health, Education & Welfare) gave further impetus to the concept of patients' rights by specifically advocating the development of patient grievance mechanisms and hospital-based ombudsmen.

Since those early stages, much has happened in this area of health care. For one thing, increasing interest in patients' rights has led many hospitals to employ full-time patient service representatives or ombudsmen who mediate between the patient and the hospital when a patient is dissatisfied with some aspect of his or her treatment. (We discuss this issue at length in the following section.) In addition, a host of written documents—some legislative, others not—have clarified the basic rights of individuals with regard to their receipt of health care in various clinical and home settings. As of today, a patient's bill of rights has been promulgated by numerous health care organizations, including the American Hospital Association, the American Civil Liberties Union, the Hospice Association of America, the American Nurses Association, and the National League for Nursing. Although the bills of rights issued by these various bodies aren't legally binding, practically speaking they set the standards for patients' rights by which court cases are or will be judged. Moreover, hospitals that violate or ignore patients' rights may jeopardize their federal funding under Medicare and Medicaid. Giving strength to the latter was the inclusion within the Omnibus Budget Reconciliation Act of 1990 of the Patient Self-Determination Act, 42 U.S.C. § 1395cc(a)(1). This law provides that, in order to receive federal funding under Medicare and Medicaid, hospitals, skilled nursing facilities, home health care agencies, and hospice programs must maintain written policies and procedures governing advance directives and the patient's right to accept or refuse treatment. Hospitals now are specifically required to inform patients of their right to refuse treatment if they are incapacitated, and must note in the patient's chart if the patient has, in writing, rejected various forms of life support. Needless to say, all professional nurses should become familiar with the rights of patients as set forth in the patient's bill of rights applicable in their own institutions and should adhere to them meticulously.

THE NURSE AS THE PATIENT'S ADVOCATE

Within recent years, much has been written about the role of the professional nurse as the patient's advocate, with a wide variety of perspectives as to what advocacy is and how it should be implemented. Some writers, for example, have suggested that the nurse's advocacy role should be that of mediator and intermediary between the patient and various health care providers to resolve conflicting interests between the parties. Others have suggested that the nurse's advocacy role should be that of protector of the patient's right to self-determination, specifically the right to make autonomous choices and decisions. However, everyone agrees that the nurse must be an advocate for patient safety, a role that is consonant with the fundamental purpose and thrust of professional nursing care.

In 1985, the American Nurses Association set forth in its revised Code for Nurses the following fairly comprehensive vision of the nurse as patient advocate:

> Since clients themselves are the primary decision makers in matters concerning their own health, treatment, and well-being, the goal of nursing actions is to support and enhance the client's responsibility and self-determination to the greatest extent possible.

Truth telling and the process of reaching informed choice underlie the exercise of self-determination, which is basic to respect for persons.

The nurse's primary commitment is to the health, welfare and safety of the client. As an advocate for the client, the nurse must be alert to and take appropriate action regarding any instances of incompetent, unethical or illegal practice by any member of the health care team or the health care system, or any action on the part of others that places the rights or best interests of the client in jeopardy.

In its broadest sense, advocacy is the act of defending or pleading the case or cause of another. As related to nursing care, the term most often is used to describe the nurse as an actor or intercessor on behalf of the patient. It is in this sense that advocacy takes on important legal overtones. As mentioned throughout this course, the nurse has the legal responsibility to safeguard the patient at all times. Moreover, it is deemed negligent conduct for a nurse to fail to do what other reasonable and prudent nurses would have done under similar circumstances; hence, a nurse's failure to report a dangerous practice, or incompetence, or negligence of another member of the health care team, is negligence by omission and represents a clear basis for holding the nurse liable for malpractice.

Understanding the concept of advocacy is considerably easier than understanding how it should be implemented. Nurses who choose to become advocates of patients' rights must be willing to take risks while espousing such rights. More often than not, the nurse is part of a larger organization such as a hospital, clinic, or nursing facility—environments in which the threats to patient safety may arise from a variety of sources including prescribed treatments, physical abuse of patients, unsafe equipment, inadequate staffing patterns, or illegal or unethical conduct of nurses or other professional colleagues. Deciding how to protect the patient's rights under these circumstances is never easy, since it places the nurse in the position of an informer or whistle blower, types not particularly admired in our society. To make matters even more difficult, there is always the possibility that the accused colleague might later sue the nurse for defamation of character, or that the accused institution will take steps to bring about the nurse's immediate discharge. Actually, retaliation of some sort is almost inevitable when a nurse blows the whistle in an effort to protect either a single patient or all patients in a particular health care facility.

Consider what happened in the following case to a head nurse employed in a private psychiatric hospital in Illinois where a special treatment program was in progress in the hospital's Orthomolecular Unit. When a patient in that unit told the nurse he wanted to end his voluntary participation in the program, she communicated this information to the physician in charge of the program. The physician became furious and threatened to have the patient committed involuntarily, information that the nurse passed along to her supervisor, together with her statement that she fully supported the patient's position.

Subsequently, the patient contacted the State Guardianship and Advocacy Commission, which ordered an immediate investigation into the matter. During the investigation, the nurse made a call from her home to the Commission, speaking to a Commission employee about various rights violations and patient care issues at the facility. Several days later, the nurse was advised by the administrator of the hospital, in the presence of the director of nursing, that she was relieved of her duties. The nurse filed an action against the hospital seeking damages for wrongful termination, claiming that the termination was solely for the reasons stated. A verdict in favor of the nurse was appealed by the hospital to the Appellate Court of Illinois, which affirmed the lower court's finding that the termination was due solely to the fact that the nurse had provided information to the Commission and not because of any apparent deficiencies in her work. Financial compensation was awarded to her; however, the court felt it would be imprudent to compel her reinstatement in view of the circumstances that led to her discharge (*Witt, R.N.* v. *Forest Hospital, et al.*, 450 N.E. 2d 811 [Ill. 1983]).

Advocacy of another sort occurred in a much discussed 1979 Idaho case. Jolene Tuma was a clinical instructor of nursing who had a special interest in the needs of dying patients. She responded to a leukemia patient's questions regarding alternatives to proposed cancer chemotherapy after the patient was told the side effects of the drugs used in such therapy. Laetrile and natural foods and herbs were among the alternatives mentioned, and the patient requested that Nurse Tuma share this information with her family when they came to visit her that evening. The ordered chemotherapy was begun, but after a family member who had talked with Tuma that evening called the doctor and informed him of nurse Tuma's discussions regarding treatment alternatives, the doctor ordered the chemotherapy stopped. Following further discussion with the patient and the family the next day, however, chemotherapy was resumed. The patient died 2 weeks later.

Although no one contended that Nurse Tuma's actions in any way contributed to the patient's death, the Board of Nursing received a complaint from the physician and the hospital alleging that Nurse Tuma had interfered with the physician-patient relationship and that her actions constituted unprofessional conduct. After a hearing, Tuma's license was suspended for 6 months. On appeal, the Supreme Court of Idaho restored her license, stating that the license could not be revoked simply because she had engaged in a discussion with the patient and the family concerning alternative treatment modalities. The court noted that Nurse Tuma could not be found guilty of unprofessional conduct in the absence of written guidelines or regulations specifically defining "unprofessional conduct" under Idaho's Nurse Practice Act (*Tuma* v. *Board of Nursing*, 593 P. 2d 711 [Ida. 1979]).

As these cases and others reflect, actions taken by nurses (acting as whistle blowers or patient advocates) to protect their patients against unsafe health care practices or to assist them in matters of self-determination or health care decision making are seldom accomplished without reprisals of one sort or another. In the first described case, the nurse was discharged from her employment, while in the second case the nurse had her license suspended by the state licensing board. One of the more common forms of retaliation is a lawsuit for defamation of character brought by the colleague who has been reported as incompetent or whose actions are otherwise alleged to be harmful to the patient.

To defame someone is to say something about him or her that will tend to injure his or her reputation. It is called *libel* when it is done in writing, and *slander* when the statement is made orally. To be actionable at law, either manner of defaming someone must be communicated to a third person. For example, it would not be slander for a nurse to make a contemptuous remark about a nurse or physician to that person alone, but it would be if the remark was made in the presence of a third person. In general, however, any slanderous or libelous statement that impugns a person in his or her professional capacity is deemed actionable without having to prove any specific damages.

The law has long provided a form of immunity against a charge of libel or slander when the person making the allegedly libelous or slanderous statement has a legal duty to report honestly on the performance of another in carrying out his or her professional responsibilities. This immunity is *qualified privilege*, and it legally negates any inference of malice on the part of the person making the libelous or slanderous statement because of the overriding public policy interest. Where the quality of medical care is concerned, the courts have held that the reputation rights of health care professionals must give way to the greater social need.

Hospitals have always had the legal responsibility to make certain that incompetent doctors and nurses are not hired or permitted to remain on their staffs, and thus, the immunity afforded by the doctrine of qualified privilege is critical to the entire personnel staffing and review process in hospitals. As pointed out earlier, both under common law principles and under the American Nurses Association's Code for Nurses, nurses have an ethical obligation to safeguard their patients against the incompetent, unethical, or illegal practices of any person. Hence, the nurse may rely on the qualified privilege against defamation when providing negative information about a co-employee or attending physician as long as the statements made are communicated pursuant to established institutional policy and through the designated reporting channels. By contrast, idle gossip about a fellow worker that reflects on his or her professional capabilities or motives, even if true, does not fall within the protection of the qualified privilege doctrine.

Procedurally, it is wise to report unsafe practices or colleague incompetence to one's immediate supervisor. "Going public" should be a last resort when everything else has failed to produce the desired result. The nurse who chooses this route should be emotionally prepared for all the negative consequences that may befall whistle blowers including harassment from supervisors and peers, verbal abuse, denial of job-related requests, demotions, firing and forced retirement.

WITNESSING WILLS

A will is a legal declaration of how one wishes to dispose of one's property upon death, as well as who is to administer the estate. Sometimes it also indicates who should act as a guardian for the testator's (will maker's) minor children. The desirability of preparing a will is beyond question, since it enables the testator to decide how his or her real and personal property is to be distributed after his or her death. When one dies without a valid will, one is said to die intestate, and under these circumstances the property will pass to family members (and sometimes even to the state) in accordance with the state's intestacy succession law—often in a manner that the individual would not have wanted. In addition, the costs of administering an estate invariably are greater when an individual dies intestate.

In the course of a nursing career a nurse will probably be asked on at least one occasion to be a witness to a patient's last will and testament. Indeed, a patient may even request that a nurse prepare the will in accordance with his or her instructions. Since these matters are not normally covered in nursing school, the following is presented as a general guide and source of information in these circumstances.

We begin with the proposition that unless you are named as a beneficiary therein there is nothing unethical or improper about being a witness to someone's last will simply because that person happens to be a patient under your care. In fact, agreeing to be a witness to a will can be a source of great comfort to the patient, since the desire to dispose of one's property in a planned and organized manner before one dies often presses heavily on persons who have delayed in dealing with this issue. However, refusing to be a witness to a patient's will—unless the nurse is named as a beneficiary—violates no rule or standard of conduct, and a nurse may legally refuse to do so without incurring any penalty therefor.

Preparing versus Witnessing

A will is an extremely important legal document whose preparation requires competent legal advice if it is to carry out the testator's intentions effectively. Unless a nurse has had legal training and has been admitted to the bar, he or she should not undertake to advise a patient in the drawing up of his or her will. To do so would constitute the unauthorized practice of law: a nurse has no more right to practice law without a license than to practice medicine without a license. When asked to give such advice, the nurse should respectfully decline and suggest that the patient contact a lawyer instead. Should the patient need help in finding one, the hospital's legal counsel can provide the names of local attorneys.

As mentioned earlier, it is perfectly proper, and perhaps even desirable, for the nurse to act as a *witness* to the signing of the patient's will, particularly since the nurse would be amply qualified to testify about the patient's physical and mental condition at the time of the signing should that issue arise at the time the will is offered for probate. Incidentally, when witnessing the execution of a patient's will, a nurse does not thereby attest to the wisdom of the patient's testamentary dispositions. Indeed, more than likely, he or she will not even know what those dispositions are, since the testator is not legally required to disclose them to the persons witnessing the will signing. By signing as a witness, the nurse merely attests that the patient signed a document that stated to be his or her last will and further attests to the patient's apparent soundness of mind and appreciation of the significance of his or her actions.

Legalities Associated with Wills

State laws are very specific concerning the formalities associated with the making of wills; if the statutory requirements are not met, a purported will may prove invalid, which is why a nurse should not presume to advise a patient concerning the preparation of a will. On the other hand, since nurses frequently attend patients who know that death is imminent and who sincerely desire to make proper disposition of their property, a nurse should be at least generally familiar with what the law requires so as to be able to explain to the patient the importance of getting legal assistance without delay.

Certain statutory requirements for the making of wills are virtually universal. Thus, in all states the testator must have testamentary capacity; that is, he or she must be sufficiently sound of mind to know the nature of the property and how he or she proposes to dispose of it. In short, the individual must be able to understand and appreciate the significance of what he or she is about to do. In addition, the law also requires that the testator be free from fraud, external coercion, or other undue influence at the time the will is made. If it can be shown that the testator was tricked into signing the will, or that someone close to the individual exercised pressure of some sort to force him or her to make a particular bequest, the probate court will consider the will or a part of it invalid. Obviously, a nurse who is requested to witness the execution of a will should decline to do so if there is any concern about the mental capacity of the patient.

Ordinarily a will must be in writing and must be witnessed *exactly* in accordance with the particular state law's formal signing requirements. In most states the testator must sign the will in the presence of all the witnesses (usually two or three disinterested persons) and must simultaneously declare aloud that the document he or she is signing is his or her last will and testament. The witnesses then must sign *in the testator's presence and in the presence of each other.* Any deviation from the statutory will-signing requirements can later prove disastrous, which is one of the principal reasons why it is preferable to have a lawyer not only prepare the document but also see to its proper execution.

Nearly every state law provides that the witnessing of a will by someone who is named as a beneficiary therein may void the disposition to that beneficiary—particularly if there are not a sufficient number of *disinterested* witnesses to satisfy the legal signing requirements. Thus, nurses who know that patients have made bequests to them in their wills must never agree to sign the wills as witnesses. Once again, a lawyer's presence at the will signing would guarantee that mistakes of this kind are not made.

Some states permit a testator to prepare a holographic will—one that is entirely handwritten by the testator and properly dated. In these states, a holographic will need not be attested to by subscribing witnesses. If the state in question does not recognize holographic wills, the testator's efforts to dispose of his or her property by means of a handwritten document will have been in vain. Accordingly, the nonlawyer nurse should hesitate to offer legal advice concerning the preparation of a will.

Finally, a few states recognize what is known as a nuncupative or oral will, where the proposed disposition of his or her property by one contemplating imminent death is stated orally in the presence of one or more witnesses and is reduced to writing immediately thereafter. A nurse who has been asked by a patient *in extremis* (at the point of death) to record his or her intentions concerning the disposition of property should do so faithfully, and should promptly forward the written memorandum of those intentions to the hospital administrator who should, in turn, notify the patient's family.

ADVANCE DIRECTIVES—LIVING WILLS

As all nurses know, advancements in medical and scientific technology have made it possible to keep alive patients who would not have survived previously. These advances have brought with them, however, a whole range of philosophical, legal, and ethical questions concerning the rights of individuals (or persons acting on their behalf) to refuse life-sustaining treatment. Following the national attention stirred up by the Karen Quinlan case, *In re Quinlan*, 355 A. 2d 647 (N.J. 1976), and the Saikewicz case, *Superintendent of Belchertown State School* v. *Saikewicz*, 370 N.E. 2d 417 (Mass. 1978), many state legislatures began considering passage of so-called right-to die laws—laws recognizing the right of competent adults to choose to die in dignity rather than be kept alive by means of artificial life-sustaining devices and procedures. Normally this choice is made by execution of a "living will," a formal document in which a person who has no reasonable expectation of recovery from an illness requests that he or she be allowed to die rather than be kept alive by artificial means or heroic, life-prolonging procedures. As a consequence, more than three fourths of the states and the District of Columbia now have such laws, and others are actively considering such legislation.

Nurses who have occasion to treat terminally ill patients are likely to encounter some who have previously executed living wills, and others who may express a desire to prepare one while hospitalized. Thus, it is important to understand the legal implications of such documents and the practical issues they present.

Although the right-to-die statutes vary greatly, in general they provide that persons over 18 years of age and of sound mind may execute a formal document declaring an intent not to be kept alive through artificial life-sustaining procedures and directing the withholding or withdrawal of such measures should they be in a terminal condition. The statutes spell out who may (or may not) be witness to such a "living will," and sometimes even mandate the actual form to be used. In addition, these laws customarily set forth the circumstances in which the will is to become effective, often stating that it does not apply until the patient "has been diagnosed and certified in writing to be afflicted with a terminal condition by two physicians who have personally examined the patient, one of whom shall be the attending physician." Finally, all of these laws provide immunity from civil or criminal liability to the health care personnel who actually withhold or withdraw treatment from patients who have executed such wills.

Under no circumstances is a living will a substitute for the express wishes of a competent adult, however old he or she may be, since the law has always given such persons the absolute right to refuse medical treatment for any reason. Thus, a patient's previously executed living will comes into play only when he or she is seriously ill and is no longer physically or mentally competent to make his or her wishes known. Moreover, once a living will exists, it may be revoked at any time by physical destruction, written revocation, or an oral declaration indicating the desire to revoke it. The nurse should understand that many of the state laws make the terms of a living will binding on the medical and nursing personnel who attend the patient, even though they may not mention any specific penalty for noncompliance. Accordingly, there should be little or no concern for legal repercussions where it is clear all the formalities have been followed.

What about the effectiveness of living wills in states that have not enacted such laws? Most legal commentators believe courts will be inclined to find them applicable, since there is no public policy against refusal of treatment by a terminally ill patient, and a living will is a clear expression of the patient's desires. Certainly, if a patient has gone to the trouble of executing such a formal document or wants assistance in preparing one, there is every reason to comply with his or her wishes. Before undertaking to assist a patient who wishes to execute a living will, however, a nurse should be reasonably familiar with the statutory requirements for preparing living wills in the particular jurisdiction (if any) or the formal requirements for the execution and witnessing of regular wills in that state. It would be advisable to check the hospital's or nursing home's guidelines on these matters before proceeding too far. The reader is referred to the material on witnessing of wills preceding this discussion.

From a practical standpoint, the nurse should understand that he or she is under a legal obligation to bring the existence of a living will to the attention of the treating physician(s) and other health care personnel treating the patient. The same is true for a patient's revocation of his or her living will. Both circumstances should be clearly recorded in the patient's chart—with a copy of the will itself, where one exists.

The legal counsel for the hospital, nursing home, or other treatment facility should be consulted regarding possibly ambiguous terms and conditions laid down in a patient's living will, and there should be no withholding or withdrawal of treatment until such matters are legally resolved. Finally, the nurse should understand that "do not resuscitate" orders based on the patient's express wishes, whether in a living will or otherwise, and properly signed by the treating physician, are legally valid and should be followed.

ADVANCE DIRECTIVES—DURABLE POWERS OF ATTORNEY

As health care practitioners and lawyers have gained more experience with living wills, they have recognized some inherent limitations in the use of such documents. Statutes authorizing living wills must be followed to the letter, which inevitably creates legal problems for those who have to make extremely difficult medical decisions on behalf of terminally ill relatives. For one thing, no living will, no matter how broadly worded, can possibly anticipate the full range of medical decisions to be made. In addition, living-will legislation has been notoriously ineffective in guaranteeing patients' rights—particularly where (as in California) only a patient diagnosed as terminally ill can execute an advance directive, and then must wait 14 days before the directive becomes operative. Finally, the courts in states without living-will laws have not been in agreement in their willingness to recognize living wills.

Thus, while the living will undoubtedly represents an affirmative step toward assuring that the patient's wishes are honored during a serous illness, it may not be sufficient to cover all major contingencies and, indeed, in some states may not be honored at all. These problems can be overcome in large part by the use of a document known as a durable power of attorney. Just as nurses who treat terminally ill patients should be familiar with the legal aspects of living wills, they should also have a basic understanding of the concept of the durable power of attorney, and particularly how such documents are used in making critical health care decisions.

At common law, a power of attorney is an agency relationship between the creator of the power, called the principal, and the holder of the power, called the agent. What is important to understand is that, under common law, the agent's authority terminates upon the death or *incapacity* of the principal. Thus, the usefulness of a standard power of attorney whereby an agent is appointed to make vital health care decisions on behalf of his or her principal would be lost at precisely the time it is most needed. To correct this situation, the legislature of a number of states, including California, Delaware, and Colorado, have adopted to one degree or another the Uniform Durable Power of Attorney Act. This model law sanctions the right of an individual to give another person a *durable* power of medical treatment decision making—one that can be exercised even while the principal is incapacitated and legally incompetent to act on his or her own behalf.

Under the typical durable power of attorney statute, the appointed agent may make medical care decisions on behalf of an incompetent (generally incapacitated) principal as an extension of the principal's right to determine his or her own medical treatment. This power includes the right to ask questions, assess risks and costs, select and remove physicians, seek the opinions of family members and other physicians, and select the preferred treatment from a variety of therapeutic options including the option to refuse life-sustaining treatment entirely. Health care providers are protected from liability if they rely in good faith on the authority of the agent. The California statute specifically provides, however, that the physician must first attempt to communicate with the patient and then note in the medical record that obtaining an informed consent from him or her is impossible.

An agent acting under a durable power of attorney has the legal authority to *enforce* the patient's treatment preferences (by going into court) to make sure they are not disregarded either by family members or physicians. Most living wills, on the other hand, are advisory at best and can be (and often have been) disregarded. The appointment of a clearly designated agent also provides the hospital, physician(s), and other health care personnel with a measure of legal protection they do not have where a living will is involved or where the physician must seek the informal consent of the patient's spouse or relatives. In short, the durable power of attorney constitutes the best form of "substituted judgment" available for an otherwise incapacitated patient.

It is highly unlikely that nurses employed by a hospital, nursing home, sanitarium, or other comparable medical treatment facility will become directly involved in deciding whether to follow the directives of duly appointed agents acting under a durable power of attorney. They should understand, however, that this legal mechanism is perfectly appropriate where sanctioned by the state's law. Here, again, the attorney representing the hospital, clinic, sanitarium, or nursing home should be consulted for authoritative advice regarding the status of local law.

ADVANCE DIRECTIVES—THE MEDICAL OR PHYSICIAN'S DIRECTIVE

Another form of advance directive is one that lists various treatments from resuscitation to antibiotic injection and lets patients indicate whether they want each treatment, in scenarios that range from irreversible coma to whatever the patient's condition may be when adopting the directive. This type of directive—often referred to as a medical directive or physician's directive—differs from a living will in that it enables patients to indicate the treatment(s) they want, as well as those they do not want. Nurses should be familiar with this and all other types of written statements of patients' preferences, the existence of which should always be noted in the patient's chart.

MALPRACTICE INSURANCE FOR NURSES

Not too many years ago an attorney representing an injured patient would have summarily rejected the notion of filing suit against a professional nurse for alleged malpractice because it was common knowledge that only a handful of nurses carried their own malpractice insurance, and in the absence of such insurance, the limited incomes and financial resources of most nurses made them essentially judgment-proof. Rather than sue the nurse, the attorney would file suit against the nurse's hospital-employer, all physicians involved in the patient's treatment, possibly an equipment or drug manufacturer, and anyone else directly or indirectly involved in the treatment process who might be financially able to respond to damages.

Much has changed, and nurses now find themselves the targets of malpractice litigation with increasing frequency. In part this change is due to the overall increase in medical malpractice litigation over the past several years, with more such cases being tried and bigger verdicts and pretrial settlements being obtained. Also, many attorneys are firm believers in the practice of naming as defendants in a malpractice case every health professional whose name appears on the patient's chart. The theory under which they work is that the more defendants there are, the more insurance carriers there are likely to be involved and available to share in paying any verdict or settlement reached. As this indiscriminate practice has flourished, more nurses inevitably have found themselves forced to defend their actions in the legal arena.

Another important reason why nurses have become fair game for malpractice suits is their assumption of greater responsibilities as clinical nurse-specialists. It is almost axiomatic that the greater the responsibility, the greater the nurse's liability; hence, it stands to reason that the OR nurse, the Critical Care Unit (CCU) and Intensive Care Unit (ICU) nurse, the ER nurse, the nurse anesthetist, and other nursing specialists have been singled out by astute malpractice lawyers as logical defendants in many malpractice cases.

Finally, we must not forget that there are still a few states in which a governmental or charitable hospital cannot be held liable for negligence causing injury to a patient, and in these states the numbers of suits brought against individual nurses are bound to continue as they have in the past.

Is Malpractice Insurance Necessary?

Given the present litigation environment, no prudent nurse should even *consider* practicing without the protection of a personal malpractice insurance policy. As noted previously, there is a growing trend to hold nurses personally liable for their acts of negligence, particularly where they have assumed added responsibilities as clinical nurse-specialists or nurse-practitioners and exercise a considerable degree of professional autonomy. However, even when providing general-duty nursing services in a hospital, clinic, or nursing home, there are substantial reasons why *every* nurse should have his or her own malpractice coverage. These reasons are now reviewed in question-and-answer format.

Q—Why should I carry malpractice insurance if my institutional employer assures me that I am covered under the institution's policy?

A—There are several reasons. To begin, the cost of the typical malpractice policy for nurses is less than 100 dollars a year for coverage up to 2 million dollars. Not only is that degree of protection ridiculously inexpensive, but the cost is fully tax deductible. If nothing else, you will be guaranteed the services of legal counsel in case you are sued—at a time when experienced trial attorneys are charging as much as 500 dollars an hour for court appearances.

There are more substantial reasons for having your own malpractice coverage, however. While it is true that the institution's policy will probably cover your normal activities as an employee, their liability is secondary in nature, based on the doctrine of *respondeat superior*. Your liability, on the other hand, is primary in nature, which is why you are sure to be named as a defendant if the suit is predicated on your allegedly negligent conduct. If your employer decides to defend the suit by claiming you were not negligent, so much the better. In that particular instance you probably would not need a separate insurance policy. However, suppose the hospital, clinic, or nursing home took the position that what you did was either (a) a violation of their written policy guidelines or direct orders, (b) beyond the scope of your nursing license, or (c) a knowing violation of law. In those circumstances the institution's insurance carrier might decide not to defend you on the grounds that what you did was not covered by the institution's malpractice policy. As a matter of fact, they may take an adversary position and go to great lengths to prove that *you and you alone are the legally responsible party*, forcing you to defend yourself in court on that issue. Needless to say, at that point you are strictly on your own, which is precisely what happened to Nurse Bobbie Sullivan in *Sullivan* v. *Sumrall By Ritchley*, 618 So. 2d 1274 (Miss. 1993). In this case the nurse ignored the physician's orders for Demerol to be administered every 4 hours and overmedicated her patient, causing cardiac arrest and coma. Both the hospital and Nurse Sullivan were sued, but the hospital's insurer settled out of court, leaving the nurse as the sole defendant. She filed a motion for summary judgment, which was denied, forcing her to defend the suit entirely on her own. The need for nurses to have their own personal liability insurance is amply demonstrated by this type of case.

There are other reasons why individual malpractice coverage is important. For example, ordinarily, a hospital's insurance carrier has "primary" coverage for liability arising out of a nurse's negligence, based on the *respondeat superior* doctrine. Conversely, the typical nurse's policy provides only "excess coverage," i.e., coverage for amounts awarded that are in excess of the coverage afforded by the hospital's policy. Sometimes, however, the hospital isn't really insured at all. Take the case of *Wake County Hospital System* v. *National Casualty Co*, 804 F. Supp. 768 (N.C. 1992), involving alleged nursing malpractice in neonatal care. In this case, the hospital had a self-insured retention (in essence, a deductible) up to 750,000 dollars per person/per event before its commercial insurance coverage with St. Paul became operative, while the defendant nurse's policy had no deductible and was deemed to be excess coverage over "other valid and collectible insurance." The U.S. District Court held that the hospital's self-insured retention of 750,000 dollars did *not* constitute "other valid and collectible insurance," and ruled that the nurse's insurer had to pay the full amount awarded in this case, which was an amount less than the hospital's 750,000 dollar self-insured retention. In short, self-insurance by a hospital is not really "insurance" in the legal sense, once again emphasizing the need for nurses to have their own malpractice coverage.

Remember, also, that when the insurance carrier makes payment to a plaintiff based on the clear-cut negligence of a nurse, the insurer is legally entitled to sue the nurse to obtain reimbursement from him or her for the amount paid. Such cases are rare, to be sure, but your only salvation in a situation such as that would be to have your own malpractice coverage.

Finally, no institutional policy affords coverage to you for acts or omissions occurring outside your normal work environment. A malpractice suit can result from a wide variety of nursing activities having nothing at all to do with hospital, clinic, or nursing home care—volunteer work, immunization programs, special-duty care, Good Samaritan situation—and in all of these instances you cannot possibly expect the institution's malpractice policy to cover your actions. Again, bear in mind that even if a claim brought against you is successfully defended, the costs of an attorney can be enormous. Having your own malpractice coverage will not only provide you with legal counsel but with indemnity protection as well.

Q—Suppose I work for a solo practitioner or for a group of physicians; won't I be automatically covered under the practitioner's or group's policy?

A—While it is true that most physicians have policies that automatically cover their employees, this is not always the case. Many policies provide that unless the nurse-employee is specifically named as an insured party, such coverage does not exist. That is exactly what happened in the case of an office-based nurse in New York, whose employer told her she was covered, but his insurance carrier contended otherwise, and the court agreed with the carrier (*National Union Fire Insurance Co.* v. *Medical Liability Mutual Insurance Co.*, 446 N.Y.S. 2d 480 [1981]). Again, most of the discussion concerning institutional coverage is equally applicable to nurses who are employed by individual physicians or groups of physicians in a clinic setting. Thus, if your employer (meaning its insurance carrier) decides that what you did was not within the scope of your nurse's license or was a direct violation of law, the employer may decide to disavow coverage.

Q—If I purchase my own liability coverage, won't that relieve my employer of responsibility if I am sued?

A—To begin, it is highly unlikely that a plaintiff's attorney will sue a nurse employed by a hospital or nursing home and *not* sue the employer. That would be tantamount to *legal malpractice*, and would be a rare event indeed. Why worry about the hospital or nursing home at this juncture? When more than one insurance company is involved in defending a malpractice suit, they usually work out some sharing arrangement among themselves in case they decide to settle or have to pay an amount awarded by a jury. However, these arrangements are the insurers' business, not yours. You need only be concerned that *your* liability is covered.

Q—I have no substantial personal assets, so why should I be concerned about being sued personally?

A—You should be greatly concerned, because a judgment against you can remain outstanding for as long as 20 years. You may be financially at a low ebb right now, but some time within the next 20 years you might well have acquired property interests on which an attorney will be able to levy. Note, also, that in most states an individual's interest in jointly owned property can be taken to satisfy a judgment. Thus, if you own a house or a car jointly with your spouse, your interest in it can be seized through supplementary judgment proceedings. In some states your wages may be garnisheed, as well. Finally, putting all your assets in your spouse's name can be a dangerous game, particularly if there is a later divorce, or if you have specific personal property you'd like to will to your children or other close relatives.

Q—I'm only a nursing student, so why do I need malpractice coverage?

A—The point has been stressed throughout this book that when a nursing student performs duties customarily performed only by a professional nurse, he or she is held to the standard of care of the latter. Today, it is quite common for the plaintiff's attorney to file suit against everyone whose name appears anywhere on the patient's chart, so you cannot escape being sued simply because you are a student. Moreover, you cannot rely on your employer's insurance to cover any award made against you personally, even though it is more than likely that you will be afforded legal representation under your employer's policy. Why incur the risk or the anxiety involved in these situation when for about 70 dollars a year you can obtain proper insurance protection that guarantees legal representation and payment of any claims against you because of some act of negligence on your part?

Protection Afforded

The principal benefits of an individual malpractice policy are the insurer's agreement to defend all claims filed against the insured nurse for nursing malpractice and its agreement to pay on behalf of the insured all sums of money the latter is legally liable to pay the plaintiff, up to the limits of coverage stated in the policy. Should there be an appeal of an adverse verdict, the policy also provides for covering all the costs associated with such appeal.

It is important to note that under the typical malpractice policy the insurer agrees to defend *all* claims against the nurse-policyholder, even if they seem baseless on their face (e.g., directed against the wrong person). In addition to the usual claims for negligence in treatment, the policy generally provides for the defense of claims alleging assault, battery, invasion of privacy, defamation of character, and (except in unusually outrageous circumstances) claims that the nurse exceeded the scope of his or her license to practice nursing.

Coverage is normally provided for claims arising out of off-duty and non–hospital-related nursing activities such as volunteer work and Good Samaritan assistance, and also includes instructional and supervisory activities—the latter being of particular interest to clinical nursing instructors and supervisory nursing personnel, none of whom should be without personal liability insurance in the present legal climate.

HEALTH CARE REFORM, NURSES, AND MANAGED CARE

Managed care and case management are acute care models that were originally developed by nurses but have taken on new meaning as cost and quality considerations are being scrutinized by the various proponents of national health care reform. The basic purpose of managed care is to achieve a proper balance between access to care, quality of care, and cost. It encompasses treatment planning from preadmission to postdischarge, with nurses playing a major role in the process. It is clear that managed care and case management in one form or another will be essential ingredients in any comprehensive national health legislation that is eventually enacted.

We are already beginning to see significant revamping of the current system, as many payers, providers, and other corporate entities—anticipating the legislative changes on the horizon—are pursuing competitive positioning strategies to enhance their per-unit revenues, lower their per-unit costs, and still provide quality health care services. In some institutions, primary nursing has already evolved into a managed care delivery model in which the primary nurse uses a predetermined critical pathway to establish and monitor the extent and timing of care within an anticipated length of hospital stay. Nurses and physicians are jointly developing standard plans of care for commonly treated conditions, individualizing the plan to reflect unique patient circumstances. The primary nurse—an RN who is assisted by LPNs and other ancillary health personnel—manages and controls patient care, using the critical pathways to evaluate patient progress and institute necessary corrective action(s).

A distinctive characteristic of managed care/case management is the increasing emphasis on information management and the use of new information technology. It is theorized that by the turn of the century such technological innovations as electronic documentation and the computer-based patient record will be realities that establish new standards throughout the health care system. It is too early to say how the courts will react to new modes of patient care and technological innovation, but one thing is certain: they will continue to hold nurses to standards of care that are not compromised by purely cost considerations or arbitrarily made subservient to new technology. Poorly designed systems can create harm as readily as incompetent medical and nursing personnel. For example, short staffing has been rejected by courts as a defense in cases in which the available nursing personnel could have been juggled to achieve closer supervision of a problem patient. See, for example, *Douglas v. Freeman*, 587 P. 2d 76 (Wash. 1990); *Horton v. Niagara Falls Memorial Medical Center*, 380 N.Y.S. 2d 116 (N.Y. 1976). When a problem can be managed to achieve better results, the courts have been quite willing to impose such standards on a hospital. See, for example, *Marks v. Mandel*, 477 So. 2d 1036 (Fla. 1985); *Habuda v. Trustees of Rex Hospital*, 164 S.E. 2d 17 (N.C. 1968); *Herrington v. Miller*, 883 F. 2d 411 (Texas 1989).

Accordingly, whether the nursing care is called *managed care, case management*, or something else, when medical injury occurs, the legal issue will not be the name of the nursing care model or system within which the patient's injury occurred, but whether professional negligence (malpractice) was the proximate cause of the injury. Managed care/case management clinical systems that utilize specific quality outcomes as benchmarks, such as those established in CareMaps, undoubtedly will give plaintiffs' attorneys additional grounds for alleging breaches of standards of care, for which nurses—and, of course, their employers—can be held responsible in given circumstances. These issues should be discussed by nursing administrators with their hospital legal counsels before they begin implementation of such programs. From a liability standpoint, the entity who employs the nurse—whether a hospital, HMO, insurance company, or other "player" in the managed care field—will still be primarily responsible for job-related errors or omissions that can be shown to have proximately caused injury to a patient, under the doctrine of *respondeat superior*. The nurse will, of course, continue to be held personally liable for his or her own negligent conduct, once again pointing to the need for personal malpractice insurance coverage.

SELECTED REFERENCES—PART EIGHT

Importance of Maintaining Accurate Medical Records

22 *Am Jur Proof of Facts (2d)*, Medical Malpractice—Use of Hospital Records

Fiesta J, *20 Legal Pitfalls for Nurses to Avoid*, Delmar Publishers, Inc., Albany, N.Y., 1994.

Tomes JP, *Healthcare Records: A Practical Legal Guide*, Healthcare Financial Management Association, Westchester, ILL., 1990.

Mech AB, "Quality Assurance and Documentation." In *Legal Issues in Nursing*, Northrop CA and Kelly ME, editors, The C.V. Mosby Company, St. Louis, 1987, Ch. 28.

Martin F, "Documentation Tips to Help You Stay Out of Court," *Nursing '94* 24(6):63, 1994.

"Computer Charting: Minimizing Legal Risks," *Nursing '93* 23(5):86, 1993.

Fiesta J, "Charting—One National Standard, One Form," *Nurs Management* 24(6):22, 1993.

"Fraudulent Charting," *Nursing '92* 22(12):23, 1992.

Hurr WL, "Lost, Destroyed and 'Doctored' Medical Records," *Trial* 28:46, 1992.

Fiesta J, "If It Wasn't Charted, It Wasn't Done," *Nurs Management* 22(8):17, 1991.

Roach WH Jr., "Legal Review: Incentives for Completing Medical Records—The Legal Risks," *Topics in Health Records Management* 10(3):78, 1990.

Gruber M and Gruber JM, "Nursing Malpractice: The Importance of Documentation, or Saved by the Pen," *Gastroent Nurs* 12(4):255, 1990.

Morrissey-Ross M, "Documentation: If You Haven't Written It, You Haven't Done it," *Nurs Clin N Am* 23(2):363, 1988.

Staggers N, "Using Computers in Nursing: Documented Benefits and Needed Studies," *Computers in Nursing* 6(4):164, 1988.

Bergson SB, "Charting with a Jury in Mind," *Nursing '88* 18(4):50, 1988.

Mandell M, "Charting: How It Can Keep You Out of Court," *Nurs Life* 7:46, 1987.

Greenlaw J, "Documentation of Patient Care: An Often Underestimated Responsibility," *Law Med Health Care* 10(3):125, 1982.

Harris County Hospital District v. *Estrada*, 872 S.W. 2d 759 (Texas 1993)

Davenport v. *St. Paul Fire & Marine Ins. Co.*, 978 F. 2d 97 (Miss. 1992)

Delaughter v. *Lawrence City Hospital*, 601 So. 2d 818 (Miss. 1992)

University of Texas Medical Branch at Galveston v. *York*, 808 S.W. 2d 106 (Texas 1991)

Roberts v. *Sisters of Saint Francis*, 556 N.E. 2d 662 (Ill. 1990)

St. Francis Regional Medical Center v. *Hale*, 752 P. 2d 129 (Kan. 1988)

Coleman v. *Touro Infirmary of New Orleans*, 506 S. 2d 571 (La. 1987)

Henry by Henry, v. *St. John's Hospital*, 512 N.E. 2d 1044 (Ill. 1987)

Ahrens v. *Katz*, 575 F. Supp. 1108 (Ga. 1985)

Kenyon v. *Hammer*, 688 P. 2d 961 (Ariz. 1984)

Dincau v. *Tamayose*, 182 Cal. Rptr. 855 (Cal. 1982)

Fox v. *Cohen*, 406 N.E. 2d 178 (Ill. 1980)

Pisel v. *Stamford Hospital*, 430 A. 2d 1 (Conn. 1980)

North Miami General Hospital v. *Gilbert*, 360 So. 2d 426 (Fla. 1979)

St. Paul Fire & Marine Ins. Co. v. *Prothro*, 590 S.W. 2d 35 (Ark. 1979)

Wanger v. *Kaiser Foundation Hospitals*, 589 P. 2d 1106 (Ore. 1979)

People v. *Smithtown General Hospital, Lorna Salzarullo, et al.*, 402 N.Y.S. 2d 318 (N.Y. 1978)

Hiatt v. *Groce*, 523 P. 2d 320 (Kan. 1978)

Ramsey v. *Physicians Memorial Hospital*, 373 A. 2d 26 (Md. 1977)

The Right to Privacy and Confidentiality

Restatement (Second) TORTS § 652A

Fiesta J, *20 Legal Pitfalls for Nurses to Avoid*, Delmar Publishers, Inc., Albany, N.Y., 1994, Ch. 10.

Nurse's Handbook of Law & Ethics, Springhouse Corporation, Springhouse, Pa., 1992, pp. 84-88.

American Nurses Association, *Code for Nurses, with Interpretive Statements*, 3, 1985.

Hemelt M and Mackert M, *The Dynamics of Law in Nursing and Health Care*, Reston Publishing, Reston, Va., 1978, pp. 104-112.

Melroe NH, "Duty to Warn vs. Patient Confidentiality: The Ethical Dilemmas in Caring for HIV-Infected Clients," *Nurse Pract* 15(2):58, 1990.

Smith J, "Privileged Communication: Psychiatric/Mental Health Nurses and the Law," *Persp in Psych Care* 26(4):26, 1990.

Tingle J, "Nurses and the Law: When to Tell . . . Patients' Rights to Confidentiality," *Nurs Times* 86(35):58, 1990.

Dimond B, "When Should You Disclose Confidential Medical Information?" *Occup Health* (London) 41(11):330, 1989.

Curran W, Laska E, Kaplan H, and Bank R, "Protection of Privacy and Confidentiality," *Science* 182(114):797, 1973.

Wyatt v. *St. Paul Fire & Marine Ins. Co.*, 868 S.W. 2d 505 (Ark. 1994)

Banks v. *Charter Hospital of Long Beach*, reported in *Med Malpr Verdicts, Settlements & Experts* 8(10):19, 1992.

Verneuil v. *Poirier*, 589 So. 2d 1205 (La. 1991)

In re Doe Children, 402 N.Y.S. 2d 958 (N.Y. 1978)

Doe v. *Roe*, 345 N.Y.S. 2d 560 (N.Y. 1973)

Horne v. *Patton*, 287 So. 2d 824 (Ala. 1973)

Hammonds v. *Aetna Casualty & Surety Co.*, 243 F. Suppl 793 (Ohio 1965)

Reporting Child Abuse

Child Abuse Prevention and Treatment Act, P.I.. 93-247, 42 USC §§ 5101-5106

Cowen PS, "Child Abuse: What Is Nursing's Role?" In *Current Issues in Nursing*, ed 4, McCloskey J and Grace HK, editors, Mosby-Year Book, Inc., St. Louis, 1994, ch. 98.

Cichetti D and Carlson V, editors, *Child Maltreatment: Theory and Research on the Causes and Consequences of Child Abuse and Neglect*, Cambridge University Press, New York, 1989.

Helfer R and Kempe R, *The Battered Child*, ed 4, University of Chicago Press, Chicago, 1987.

Holder AR, *Legal Issues in Pediatrics and Adolescent Medicine*, ed 2, Yale University Press, New Haven, 1985, pp. 216-220.

Annotation, 73 ALR 4th 782, "Child Abuse Reporting Statutes."

Allen J and Hollowell E, "Nurses and Child Abuse/Neglect Reporting: Duties, Responsibilities and Issues," *J Pract Nurs* 40(2):56, 1990.

Aron J, "Civil Liability for Teacher's Negligent Failure to Report Suspected Child Abuse," *Wayne L Rev* 28:183, 1981.

Kreitzer M, "Symposium on Child Abuse and Neglect: Legal Aspects of Child Abuse; Guidelines for the Nurse," *Nurs Clin N Am* 16:149, 1981.

Gelles R, "Studies Show Factors Related to Child Abuse," *Am Fam Phys* 19:215, 1979.

McKeel N, "Child Abuse Can Be Prevented," *Am J Nurs* 78:1478, 1978.

Friedman A, "Nursing Responsibility in Child Abuse," *Nurs Forum* 15(1):95, 1976.

Capaldi v. *State*, 763 P. 2d 117 (Okla. 1988)

Kempster v. *Child Protective Services of Dep't. of Social Services*, 515 N.Y.S. 2d 807 (N.Y. 1987)

O'Keefe v. *Dr. Osorio & Osorio Medical Center*, reported in *ATLA L Rep* 27:392 (1984)

State v. *Groff*, 409 So. 2d 44 (Fla. 1982)

Landeros v. *Flood*, 551 P. 2d 389 (Cal. 1976)

Handicapped Newborns—Baby Doe Regulations

Bowen v. *American Hospital Association*, 106 S. Ct. 2101 (1986)

American Hospital Association v. *Heckler*, 585 F. Supp. 541 (N.Y. 1984)

United States v. *University Hospital of SUNY at Stony Brook*, 729 F. 2d 144 (N.Y. 1984)
United States v. *University Hospital of SUNY at Stony Brook*, 575 F. Supp. 607 (N.Y. 1983)
American Academy of Pediatrics v. *Heckler*, 561 F. Supp. 395 (D.C. 1983)
Weber v. *Stony Brook Hospital*, 469 N.Y.S. 2d 63 (N.Y. 1983)

Elder Abuse Issues

Conard AF, "Elder Choice," *Am J Law & Med* 19(3):233, 1993.
Haddad AM and Kapp MB, *Ethical and Legal Issues in Home Health Care*, Appleton & Lange, Norwalk, Conn., 1991, pp. 190–191.
Kapp M and Bigot A, *Geriatrics and the Law*, Springer Publishing Co., New York, 1985, Ch. 7.
DeRenzo EG, "Elder Abuse: Ethical Theory in Every Day Practice," *Caring* 8(3):10, 1989.
Callahan JJ, "Elder Abuse: Some Questions for Policymakers," *The Gerontologist* 28:453, 1986.
Quinn MJ, "Elder Abuse and Neglect Raise New Dilemmas," *Generations* 10(2):22, 1985.
Beck R and Phillips J, "Abuse of the Elderly," *J Geron Nurs* 9:97, 1983.
Faulkner B, "Mandating the Reporting of Suspected Cases of Elder Abuse: An Inappropriate, Ineffective and Ageist Response to the Abuse of Older Adults," *Fam L Q* 16:69 (1982).

Patients' Rights and Self-Determination

The Patient Self-Determination Act, 42 U.S.C. §§ 1395cc(a) et seq. (1990)
American Hospital Association, *A Patient's Bill of Rights*, American Hospital Association, Chicago, 1992.
Nurse's Handbook of Law & Ethics, Springhouse Corporation, Springhouse, Pa, 1992, Ch. 2.
"How Our Staff Implemented the Patient Self-Determination Act," *Nursing '92* 22(4):32, 1992.
Ramsey MK, "Patient Rights and Obligations," *Advancing Clin Care* 5(1):29, 1990.
Johnstone MJ, "Professional Ethics and Patients' Rights: Past Realities, Future Imperatives," *Nurs Forum* 24(3/4):19, 1989.

The Nurse as the Patient's Advocate

Anderson SL, "Patient Advocacy and Whistle-Blowing in Nursing: Help for the Helpers," *Nurs Forum* 25(3):5, 1990.
Fiesta J, "Whistleblowers: Heroes or Stool Pigeons?—Part I" *Nurs Management* 21(6):16, 1990.
Fiesta J, "Whistleblowers: Retaliation or Protection—Part II" *Nurs Management* 21(7):38, 1990.
Tadd V, "Where are the Whistle-Blowers?" *Nurs Times* 87(1):42, 1990.
Fry ST, "Whistle-Blowing by Nurses: A Matter of Ethics," *Nurs Outlook* 37(1):56, 1989.
Nelson ML, "Advocacy in Nursing," *Nurs Outlook* 36(3):136, 1988.
Rothrock JC, "Whistle-Blowing: Is It Worth the Consequences?" *AORN J* 48(4):757, 1988.
Luckenbrill-Brett JL and Stuhler-Sclag, "Mandatory Reporting: Legal and Ethical Issues," *J Nurs Admin* 17:37, 1987.
Winslow GR, "From Loyalty to Advocacy: A New Metaphor for Nursing," *Hastings Center Report* 14:32, 1984.
Feliu AG, "The Risks of Blowing the Whistle," *Am J Nurs*, Oct. 1983.
Price DM and Murphy P, "How and When to Blow the Whistle on Unsafe Practices," *Nurs Life* 3:53, 1983.
Warthen v. *Toms River Hospital*, 488 A. 2d 229 (N.J. 1985)
Jones v. *Memorial Hospital System*, 677 S.W. 2d 221 (Texas 1984)
Wrighten v. *Metropolitan Hospitals*, 33 FEP Cases 1714 (Cal. 1984)
Witt, R.N. v. *Forest Hospital et al.*, 450 N.E. 2d 811 (Ill. 1983)
Tuma v. *Board of Nursing*, 593 P. 2d 711 (Ida. 1979)

Wills and Matters Related Thereto

Nurse's Handbook of Law & Ethics, Springhouse Corporation, Springhouse, Pa., 1992, pp. 112-114.
Creighton H, *Law Every Nurse Should Know*, ed 5, W.B. Saunders Co., Philadelphia, 1986, pp. 243-250.

Bernzweig E, "The Patient Who Wants Help with a Will," *RN* 48(9):71, 1985.
Brent EA, "Think, Before You Witness That Will," *RN* 43(3):61, 1983.
Kerns W, "The Anatomy of a Bequest, *Mod Hosp* 109:112, 1967.
Succession of Zinsel, 360 So. 2d 587 (La. 1979)
Succession of Andrews, 153 So. 2d 470 (La. 1963)
In re Bliss' Estate, 18 Cal. Rptr. 821 (Cal. 1962)
Pollard v. *El Paso National Bank*, 343 S.W. 2d 909 (Texas 1961)
In re Cochran's Estate, 108 N.W. 2d 529 (Wis. 1961)

Advance Directives—Living Wills; Powers of Attorney

Urofsky MI, *Letting Go: Death, Dying and the Law*, Macmillan Publishing Co., New York, 1993.
Nurse's Handbook of Law & Ethics, Springhouse Corporation, Springhouse, Pa. 1992, pp. 155-179.
Meisel A, *The Right to Die*, John Wiley & Sons, New York, 1989.
Conrad AF, "Elder Choice," *Am J Law & Med* 19(3):233, 1993.
Gloe DSO, "The Right to Die and the Living Will: Missouri Status," *Critical Care Nurse* 11(1):26, 1991.
McLean ED, "Living Will Statutes in Light of *Cruzan* v. *Missouri Department of Health*: Ensuring that a Patient's Wishes Will Prevail," *Emory LJ* 40:1305, 1991.
Seckler AB et al., "Substituted Judgment: How Accurate Are Proxy Predictions?" *Annals Int Med* 115:92, 1991.
Killian WH, "Knowledge of Living Will Law Essential," *Am Nurse* 22(7):33, 1990.
Emanuel L, "Beyond the Living Will," *Harv Med Sch Health Letter* 15(8):4, 1990.
Rouse F, "Where Are We Heading After *Cruzan*?" *Law Med & Health Care* 18:353, 1990.
Emanuel L and Emanuel E, "The Medical Directive: A New Comprehensive Advance Care Document," *JAMA* 261(22):3288, 1989.
Nye CA, "Living Wills: The Ethical Dilemmas," *Critical Care Nurse* 9(8):20, 1989.
Fowler M, "Appointing an Agent to Make Medical Treatment Choices," *Colum L Rev* 84:985, 1984.
Courtright G, "The Case for a Living Will," *RN* 47(8):16, 1984.
Cohn S, "The Living Will from the Nurse's Perspective," *Law Med & Health Care* 11(3):121, 1983.
Anderson v. *St. Francis-St. George Hospital*, 614 N.E. 2d 841 (Ohio 1992)
Cruzan v. *Missouri Department of Health*, 760 S.W. 2d 408 (Mo. 1988)
In re Peter, 529 A. 2d 419 (N.J. 1987)
John F. Kennedy Memorial Hospital v. *Bludworth*, 432 So. 2d 611 (Fla. 1983)
In re Storar, 438 N.Y.S. 2d 266 9N.Y. 1981)
In re Quinlan, 355 A. 2d 647 (N.J. 1976), *cert denied* sub nom *Garger* v. *New Jersey*, 429 U.S. 922 (1976)

Need for Malpractice Insurance and Coverage Issues

Fuetz SA, "Do You Need Professional Liability Insurance" *Nursing '91* 21(1):56, 1991.
Gordon RJ, "The Effects of Malpractice Insurance on Certified Nurse-Midwives: The Case of Rural Arizona," *J Nurs Midwifery* 35(2):99, 1990.
Fuetz SA, "Professional Liability Insurance," *J Nurs Admin* 19(2):5, 1989.
George JE and Quattrone MS, "Liability Insurance Issues . . . Emergency Nurse Employed by a Hospital," *J Emerg Nurs* 5(4):340, 1989.
Tammelleo AD, "Do You Really Have Professional Liability Insurance?" *Regan Rep on Nurs L* 27(7):2, 1986.
Arbeiter J, "A Buyer's Guide to Malpractice Insurance," *RN* 49(5):22, 1986.
Bernzweig E, "Why You Need Your Own Malpractice Policy," *RN* 48(3):59, 1985.
Sandroff R, "Why You Really Ought to Have Your Own Malpractice Policy," *RN* 46(6):29, 1983.
Regan W, "Malpractice Insurance Coverage for Nurses," *Regan Rep Nurs L* 22(12):1, 1982.
Snow J, "Professional Liability Coverage: Is It Necessary?" *Emerg Med* 10(3):105 (Mar. 1981)
Mancini M, "What You Should Know About Malpractice Insurance," *Am J Nurs* 79:729, 1979.

Sullivan v. *Sumrall by Ritchley*, 618 So. 2d 1274 (Miss. 1993)

Davenport v. *St. Paul Fire & Marine Ins. Co.*, 978 F. 2d 97 (Miss. 1992)

Navarro v. *George*, 615 A. 2d 890 (Pa. 1992)

St. Paul Medical Center v. *Cecil*, 842 S.W. 2d 808 (Texas 1992)

Wake County Hospital System v. *National Casualty Co.*, 804 F. Supp. 768 (N.C. 1992)

William M. Mercer, Inc. v. *Woods*, 717 S.W. 2d 391 (Texas 1986)

American Nurses Association v. *Passaic General Hospital*, 417 A. 2d 66 (N.J. 1984)

Jones v. *Medox*, 430 A. 2d 488 (D.C. 1981)

National Union Fire Insurance Co. v. *Medical Liability Insurance Co*, 446 N.Y.S. 2d 480 (N.Y. 1981)

Argonaut Insurance Co. v. *Continental Insurance Co*, 406 N.Y.S. 2d 96 (N.Y. 1978)

Tankersley v. *Insurance Company of North America*, 216 So. 2d 333 (La. 1968)

NOTE: This completes the course on the nurse's liability for malpractice. In the remaining pages you will find test questions and answers and a glossary. The comprehensive index at the end will enable you to use this book as a future reference source.

TEST QUESTIONS*

Problem No. 1

Nurse Jones is an RN employed in a small community hospital. The state in which the hospital is located has a Narcotic Drug Act that provides: "A narcotic drug shall be dispensed only upon a written prescription of a practitioner licensed by law to administer such drug. The act of dispensing a narcotic drug contrary to the provisions of this paragraph shall be a misdemeanor."

Late one Sunday evening an auto-accident victim is admitted to the emergency room of the hospital, and Nurse Jones, the only RN on duty, observes the unusual amount of pain being experienced by the patient. While awaiting the arrival of the local physician-on-call, she decides to give the patient an injection of a narcotic drug. In her haste, she causes the needle to break, resulting in further injury to the patient.

1-1 The quoted law is an example of

☐ common law

☐ statutory law

☐ tort law

1-2 How does common law differ from statutory law?

☐ Common law is not the result of a legislative enactment.

☐ Common law is less important than statutory law.

☐ Common law does not have the legal effect of statutory law.

1-3 In what major category is the quoted law properly classified?

☐ criminal law

☐ civil law

☐ administrative law

---

* Answers begin on p. 457.

1-4 A law is classified as part of the criminal law when it is concerned with

☐ conduct that causes serious harm or injury to the person or property of another

☐ conduct that pertains to the public interest and is considered an offense against society as a whole

☐ conduct that is intentionally harmful

1-5 Which of the following is true in this case?

☐ The patient can sue Nurse Jones for negligence, and the local governmental authority can bring criminal charges against her for violation of the statute.

☐ Nurse Jones can be brought to trial on a criminal charge or can be sued for negligent conduct, but not both.

☐ If Nurse Jones is found innocent of any criminal conduct, the patient would have no legal basis for suing her for negligence.

1-6 If Nurse Jones stands trial in a criminal case for violating the quoted law and is found guilty, what will be the probable consequence?

☐ She will be held responsible for paying all the medical and hospital bills incurred by the patient in connection with the additional injury sustained.

☐ She will forfeit her license to practice nursing in that state.

☐ She will be fined, imprisoned, placed on probation, or some combination thereof.

1-7 The branch of law that deals with negligent conduct is part of the law of

☐ contracts

☐ crimes

☐ torts

1-8 If Nurse Jones is held "legally liable" in a civil case, what will be the probable consequence?

☐ She will be required to pay money damages to the injured plaintiff.

☐ She will no longer be permitted to administer narcotic drugs.

☐ She will temporarily forfeit her license to practice nursing in that state.

1-9 What can the trial court "judicially notice" in this case?

☐ Nurse Jones was the only RN on duty on the evening in question

☐ Nurse Jones was negligent in her manner of giving the injection

☐ the state law prohibits the administration of narcotic drugs without a doctor's prescription

1-10 What would be considered legally sufficient proof to hold Nurse Jones liable for the harm to the patient in this case?

☐ proof of her deviation from the standard of care normally applicable in the giving of injections

☐ proof of her violation of the statute relating to the administration of narcotic drugs

☐ proof of her deviation from the standard of care normally exercised by physicians in treating patients in similar emergency circumstances

Problem No. 2

Nurse Smith is a licensed RN who generally works as a private-duty nurse. A local hospital employs Nurse Smith to help out over a holiday weekend. While assigned to duty in the obstetrical ward, he notices an elderly woman patient in obvious respiratory distress in the adjacent hallway. Going to her aid, Nurse Smith administers improper treatment, which causes the patient's condition to worsen. The patient later sues Nurse Smith for the harm suffered, and the case is heard by a judge without a jury.

2-1   The judge's decision in this case would be an example of

□   administrative law

□   common law

□   statutory law

2-2   The patient's suit claiming damages for the harm suffered due to Nurse Smith's improper care brings the case within the general category of

□   criminal law

□   tort law

□   contract law

2-3   As indicated, Nurse Smith *normally* is employed as a private-duty nurse. *While so employed,* he can be held legally liable

□   when he fails to act as other reasonably prudent nurses would act under similar circumstances

□   when the patient's condition deteriorates substantially, or the patient dies during his period of employment

□   when he does not follow the doctor's orders exactly

2-4   The legal term for a person's failure to act in a reasonable and prudent manner is

□   negligence

□   malpractice

□   tortious misconduct

2-5   Only a person with professional training and credentials can be held liable for

☐ damages

☐ malpractice

☐ negligence

2-6   If the Court were to determine that Nurse Smith failed to conduct himself in a reasonable and prudent manner while engaged in a *nonnursing* activity, the basis of his legal liability would be

☐ ordinary negligence

☐ professional malpractice

☐ ordinary malfeasance

2-7   While employed by the hospital, Nurse Smith was legally responsible for exercising a special duty of care with respect to

☐ designated patients in his assigned ward

☐ any of the hospital's patients he might have had occasion to treat

☐ none of the hospital's patients, because of his status as a private-duty nurse

2-8   Under which of the following circumstances could Nurse Smith have entered into a nurse-patient relationship with an individual?

☐ whenever he established good rapport with that individual

☐ whenever he achieved an agreeable therapeutic relationship with that individual

☐ whenever he actually provided nursing care to that individual

2-9   A legal nurse-patient relationship is based on what necessary factor?

☐ the provision of nursing care to someone by a person with professional nurse's training

☐ the consent of the patient to receive nursing care from a particular nurse

☐ the patient's legal capacity to enter into a contract of employment

2-10 Nurse Smith ☐ entered into ☐ did not enter into a nurse-patient relationship with the elderly patient in distress because

☐ the patient was not someone within the scope of Nurse Smith's normal nursing duties

☐ the giving of nursing care in an emergency situation cannot be the basis of a nurse-patient relationship

☐ Nurse Smith undertook to provide nursing care to the patient

2-11 Whether a nurse acted with reasonable care in a given situation is judged mainly by

☐ the extensiveness of his or her experience and training in that type of care

☐ his or her conduct compared with that of other nurses with similar training under comparable circumstances

☐ the degree to which he or she adhered to a physician's orders or followed hospital protocols in giving the care in question

2-12 The standard of care applied to a nurse's conduct in emergency situations recognizes what key legal fact?

☐ The surrounding circumstances always must be considered in deciding the issue of negligence.

☐ Normal prudence need not be exercised in an emergency situation.

☐ No legal standard of care applies in emergency situations.

Problem No. 3

> Nurse Simpson is the head nurse in a state mental hospital. This state recognizes the common law rule regarding governmental immunity from tort liability. One day Nurse Simpson assigns Mr. Newby, an 18-year-old nursing student, to care for a manic-depressive patient with known suicidal tendencies. Nurse Simpson gives no instructions to Mr. Newby, and the latter's consequent inattention to the patient materially aids another suicide attempt—this time resulting in total paralysis. A malpractice suit is filed against Mr. Newby, Nurse Simpson, and the hospital for the injuries incurred.

3-1   The fact that Mr. Newby is only 18 years old

☐   is the single most legally significant fact in this case

☐   is pertinent only with respect to what could reasonably be expected of a young and inexperienced nurse

☐   is sufficient to make him not liable in this case

3-2   When a nursing student performs duties customarily performed by RNs, what standard of care applies to his or her conduct?

☐   The student is held to a diminished standard of care.

☐   The student is held to the same standard of care as an RN.

☐   The student is held to a student's standard of care.

3-3   Assuming that a court finds Mr. Newby negligent in this case, what effect (if any) might this have on Nurse Simpson's liability?

☐   As a supervisor, Nurse Simpson cannot be held liable for acts or conduct in which she did not personally participate.

☐   Nurse Simpson automatically will be held liable as Mr. Newby's supervisor.

☐   Nurse Simpson can be held liable only if she is held to be negligent in making the assignment to an inexperienced nurse.

3-4   With respect to the hospital's liability (if any), which of the following is true?

☐   The hospital cannot be held liable in this case.

☐   The hospital can be held liable only if Mr. Newby is held liable.

☐   The hospital can be held liable if either Mr. Newby or Nurse Simpson is held liable.

3-5   If Mr. Newby, when given the assignment, sincerely believed he was not sufficiently experienced to cope with a manic-depressive patient, how should he have met his legal responsibility to the patient?

☐   He should have first discussed the proper nursing care with other competent nurses.

☐   He should have first informed the patient of his inexperience and then obtained the patient's informed consent to his providing the necessary nursing care.

☐   He should have declined to carry out the assignment, explaining his reasons to his supervisor before so doing.

3-6   Which of the following factors is the *most legally significant* in this case with respect to determining the degree of care required to protect the patient from harm?

☐   Mr. Newby's age and his status as a nursing student

☐   the hospital's status as a state mental hospital

☐   the patient's known physical and mental condition

3-7   What is the principal reason a higher standard of care may be required for safeguarding mentally ill persons?

☐   mentally ill patients are the ones who most often bring lawsuits

☐   mentally ill persons frequently do not appreciate their exposure to potential harm

☐   state and provincial statutes specifically impose a higher standard of care in the treatment of mentally ill persons

3-8 It was stated that the patient had previously attempted to commit suicide. Which of the following statements is *most accurate*?

☐ Suicidally inclined persons seldom give clues to their suicidal tendencies.

☐ Suicidally inclined persons are easily identified by the fact that they are always depressed and disoriented.

☐ Suicidally inclined persons generally give verbal or behavioral clues to their suicidal tendencies.

3-9 With respect to the issue of liability in this case, which of the following is correct?

☐ Only the hospital and Nurse Simpson can be held liable.

☐ Only Mr. Newby can be held liable.

☐ Both Mr. Newby and Nurse Simpson can be held liable, but not the hospital.

3-10 The doctrine of governmental immunity is an exception to which of the following doctrines?

☐ the doctrine of *respondeat superior*

☐ the doctrine of *res ipsa loquitur*

☐ the doctrine of personal liability

Problem No. 4

Nurse Brown is an experienced RN employed as an office nurse for Dr. Swift. One particularly busy day the doctor tells Nurse Brown: "Mrs. Long is complaining about a variety
of symptoms that are indicative of mild hypertension. Take her blood pressure and reas-
sure her, and if her blood pressure seems elevated, give her a prescription for (name of
drug), the usual dose. You can sign my name on the prescription and don't worry about
anything; I'll take full responsibility."

Nurse Brown follows Dr. Swift's instructions to the letter and gives Mrs. Long a prescription for her hypertension. The next day, in discussing the case with Nurse Brown, Dr. Swift
notes that Nurse Brown erroneously wrote a prescription for a similar sounding but actually *different* drug. By the time Dr. Swift is able to contact Mrs. Long, she learns that Mrs.
Long has suffered a severe reaction to the prescribed drug and has had to be hospitalized.
Mrs. Long later sues both Nurse Brown and Dr. Swift for malpractice.

4-1   If Nurse Brown is held liable for her conduct in this case, she will be held liable under the
        doctrine of

        ☐   borrowed servant

        ☐   personal liability

        ☐   *respondeat superior*

4-2   If Dr. Swift is held liable in this case, she will be held liable under the doctrine of

        ☐   captain of the ship

        ☐   personal liability

        ☐   *respondeat superior*

4-3   The doctrine of personal liability is a legal rule that

        ☐   protects nurses against personal liability for malpractice

        ☐   makes some persons liable for the negligence of others

        ☐   holds everyone legally responsible for his or her own negligent conduct

4-4 Under which of the following circumstances would the doctrine of *respondeat superior* apply in this case?

☐ It would apply if Nurse Brown committed the act within the scope of her employment as a nurse by Dr. Swift.

☐ It would apply if a specific state law says that it applies in cases of this type.

☐ It would apply if Dr. Swift and Nurse Brown agree in advance that it will apply.

4-5 The legal doctrine of *respondeat superior* applies to the acts of

☐ employees of health care institutions only

☐ all types of employees

☐ professional employees only

4-6 In legal effect, the doctrine of *respondeat superior* provides that

☐ an employee can be held liable for the negligent acts of a supervisory co-employee

☐ an employer can be held liable for the negligent acts of his or her employees

☐ employees and their employers are deemed to be jointly liable for the negligent conduct of each other

4-7 The doctrine of *respondeat superior* comes into play only when the following three relationships are present (select one):

☐ nurse-patient-physician

☐ employer-employee-negligent conduct

☐ hospital-nurse-physician

4-8   If Mrs. Long sues Dr. Swift alone and is successful in recovering damages, which of the following is true?

   ☐ Dr. Swift legally can recover from Nurse Brown the amount she is required to pay Mrs. Long.

   ☐ Dr. Swift legally cannot recover from Nurse Brown the amount she is required to pay Mrs. Long.

   ☐ Nurse Brown's license to practice automatically will be suspended.

4-9   What legal effect (if any) resulted from Dr. Swift's statement that she would take "full responsibility" for Nurse Brown's conduct?

   ☐ It provided Nurse Brown with a valid legal defense to any lawsuit that might be brought against her personally.

   ☐ It did not alter the rule of personal liability insofar as Nurse Brown's conduct was concerned.

   ☐ It altered the rule of personal liability insofar as Nurse Brown's conduct was concerned.

4-10   In what significant manner (if any) did Nurse Brown's conduct constitute unreasonable care?

   ☐ She signed the prescription form without showing it to the doctor.

   ☐ She undertook to diagnose the patient's condition and prescribe for her.

   ☐ She was *not* unreasonable since she followed the doctor's orders in all respects.

4-11   What conduct on Nurse Brown's part would have constituted reasonable care under the given facts?

   ☐ She should have declined to carry out Dr. Swift's request on the grounds that it would place her in the position of performing acts only a physician is authorized to perform.

   ☐ She should have requested Dr. Swift to put her instructions in writing.

   ☐ She should have asked the patient many more questions about her condition and not simply have taken her blood pressure and prescribed medication.

Problem No. 5

P, a 30-year-old pastry chef, agrees to undergo an elective appendectomy. In the course of the operation, her surgeon, Doctor D, discovers large stones in P's gallbladder and performs a cholecystectomy. P has an uneventful recovery, but after learning about the gallbladder operation, files suit against Doctor D.

5-1 What legal element did Doctor D fail to take into consideration in this case?

☐ the captain of the ship doctrine

☐ the doctrine of informed consent

☐ the doctrine of *res ipsa loquitur*

5-2 If a patient is given treatment to which she has not consented, the physician or nurse who gives the treatment may be held liable for

☐ civil battery

☐ unethical professional conduct

☐ willful misconduct

5-3 P's consent to the appendectomy would not extend to the cholecystectomy because

☐ there was no agreement as to the additional costs of a cholecystectomy

☐ there was no emergency requiring an immediate cholecystectomy

☐ consent can be given to only one operation at a time

5-4 The fact that both surgical procedures were successful and benefited the patient

☐ is legally relevant on the issue of battery

☐ is not legally relevant on the issue of battery

☐ may be legally relevant on the issue of battery

5-5   To be legally effective, P's agreement to undergo the appendectomy

☐   would have to be in writing

☐   would have to be witnessed by two persons

☐   could be either in writing or verbal

5-6   A patient's consent to a surgical procedure is legally ineffective unless

☐   the patient's spouse or legal representative also gives approval

☐   the patient's consent is given in writing

☐   the patient fully understands to what he or she is consenting

5-7   If P had been a child of 13, her consent to the appendectomy

☐   would have been legally effective if it was known that she had run away from home

☐   would not have been legally effective under the given circumstances

☐   would have been legally effective provided her parents could not be located promptly

5-8   A patient's consent to a surgical procedure is said to be informed when

☐   the patient understands the nature and consequences of the procedure, and the alternatives thereto

☐   the patient understands how much he or she will benefit therefrom

☐   the patient is an adult and otherwise competent to understand medical procedures

5-9   Consent is not required when

☐   routine diagnostic procedures are being employed

☐   the patient is unconscious and the procedure is necessary to save his or her life

☐   the patient does not speak English and accordingly would not comprehend what is being explained to him or her

5-10 Consent to elective treatment of a person who is legally under age and living at home can be given

- ☐ only by the minor's parents or legal guardian

- ☐ either by the minor or by his or her parents

- ☐ only upon the order of a court

5-11 The giving of nonemergency medical treatment to a minor without first obtaining the consent of a parent or guardian is permissible if

- ☐ the minor lives away from home and is financially independent

- ☐ the parent or guardian cannot be located without difficulty

- ☐ the proposed treatment has only a minimal risk of adverse results

5-12 Consent to a procedure, once validly given by a patient,

- ☐ may be revoked only in emergency circumstances

- ☐ may be revoked only if in writing

- ☐ may be revoked at any time before the procedure

5-13 In order to prove he or she has sustained a civil battery, a patient must show

- ☐ serious bodily harm or other substantial damages

- ☐ anger or violent conduct on the part of the physician

- ☐ the touching of his or her person without the patient's consent

5-14 In the eyes of the law, whether specific treatment should be rendered to a competent adult patient is

- ☐ the patient's decision exclusively

- ☐ the doctor's decision, based on his or her professional judgment

- ☐ a decision that can be arrived at objectively by reference to medical standards

Problem No. 6

Mr. Green sustains an eye injury while at work and immediately seeks medical aid from the company nurse, Mr. Owen. The latter inspects the injury, concludes it is only a superficial laceration, and gives only minimal treatment. One week later, Mr. Green's eye becomes extremely painful and an ophthalmologist discovers a piece of metal embedded in the eye. The delay in the discovery and removal of the metal results in blindness of the eye, and Mr. Green promptly sues Nurse Owen for the permanent disability thus sustained.

6-1   The plaintiff in this lawsuit is

□   Mr. Green

□   Nurse Owen

□   Mr. Green's employer

6-2   What fact (if any) would show the existence of a nurse-patient relationship between Mr. Green and Nurse Owen?

□   No nurse-patient relationship could have existed.

□   Both parties were employed by the same company.

□   Nurse Owen treated Mr. Green for his injury.

6-3   If this case is tried before a jury, who would *normally* decide whether Nurse Owen's conduct was negligent?

□   the judge alone

□   the jury alone

□   either the judge or the jury, depending on the facts

6-4   How will the issue of Nurse Owen's negligence have to be proved?

□   by Mr. Green's testimony about what occurred and the treatment that was rendered

□   by medical records of the treatment given by Nurse Owen and by the ophthalmologist

□   by the testimony of experts concerning the standard of care applicable in the case

6-5   With respect to the question of proof, which of the following is true?

☐   Mr. Green has the burden of proving Nurse Owen's negligence.

☐   Nurse Owen has the burden of proving that no negligence occurred.

☐   The burden of proof will depend entirely on the facts of the case.

6-6   If the trial judge determines that no nurse-patient relationship existed, what legal effect will this have, if any?

☐   The case will be dismissed.

☐   The case will proceed, but the plaintiff will be limited to nominal damages.

☐   Mr. Green automatically will be entitled to recover damages from his employer.

6-7   Which of the following items might the trial judge *judicially notice* in this case?

☐   the general qualifications of a nurse to render first aid

☐   Nurse Owen's negligent conduct

☐   the degree of Mr. Green's disability

6-8   If Mr. Green wins his case, which of the following will be the result?

☐   Nurse Owen probably will lose his license to practice nursing.

☐   Nurse Owen will be required to pay money damages to Mr. Green.

☐   Nurse Owen's employer will be required to pay money damages to Mr. Green.

6-9   Mr. Green and Nurse Owen work for the same employer. What legal effect (if any) does this have with respect to the question of liability?

☐   It has no legal effect.

☐   The employer can be held liable along with Nurse Owen.

☐   The employer cannot be held liable because of state workers' compensation laws.

Problem No. 7

> Nurse Grady is an experienced nurse in charge of the obstetrical ward of a large hospital. She is considered an expert technically, but has a reputation for being on the "cold" side. One day Nurse Grady brusquely informs a young maternity patient, "We have to give you a predelivery enema." The patient, obviously somewhat concerned, begins to question Nurse Grady about the procedure but is cut short with the following remark: "Don't carry on like a baby. No one has ever died from an enema, and besides, it's a standard hospital procedure."
>
> During the administration of the enema, Nurse Grady turns to give instructions to another nurse, and while so doing she accidentally punctures the patient's anal membrane, causing serious injury. The patient later sues Nurse Grady for malpractice.

7-1   Nurse Grady is described as being technically proficient but impersonal and cold. What relationship is there (if any) between a nurse's attitude and the prevention of malpractice claims?

☐   There is little or no relationship whatever.

☐   Malpractice claims often can be prevented by giving recognition to the interpersonal and emotional aspects of patient care.

☐   Malpractice claims can be prevented only by giving proper attention to the patient's physical needs.

7-2   Which type of nurse is most likely to be sued for an act of malpractice, following some adverse medical event?

☐   the nurse who is technically proficient but tends to be very impersonal

☐   the nurse who is not afraid to challenge doctors' orders

☐   the nurse who is adept at concealing her nursing errors or omissions

7-3 With respect to the likelihood of a lawsuit in this case, which of the following is *more nearly* correct?

☐ Nurse Grady probably would have been sued *regardless* of her attitude toward the patient, once the latter sustained the described injury.

☐ Nurse Grady probably would have been sued even if *no* injury was sustained because of her impersonal and indifferent treatment of the patient.

☐ Nurse Grady might *not* have been sued if, before the injury, she had treated the patient with respect and made a sincere attempt to allay her fears.

7-4 What role (if any) do psychological factors play as causes of malpractice suits?

☐ They play only a minor role, if any at all.

☐ They play the single most important role.

☐ The play an extremely important role.

7-5 All other things being equal, which of the following factors are the *principal* causes of malpractice suits?

☐ sociological factors, such as TV programs that highlight the frequency of medical malpractice

☐ unfavorable medical events that occur to patients in the course of treatment

☐ psychological factors that upset patients and make them want to seek revenge

7-6 Nurse Grady's remarks indicate that she ☐ is ☐ is not a believer in the patient-centered approach to nursing. This approach is based on the theory that

☐ the patient wants to and should be encouraged to participate in his or her care

☐ the patient's cooperation in the treatment process can do no harm but is not significant

☐ the patient's participation in the treatment process tends to interfere with more important nursing activities

7-7   What would be the *best* way to cope with the patient's apprehensiveness in this case?

☐ Assure her that the predelivery enema is a standard hospital procedure given to all maternity patients.

☐ Give her a chance to understand and cooperate in the procedure to the greatest extent possible.

☐ Tell her as little as possible so that she will have less cause for anxiety.

7-8   All other things being equal, what is the best thing nurses can do to reduce the possibility of malpractice claims?

☐ They should place emphasis on meeting all their patients' physical needs in an efficient and objective manner.

☐ They should stress the emotional aspects of patient care, even if this results in a certain degree of inattention to physical needs.

☐ They should regard patients as persons with equally important physical and emotional needs, both of which they should treat in a competent manner.

7-9   What is the *best* reason why someone like Nurse Grady should become concerned about malpractice claims prevention?

☐ She can minimize the chances that her malpractice insurance will be cancelled.

☐ She can learn how to avoid lawsuits and give better patient care at the same time.

☐ She can reduce the likelihood of disciplinary action against her for negligent acts she may commit.

7-10   Nurse Grady is an experienced nurse with many years of nursing service. What psychological consequence is this lawsuit *likely* to have on her?

☐ Because she is experienced and professionally competent, it is not likely that she will suffer *any* adverse psychological consequence.

☐ The lawsuit probably will prove disturbing to her only if she has to pay money damages to the patient.

☐ The lawsuit probably will prove to be a threat to her professional reputation even though she is experienced, and she will probably suffer some psychological tension pending the outcome of the case.

Problem No. 8

> Consider the following two hospitalized patients:
>
> Patient A is a 55-year-old artist admitted to the hospital for elective surgery. She is aloof, impatient, and generally critical of others.
>
> Patient B is a 30-year-old unemployed man who has been in and out of mental hospitals for many years, seeking treatment for a personality disorder that has incapacitated him.

8-1   Which of these two patients (if either) exhibits traits calculated to make him or her "suit-prone"?

      ☐ Patient A

      ☐ Patient B

      ☐ both patients

      ☐ neither patient

8-2   Which of the following is a good description of suit-prone patients?

      ☐ They generally prefer to deal with persons who antagonize them by suing them.

      ☐ They tend to be familiar with legal matters and courtroom procedures.

      ☐ They tend to have great respect for doctors, lawyers, and other professionals.

8-3   What threat (if any) is posed to the nurse by suit-prone patients?

      ☐ They are generally nuisances but do not pose any significant threat.

      ☐ Their conduct is generally violent, which creates the possibility they may cause the nurse physical harm.

      ☐ Their constant need to blame others when something goes wrong marks them as individuals who may eventually sue a nurse.

8-4   Which of the following personality traits *best* describes suit-prone patients?

☐   They are emotionally immature and tend to avoid responsibility.

☐   They are socially mature and have a well-defined sense of personal responsibility.

☐   They are independent, secure, and forthright in their dealings with others.

8-5   Of the two patients described, which of them (if either) is *more likely* to be suit prone than the other?

☐   Patient A

☐   Patient B

☐   Both are about equally suit prone.

8-6   If a nurse recognizes a patient as being suit prone, how should the nurse react to the patient in order to avoid the threat he or she represents?

☐   The nurse should be polite but impersonal and try to avoid the patient as much as possible.

☐   The nurse should be sympathetic and attentive to all the patient's physical and emotional needs, even if it means spending a little more time with him or her than with other patients.

☐   The nurse should be aggressive and forceful in dealing with the patient, concentrating on meeting all the patient's physical needs but not catering to his or her emotional demands.

8-7   Assuming some relationship between a nurse's attitude toward patients and their later likelihood of suing the nurse for an act of malpractice, the nurse who is impersonal, impatient, and inflexible is

☐   more likely

☐   less likely

☐   neither more nor less likely

to be sued for malpractice than a nurse who is personal, patient, and flexible in his or her attitudes toward patients.

8-8   Assume that Nurse N has occasion to treat both Patient A and Patient B while they are hospitalized and openly displays hostility and antagonism toward both of them. What additional element is necessary before Nurse N can be sued by either or both of them?

☐   Nurse N would have to have one or more serious arguments with either patient, leading to direct threats of a lawsuit.

☐   Nurse N would have to cause some physical injury to either patient.

☐   There would have to be evidence that either patient's condition worsened while he or she was being attended by Nurse N.

8-9   Assuming that Nurse N commits acts amounting to malpractice while treating Patient A and Patient B, which of the following factors probably would be the *most important* in each patient's decision whether or not to sue?

☐   the patient's prior rapport and relationship with respect to Nurse N

☐   the patient's prior feelings about doctors, nurses, and health care personnel in general

☐   the patient's personal knowledge of medical matters and how to bring a lawsuit

8-10 Which of the following expresses the most reasonable and most probable rule regarding the *likelihood* of malpractice claims?

☐   A malpractice claim will usually result whenever there is an unfavorable medical event causing harm or injury to the patient.

☐   A malpractice claim will usually result when a nurse's conduct causes harm or injury to the patient and the nurse's prior relationship with the patient has been a poor one.

☐   A malpractice claim will result whenever there is poor rapport and a breakdown in the personal relationship between nurse and patient.

Problem No. 9

> Nurse Harvey is assigned to keep track of all pads and sponges used during a gallbladder operation, and the operating surgeon closes the incision only after being assured by Nurse Harvey that all sponges are accounted for. After the operation, the patient's complaint of continued abdominal pain causes the surgeon to suspect a foreign object. The surgeon reopens the incision the following day and finds a lap pad that had been overlooked during the first operation. The patient later sues Nurse Harvey for his negligence in counting the sponges and pads.

9-1   In order to win this case, what character of evidence will the plaintiff be required to offer?

☐   evidence more likely true than not

☐   evidence beyond all reasonable doubt

☐   evidence convincing to a majority of the jury

9-2   What initial presumption of law exists in every malpractice case?

☐   the presumption that the defendant is free from negligence

☐   the presumption that the plaintiff's injury was due to the defendant's negligence

☐   the presumption that a certain number of injuries to patients are inevitable in the normal course of medical treatment

9-3   How does the so-called burden-of-proof rule affect Nurse Harvey in this case?

☐   He is presumed to be blameless and therefore has the jury's sympathy

☐   He does not have to prove his freedom from negligence until the plaintiff produces evidence of his negligence.

☐   He has the burden of proving he was not negligent in the circumstances alleged.

9-4 Which *two* of the following items are *essential* for the plaintiff to prove in order to win this case?

☐ proof of a nurse-patient relationship

☐ proof of Nurse Harvey's qualifications and license to practice nursing

☐ proof of Nurse Harvey's employment relationship with the hospital

☐ proof of the act constituting negligence

9-5 Under ordinary circumstances, how must the question of whether a nurse acted with reasonable care be proved?

☐ by the defendant's explanation of what he or she did

☐ by the testimony of medical or nursing experts

☐ by the trial judge, after checking the outcome of prior similar court cases

9-6 Assume that the doctrine of *res ipsa loquitur* applies in this case. What effect does it have on the question of proof of negligence?

☐ The plaintiff does not have to introduce the testimony of experts to prove the defendant's negligence.

☐ Evidence of the defendant's negligence can be dispensed with entirely.

☐ The defendant is not required to prove his freedom from negligence.

9-7 What is the legal effect of the doctrine of *res ipsa loquitur*?

☐ The defendant is considered liable whether or not he or she can prove due care or lack of negligence.

☐ The nurse's negligence becomes a legal question to be decided solely by the trial judge.

☐ The circumstances under which the injury occurred create an inference that the nurse was negligent, which the nurse must then disprove.

9-8   Under what factual circumstances does the doctrine of *res ipsa loquitur* not apply?

☐   when the extensiveness of the injury sustained by the plaintiff is in doubt

☐   when the cause of the injury was in the exclusive control of the defendant

☐   when the injury sustained was caused in part by the plaintiff's own conduct

9-9   Whether or not the doctrine of *res ipsa loquitur* applies in a particular case is determined by

☐   the judge, pursuant to a motion therefor by the plaintiff

☐   the jury, after hearing all the evidence

☐   the plaintiff's attorney, at the time the suit is commenced

9-10   A trial Court will *direct a verdict* in favor of one party or the other when

☐   the Court believes the testimony offered by a particular party supports that party's position on all the legal questions raised

☐   the Court believes the jury is not capable of deciding issues of negligence

☐   the Court believes there is no substantial dispute about what occurred, and reasonable minds could not arrive at a conclusion different from that of the Court's

Problem No. 10

> Patient P, elderly and infirm but otherwise of sound mind, tells private-duty Nurse N he wishes to prepare a will as quickly as possible and without his (second) wife's knowledge. He tells Nurse N he plans to leave 80% of his rather extensive estate to his favorite niece, 15% to his wife, and 5% to Nurse N out of gratitude for her attentive care during the past year. He asks Nurse N to help him prepare the document, employing a preprinted will form in order to assure that "all necessary legal language" is included in the document. State law requires two witnesses to the execution of a will.

10-1 Nurse N will be acting both ethically and legally if she tells Patient P

- ☐ that he must leave a greater share of his estate to his wife if a will contest is to be avoided

- ☐ that she can prepare the will but cannot be a witness to its signing

- ☐ that P should seek the advice of a lawyer before attempting to proceed on his own in the matter

10-2 If Nurse N follows P's instructions to the letter and he subsequently dies, the Probate Court will not admit the will to probate if it appears that

- ☐ no attorney was involved in its preparation

- ☐ insufficient or ineligible persons were witnesses to the will

- ☐ the will was signed in pencil rather than in ink

10-3 What is the legal significance of the fact that Nurse N is shown to have assisted P in the preparation of his will?

- ☐ It indicates her undue influence over him and will thereby void the will.

- ☐ It has no legal significance in the absence of other facts.

- ☐ It automatically voids any bequest made to Nurse N.

10-4 If Nurse N and a fellow nurse were the only witnesses to P's will, how would this affect the probate of the will?

☐ The bequest to Nurse N would be declared null and void.

☐ The will would be declared null and void in its entirety.

☐ The will would be declared valid in all respects.

10-5 When a decedent's purported will is not admitted to probate because it has not been prepared or executed in accordance with law,

☐ the decedent's property becomes the property of the state

☐ the decedent's property automatically passes in its entirety to his or her surviving spouse

☐ the decedent's property is distributed in accordance with the state law on succession of decedents' estates or in accordance with a valid prior will

10-6 A holographic will is one prepared

☐ when the testator is *in extremis* and there is no time to call a lawyer

☐ in a person's own handwriting

☐ by a minister, priest, or other clergy member

Problem No. 11

Patient P, a 71-year-old man, was admitted to Hospital H suffering from chest pain. After initial treatment in the ER, he was transferred to the hospital's coronary care unit (CCU). In a discussion with his family and his private physician, P expressed his wish that heroic efforts not be used to keep him alive in the event his cardiopulmonary status worsened and he was no longer able to make treatment choices on his own. Following this discussion, Doctor D placed instructions in P's chart that he was to be treated as a "No Code Blue," which was the hospital's description for a Do-Not-Resuscitate (DNR) order. Two days later, P suffered ventricular fibrillation and CCU Nurse N, seeing this as a medical emergency, immediately undertook to resuscitate P by shocking his heart with an electric current. Although P's heartbeat was restored, he died 1 week later from the sequelae of a paralyzing stroke and other complications of his compromised cardiopulmonary condition. His family subsequently brought suit against the hospital, Doctor D, and Nurse H claiming damages for pain, suffering, emotional distress, and disability and alleging, among other things, the tort of "wrongful life," as well as battery.

11-1 In the given circumstances, Nurse N   ☐ acted properly   ☐ acted improperly because

   ☐ an emergency existed, and an emergency always takes precedence over a DNR order

   ☐ a DNR order takes precedence over normal treatment even in an emergency

   ☐ the CCU nurse's legal responsibility is to do whatever is necessary to keep his or her patients alive

11-2 The fact that Doctor D's DNR order was not followed by Nurse N

   ☐ would absolve Doctor D of any liability for the charge of "wrongful life"

   ☐ would absolve Hospital H of any liability for the charge of "wrongful life"

   ☐ would absolve Nurse N of any liability for the charge of "wrongful life," as long as she met the applicable standard of care under the given emergency circumstances

11-3 If the state in question does not recognize claims for "wrongful life," either by statute or common law, the trial judge more than likely would

   ☐ rule in favor of a motion to dismiss the plaintiff's entire claim

   ☐ take judicial notice thereof in open court

   ☐ refrain from ruling on this issue so that it could be decided by an appellate court

11-4 If the trial judge were to disallow the plaintiff's claim for "wrongful life,"

☐   the claim for battery could still be pursued at the trial

☐   the amount of damages recoverable would be significantly reduced

☐   that claim could not be heard on any subsequent appeal

11-5 If, after requesting the DNR order noted above, Patient P informed the nurses in the CCU that he had a change of heart, his wishes

☐   could be honored, but only with the express concurrence of his family and Doctor D

☐   would take precedence over Doctor D's written DNR order and the family's wishes

☐   would be legally binding, but only if they were reduced to writing

11-6 A claim alleging battery in this case

☐   would have to be based on the patient's lack of consent to any further treatment

☐   would not be allowed, since the patient's consent is always implied in an emergency

☐   would have to be based on the willful or negligent violation of the DNR order

11-7 Doctor D could be held liable in this case

☐   only if he had personally participated in the resuscitative procedure

☐   only if he had improperly instructed Nurse N in cardiopulmonary resuscitation

☐   only if he were to have written the DNR order without the family's concurrence

11-8 All things considered, the party or parties most likely to be held liable in this case is (are):

☐   Nurse N and Hospital H, but not Doctor D

☐   Nurse N alone

☐   Nurse N, Doctor D, and Hospital H

11-9 Which of the following doctrines could *not* be applicable in this case?

☐   the captain of the ship doctrine

☐   the doctrine of *stare decisis*

☐   the *respondeat superior* doctrine

Miscellaneous Test Questions

12-1 The existence of a nurse-patient relationship is dependent on

☐ the mere fact of giving nursing care

☐ the specific nature of a nurse's duty assignments

☐ contractual arrangements to care for someone in particular

12-2 When a nurse offers his or her services to an individual as a private-duty nurse, which of the following legal doctrines *cannot* apply to the nurse's conduct?

☐ the rule of personal liability

☐ the rule of *respondeat superior*

☐ *res ipsa loquitur*

12-3 What is the usual rule with respect to the giving of emergency care outside the nurse's normal work duties?

☐ The nurse has an *ethical* but not a *legal* obligation to render such care.

☐ The nurse has an ethical and legal obligation to render such care.

☐ The nurse has a *legal* but not an *ethical* obligation to render such care.

12-4 If a nurse renders emergency care to someone not within his or her normal work responsibilities, what standard of care is applicable to the nurse's conduct?

☐ The nurse is held to the standard of care applicable to all private citizens.

☐ The nurse is held to the highest standard of care because of the unusual circumstances.

☐ The nurse is held to the standard of care applicable to other nurses acting under similar conditions.

12-5 Which of the following "surrounding circumstances" would *most likely* relieve a nurse of liability for his or her conduct?

☐ the nurse is a student and not yet licensed

☐ the care was given under emergency conditions

☐ the nurse was on a temporary float assignment in a short-staffing situation

12-6 Nurse N admits to an act of malpractice. He can avoid liability if he can show

☐ that the patient contributed to his or her own injury

☐ that his supervisor was negligent in making the assignment to him

☐ that other nurses have committed similar acts of malpractice and avoided liability

12-7 Under what circumstances (if any) may a nurse make a diagnosis?

☐ under no circumstances, since this is the physician's sole responsibility

☐ whenever the nurse believes he or she has sufficient experience to do so

☐ whenever the nurse is required to evaluate the patient's condition to determine his or her specific needs for nursing care

12-8 What is the nurse's legal duty with regard to carrying out a physician's order?

☐ The nurse must follow the order to the letter unless in his or her professional judgment some other course of treatment would be more effective.

☐ The nurse must follow the order without question unless he or she has reason to believe some harm may result to the patient.

☐ The nurse must always review the order with the physician to make sure it is correct before carrying it out.

12-9 In which of the following instances is there no basis for a *malpractice* suit?

☐ Nurse A negligently injures a neighbor's child while attempting to remove a splinter from her eye.

☐ Nurse B injures a visitor to the hospital when he negligently manipulates a wheelchair.

☐ Nurse C negligently burns a patient in a ward to which she is not normally assigned.

12-10 Which of the following classes of nurses is exposed to the *greatest* risk of liability for malpractice because of the nature of the employment relationship?

☐ the government-employed nurse

☐ the occupational health nurse

☐ the hospital nurse

12-11 Nurse P is employed by a private physician. Which of the following legal doctrines makes the physician liable for Nurse P's conduct while so employed?

☐ the captain of the ship doctrine

☐ *respondeat superior*

☐ borrowed servant doctrine

12-12 In what way (if any) does the doctrine of *respondeat superior* alter the liability of a nurse for his or her negligent conduct?

☐ It shifts the nurse's liability to another person and eliminates his or her liability altogether.

☐ It makes the nurse liable to his or her employer.

☐ It does not alter the nurse's liability at all.

12-13 In which of the following instances of nursing care does the doctrine of *respondeat superior* not apply?

☐ care given by a licensed practical nurse

☐ care given under emergency circumstances

☐ care given outside the scope of the nurse's regular employment

12-14 What is the most important reason for keeping accurate medical records by nursing personnel?

☐ to keep track of the patient's condition

☐ to assist in treating the patient

☐ to provide a good defense against a legal claim

12-15 Why should a nurse refrain from inserting in a patient's chart derogatory remarks about the patient's quirks or idiosyncracies?

☐ they might prove embarrassing or libelous in later litigation

☐ they might not accurately describe the patient's quirks or idiosyncracies

☐ they might give rise to a malpractice action

12-16 In reviewing a patient's chart, Nurse N discovers that he had erroneously recorded the administration of 30 ml of a particular drug when the correct amount (which he had administered) should have been 3 ml. What action should Nurse N take to correct this discovered error?

☐ He should ink out the error on the chart and insert the correct information in its place.

☐ He should immediately notify his nursing supervisor so the latter can record the proper entry.

☐ He should enter a new note referring to the prior error and giving the correct information.

12-17 Surgeon S instructs OR Nurse N to omit in her nursing notes any reference to a cardiac arrest that occurred during a surgical procedure. What is Nurse N's legal position in this situation if she follows the surgeon's order?

☐ She could be held liable to the patient for any harm resulting from the cardiac arrest.

☐ She could risk the suspension or revocation of her license by the state licensing authority.

☐ She is fully protected against any legal action or disciplinary action, since she followed the doctor's order explicitly.

12-18 Nurse S is a clinical nursing supervisor at a teaching hospital. What is the legal effect of his countersigning entries in patients' charts made by nursing students?

☐ It places Nurse S in the position of endorsing and authenticating the entries made in the charts.

☐ It makes Nurse S personally liable for any subsequent harm to the patients in question.

☐ It gives legal proof of Nurse S's authority as a clinical nursing supervisor.

12-19 The general rule holds that information in a patient's chart may be released to an outside (nonhospital) party without the patient's consent

- ☐ if the requesting party is an attorney seeking the information for litigation purposes

- ☐ if such release is authorized by law or pursuant to a court order

- ☐ if the patient is a recognized public figure whose comings and goings are considered public information

12-20 In a civil or criminal trial, statements contained in a patient's medical record are given credence for evidentiary purposes because

- ☐ they represent the unbiased observations of health professionals

- ☐ they have been recorded pursuant to hospital rules and regulations

- ☐ they represent the contemporaneous recording of events in the course of treating the patient

12-21 The right of privacy is a legal right that assures freedom from unwarranted public scrutiny to

- ☐ everyone

- ☐ well-known public figures

- ☐ hospitalized patients only

12-22 If a former patient brings a legal action in which his or her physical condition is a major issue, in the eyes of the law the patient's medical record

- ☐ is no longer confidential for purposes of that legal action

- ☐ is presumed to be a biased document that should be given little legal weight

- ☐ is deemed confidential and cannot be used to refute his or her claim

12-23 State laws enacted pursuant to the federal Child Abuse Prevention and Treatment Act of 1973 generally grant to health professionals who report suspected cases of child abuse

☐   immunity from being sued for malpractice

☐   immunity from professional disciplinary proceedings

☐   immunity from invasion of privacy and defamation of character suits

12-24 Child abuse reporting statutes are important because they give nursing personnel the opportunity to

☐   prevent further injuries to defenseless children

☐   make sure that abusers of children are appropriately punished

☐   have abused children removed from their home environments

12-25 When a nurse who is not named as a beneficiary is asked by a patient to witness the signing of his or her will, the nurse should understand that this act is

☐   frowned on as unprofessional nursing practice

☐   unethical, as well as a violation of the state nurse practice act

☐   ethical, legal, and the compassionate thing to do

12-26 Living wills are a mechanism used by persons who wish to

☐   indicate their willingness to be allowed to die in designated conditions such as terminal illness or irreversible coma

☐   circumvent the legalities of regular wills

☐   add health care directives to earlier-executed wills

12-27 Once a competent adult patient has executed a valid living will,

☐ it takes precedence over his or her express wishes that may be in direct conflict therewith

☐ it is legally binding on all the doctors and nurses who attend the patient

☐ it can be revoked only by the patient's execution of another living will meeting all statutory formalities

12-28 As the law currently exists, most legal commentators believe that a durable power of attorney is

☐ an ineffective way of implementing a patient's wishes regarding the making of critical health care decisions

☐ superior to the living will as a device for authorizing the making of critical health care decisions

☐ relatively ineffective, since it is no longer binding once a patient becomes incapacitated

12-29 Becoming an advocate for the patient's interests in the health care setting is a role that

☐ is vigorously opposed by professional nursing codes of ethics

☐ nurses should avoid, unless they are required to carry out such responsibilities by statute

☐ often results in litigation and other forms of retaliation against the nurse

12-30 In the absence of personal liability insurance coverage, a hospital-based nurse who is sued for malpractice

☐ is considered judgment proof and can't be required to pay any damages assessed

☐ can be held personally responsible for all damages assessed

☐ can rely on the coverage afforded by the hospital's policy as protection from personal financial responsibility

12-31 In the present legal environment, nurses as a class are being sued for malpractice

☐   with greater frequency than a decade ago

☐   with less frequency than a decade ago

☐   with about the same frequency as a decade ago

12-32 Clinical nursing specialists run a higher risk of being sued for malpractice because

☐   they deal with seriously ill patients who are more likely to suffer injury in the course of treatment

☐   they assume greater legal responsibilities by virtue of their specialist credentials

☐   they enjoy higher incomes and are therefore considered good litigation targets

12-32 When a nurse has a personal malpractice policy, the nurse's insurance carrier agrees

☐   to pay all malpractice claims filed against him or her, within policy limits

☐   to pay only those malpractice claims for which he or she is deemed legally liable

☐   to pay only those malpractice damages in excess of the hospital's coverage limits

12-34 Under the typical nursing malpractice policy, coverage generally is provided

☐   for all types of nursing care given

☐   for normal nursing care, but not volunteer or Good Samaritan care

☐   for hospital care, but not private-duty care

12-35 Nursing student S does not know whether to purchase personal malpractice coverage. The best rationale for doing so is that

☐   the law requires nursing students to maintain personal malpractice coverage

☐   nursing students are just as liable as graduate nurses for their acts of malpractice

☐   the costs of such coverage are nominal and are fully tax deductible

ANSWERS TO TEST QUESTIONS

1-1 statutory law

1-2 Common law is not the result of a legislative enactment.

1-3 criminal law

1-4 conduct that pertains to the public interest and is considered an offense against society as a whole

1-5 The patient can sue Nurse Jones for negligence, and the local governmental authority can bring criminal charges against her for violation of the statute.

1-6 She will be fined, imprisoned, placed on probation, or some combination thereof.

1-7 torts

1-8 She will be required to pay money damages to the injured plaintiff.

1-9 the fact that the state law prohibits the administration of narcotic drugs without a doctor's prescription

1-10 proof of her violation of the statute relating to the administration of narcotic drugs

2-1 common law

2-2 tort law

2-3 when he fails to act as other reasonably prudent nurses would act under similar circumstances

2-4 negligence

2-5 malpractice

2-6 ordinary negligence

2-7 any of the hospital's patients he might have had occasion to treat

2-8 whenever he actually provided nursing care to that individual

2-9 the provision of nursing care to someone by a person with professional nurse's training

2-10 entered into

Nurse Smith undertook to provide nursing care to her

2-11 his or her conduct compared with that of other nurses with similar training under comparable circumstances

2-12 The surrounding circumstances always must be considered in deciding the issue of negligence.

3-1 is pertinent only with respect to what could be reasonably be expected of a young and inexperienced nurse

3-2 The student is held to the same standard of care as an RN.

3-3 Nurse Simpson can be held liable only if she is held to be negligent in making the assignment to an inexperienced nurse.

3-4 The hospital cannot be held liable in this case.

3-5 He should have declined to carry out the assignment, explaining his reasons to his supervisor before so doing.

3-6 the patient's known physical and mental condition

2-7 because mentally ill persons frequently do not appreciate their exposure to potential harm

3-8 Suicidally inclined persons generally give verbal or behavioral clues to their suicidal tendencies.

3-9 Both Mr. Newby and Nurse Simpson can be held liable, but not the hospital.

3-10 the doctrine of *respondeat superior*

4-1 personal liability

4-2 *respondeat superior*

4-3 holds everyone legally responsible for his or her own negligent conduct

4-4 It would apply only if Nurse Brown committed the act within the scope of her employment as a nurse by Dr. Swift.

4-5 all types of employees

4-6 an employer can be held liable for the negligent acts of his or her employees

4-7 employer-employee-negligent conduct

4-8 Dr. Swift legally can recover from Nurse Brown the amount she is required to pay Mrs. Long.

4-9 It did not alter the rule of personal liability insofar as Nurse Brown's conduct was concerned.

4-10 She undertook to diagnose the patient's condition and prescribe for her.

4-11 She should have declined to carry out Dr. Swift's request on the grounds that it would place her in a position of performing acts only a physician is authorized to perform.

5-1 the doctrine of informed consent

5-2 civil battery

5-3 there was no emergency requiring an immediate cholecystectomy

5-4 is not legally relevant on the issue of battery

5-5 could be either in writing or verbal

5-6 the patient fully understands to what he or she is consenting

5-7 would not have been legally effective under the given circumstances

5-8 the patient understands the nature and consequences of the procedure, and the alternatives thereto

5-9 the patient is unconscious, and the procedure is necessary to save his or her life

5-10 only by the minor's parents or legal guardian

5-11 the minor lives away from home and is financially independent

5-12 may be revoked at any time before the procedure

5-13 the touching of his or her person without his or her consent

5-14 the patient's decision exclusively

6-1 Mr. Green

6-2 Nurse Owen treated Mr. Green for his injury.

6-3 the jury alone

6-4 by the testimony of experts concerning the standard of care applicable in the case

6-5 Mr. Green has the burden of proving Nurse Owen's negligence.

6-6 The case will be dismissed.

6-7 the general qualifications of a nurse to render first aid

6-8 Nurse Owen will be required to pay money damages to Mr. Green.

6-9 The employer cannot be held liable because of state workers' compensation laws.

7-1 Malpractice claims often can be prevented by giving recognition to the interpersonal and emotional aspects of patient care.

7-2 the nurse who is technically proficient but tends to be very impersonal

7-3 Nurse Grady might *not* have been sued if, before the injury, she had treated the patient with respect and made a sincere attempt to allay her fears.

7-4 They play an extremely important role.

7-5 unfavorable medical events that occur to patients in the course of treatment

7-6 is not

the patient wants to and should be encouraged to participate in his or her care

7-7 Give her a chance to understand and cooperate in the procedure to the greatest extent possible.

7-8 They should regard patients as persons with equally important physical and emotional needs, both of which they should treat in a competent manner.

7-9 She can learn how to avoid lawsuits and give better patient care at the same time.

7-10 The lawsuit will probably prove to be a threat to her professional reputation even though she is experienced, and she will probably suffer some psychological tension pending the outcome of the case.

8-1 both patients

8-2 They generally prefer to deal with persons who antagonize them by suing them.

8-3 Their constant need to blame others when something goes wrong marks them as individuals who may eventually sue a nurse.

8-4 They are emotionally immature and tend to avoid responsibility.

8-5 Both are about equally suit prone.

8-6 The nurse should be sympathetic and attentive to all the patient's physical and emotional needs, even if it means spending a little more time with him or her than with other patients.

8-7 more likely

8-8 Nurse N would have to cause some physical injury to either patient.

8-9 the patient's prior rapport and relationship with respect to Nurse N

8-10 A malpractice claim will usually result when a nurse's conduct causes harm or injury to the patient and the nurse's prior relationship with the patient has been a poor one.

9-1 evidence more likely true than not

9-2 the presumption that the defendant is free from negligence

9-3 He does not have to prove his freedom from negligence until the plaintiff produces evidence of his negligence.

9-4 proof of a nurse-patient relationship

proof of the act constituting negligence

9-5 by the testimony of medical or nursing experts

9-6 The plaintiff does not have to introduce the testimony of experts to prove the defendant's negligence.

9-7 The circumstances under which the injury occurred create an inference that the nurse was negligent, which the nurse must then disprove.

9-8 when the injury sustained was caused in part by the plaintiff's own conduct

9-9 the judge, pursuant to a motion therefor by the plaintiff

9-10 the Court believes there is no substantial dispute about what occurred and reasonable minds could not arrive at a conclusion different from that of the Court's.

10-1   that P should seek the advice of a lawyer before attempting to proceed on his own in the matter

10-2   insufficient or ineligible persons were witnesses to the will

10-3   It has no legal significance in the absence of other facts.

10-4   The bequest to Nurse N would be declared null and void.

10-5   the decedent's property is distributed in accordance with the state law on succession of decedents' estates or in accordance with a valid prior will.

10-6   in a person's own handwriting

11-1   acted improperly

a DNR order takes precedence over normal treatment even in an emergency

11-2   would absolve Doctor D of any liability for the charge of "wrongful life"

11-3   take judicial notice thereof in open court

11-4   the claim of battery could still be pursued at the trial

11-5   would take precedence over Doctor D's written DNR order and his family's wishes

11-6   would have to be based on the willful or negligent violation of the DNR order

11-7   only if he had personally participated in the resuscitative procedure

11-8   Nurse N and Hospital H, but not Doctor D

11-9   the captain of the ship doctrine

12-1   the mere fact of giving nursing care

12-2   the rule of *respondeat superior*

12-3   The Nurse has an *ethical* but not a *legal* obligation to render such care.

12-4   The nurse is held to the standard of care applicable to other nurses acting under similar conditions.

12-5   the care was given under emergency conditions

12-6   that the patient contributed to his or her own injury

12-7 whenever the nurse is required to evaluate the patient's condition to determine his or her specific needs for nursing care.

12-8 The nurse must follow the order without question unless he or she has reason to believe some harm may result to the patient.

12-9 Nurse B injures a visitor to the hospital when he negligently manipulates a wheelchair.

12-10 the occupational health nurse

12-11 *respondeat superior*

12-12 It does not alter the nurse's liability at all.

12-13 care given outside the scope of the nurse's regular employment

12-14 assist in treating the patient

12-15 they might prove embarrassing or libelous in later litigation

12-16 He should enter a new note referring to the prior error and giving the correct information.

12-17 She could risk the suspension or revocation of her license by the state licensing authority.

12-18 It places Nurse S in the position of endorsing and authenticating the entries made in the charts.

12-19 if such release is authorized by law or pursuant to a court order

12-20 they represent the contemporaneous recording of events in the course of treating the patient

12-21 everyone

12-22 is no longer confidential for purposes of that legal action

12-23 immunity from invasion of privacy and defamation of character suits

12-24 prevent further injuries to defenseless children

12-25 ethical, legal, and the compassionate thing to do

12-26 wish to indicate their willingness to be allowed to die in designated conditions such as terminal illness or irreversible coma

12-27 it is legally binding on all the doctors and nurses who attend the patient

12-28 superior to the living will as a device for authorizing the making of critical health care decisions

12-29 often results in litigation and other forms of retaliation against the nurse

12-30 can be held personally responsible for all damages assessed

12-31 with greater frequency than a decade ago

12-32 they assume greater legal responsibilities by virtue of their specialist credentials

12-33 to pay only those malpractice claims for which he or she is deemed legally liable

12-34 for all types of nursing care given

12-35 nursing students are just as liable as graduate nurses for their acts of malpractice

GLOSSARY

Abortion   The interruption of a pregnancy resulting from premature stoppage of normal processes within the uterus, not necessarily of a premeditated or deliberate character.

Administrative Law   The branch of law that deals with organs of government and their powers such as the State Board of Nurse Examiners.

Advance Directives   The various methods used by competent adults to indicate their choices in health care treatment decisions. These include but are not limited to express verbal communications, living wills, durable powers of attorney, and trust agreements.

Age of Majority   Statutory or legal age of adulthood, generally 18 years of age.

Agency   The relationship in which one person acts for or represents another, such as employer and employee.

Agent   The person authorized by another to act for him or her.

Allegation   A statement, charge, or assertion that a person expects to be able to prove.

Appeal   A legal proceeding in which a higher court is asked to reverse or correct the decision of a lower court.

Appellant   The party who files the appeal seeking to reverse the decision of a lower court.

Appellee   The party against whom an appeal to a higher court is taken.

Assault   An intentional threat to cause bodily harm to another, designed to intimidate or place the person in reasonable apprehension of harm.

Attestation   The act of confirming that a document has been duly signed in accordance with law.

Battery   The intentional touching of another person either without permission (consent) or with consent that has been exceeded or fraudulently obtained.

Borrowed Servant Rule   The legal doctrine that holds that a hospital employee (e.g., a nurse) may be considered a temporary employee of someone else (usually the operating surgeon) while acting under the latter's direct control. The rule states that while so engaged, the temporary employer (surgeon) will be held liable for the negligence of the borrowed servant. This is a special application of the doctrine of *respondeat superior*.

Cause of Action   The legal ground(s) for a party to bring suit against another.

Charitable Immunity   The legal doctrine that holds that a nonprofit, charitable hospital is immune from suit for acts or negligence by its employees.

Civil Action   A lawsuit dealing with some private legal right or duty, as opposed to a criminal action.

Civil Immunity   Immunity from suit alleging breach of confidentiality, granted by statute to someone who is required by law to report a particular activity such as child abuse.

Common Law   Judge-made or decisional law, as opposed to law enunciated through statutes enacted by legislative bodies.

Comparative Negligence   The legal doctrine that compares the negligence of the plaintiff and the defendant and apportions damages to the plaintiff based on the relative degrees of negligence found.

Compensatory Damages   See *damages*.

Confidential Communication   A statement made to someone in a position of trust who has a legal duty not to disclose the information thus communicated. Applies to information revealed by a patient to a physician or nurse in the course of treatment that the law protects from being revealed, even in court (except when the patient consents to such release or the court orders it).

Consent   In the medical context, the patient's voluntary act of agreeing to allow someone else (usually a doctor) to do something to him or her that would otherwise be considered an unauthorized touching or battery.

Contract   A promissory agreement between two or more persons that creates, modifies, or destroys a legal relation. It is a legally enforceable promise between two or more persons to do or not to do something. May be express (written) or implied from the behavior of the parties.

Contributory Negligence   In the medical context, a patient's failure to exercise reasonable care that aggravates an injury initially caused by someone else. Such conduct may negate the patient's right to recover damages against the party who caused the original injury.

Corporate Negligence Doctrine   The doctrine that holds a health care corporation liable for negligence on its own part in failing to provide the requisite facilities and personnel necessary to assure the provision of quality health care in accordance with accepted standards.

Crime   A public offense; the breach of any law established for the protection of society as a whole. Crimes are prosecuted by and in the name of the state.

Criminal Law   The branch of law dealing with crimes and their punishment, as opposed to civil law, which deals with private legal interests.

Cross Examination   Examination of a witness in a court case by the opposing attorney to challenge the truth or credibility of the testimony given by that witness earlier.

Damages   Monetary compensation for one who has sustained loss, detriment, or injury to his or her person or property through the unlawful conduct of another.

Defamation   The injury of a person's reputation or character by willful and malicious statements made to a third person. Defamation includes both written and oral statements (libel and slander).

Defendant   The person against whom a civil action or criminal action is instituted.

Delegation   The assignment by one person of specified tasks to another, often to a person who is lower in rank and theoretically less qualified.

Deposition   An oral interrogation of someone before trial regarding issues involved in a matter, given under oath and transcribed by a court reporter who is usually a notary public.

Diagnosis   See *nursing diagnosis*.

Directed Verdict   A verdict that a trial judge has directed a jury to make in favor of one party to the action because the evidence and/or law so clearly favors that party.

Due Care   That degree of care or concern expected of an ordinary person in the given circumstances.

Emancipated Minor   See *mature minor or emancipated minor*.

Emergency   A sudden, unexpected occurrence or event causing a threat to life or health.

Emergency Rule   A legal doctrine that relaxes the standard of care normally applicable to the conduct of a physician or nurse because of the emergency circumstances.

Evidence   Any probative matter submitted to a tribunal by a party to a proceeding for the purpose of persuading the tribunal of the validity of a particular contention. Evidence may be of a physical nature, such as documents, physical objects, and so on, or an oral nature, such as the testimony of some person.

Executor   The person chosen by an individual to carry out the provisions of his or her will.

Expert Witness   One who has special training, experience, or skill in a relevant area and who is allowed by the court to offer an *opinion* on some issue within his or her area of expertise as opposed to firsthand testimony or evidence thereon.

Express Consent   Consent to treatment given expressly, i.e., either orally or in writing.

False Imprisonment   Restraining a person's freedom of movement without lawful authority and thereby giving rise to a civil action by the person so restrained. False imprisonment usually involves constricting someone to a confined area by force or threat of force, even though there may be no physical contact.

Foreseeability Doctrine   The legal doctrine that holds an individual liable for all the natural and proximate consequences of his or her negligent conduct with respect to another.

Good Samaritan Law   A statute enacted to provide legal protection to someone who stops and renders emergency aid to another in good faith and without compensation.

Govermental Immunity   The legal doctrine that holds that a sovereign government cannot be sued without its consent thereto. The federal government has given its consent to be sued in specified instances, including the filing of actions for the negligence of its employees (including medical negligence).

Guardian ad Litem   A person officially appointed to prosecute or defend a lawsuit on behalf of a person who is deemed legally incapacitated due to infancy or otherwise.

Harm   Damage or injury to a person sufficiently measurable to constitute the legal basis for a claim against the party who caused the harm.

Hearsay Evidence   Any evidence that is not based on the personal knowledge of the witness; such evidence is admissible in a court case only under strict rules.

Holographic Will   A handwritten will; one that is deemed valid in most states provided it is properly executed and witnessed.

Immunity   See *charitable immunity, governmental immunity.*

Implied Consent   Consent to treatment based on the emergency nature of the situation rather than the patient's direct consent; also called constructive consent.

Indemnify   To make whole financially; to reimburse.

Independent Contractor   One who is hired to perform a job without supervision, i.e., not under the direct control or supervision of the hiring party.

In extremis   At the point of death.

Informed Consent Doctrine   The legal doctrine that holds that a patient's consent to treatment is not valid unless the patient fully understands (1) the nature of his or her condition, (2) the nature of the proposed treatment or procedure, (3) the alternatives to such course of action, (4) the risks involved in both the proposed and the alternative procedures, and (5) the relative chances of success or failure of the proposed and alternative procedures.

In Loco Parentis   Literally "in the place of a parent." Applied to a person acting temporarily with parental authority to give substituted consent to treatment of a minor.

Intentional Tort   Wrongful conduct that is intentional in nature and designed to cause harm or damage to another; examples include assault, battery, false imprisonment, libel, and invasion of privacy.

Interrogatories A set of written questions propounded to parties involved in a lawsuit by the opposing attorneys in an effort to discover the facts and narrow the issues in the suit.

Intestate Without a valid will. The property of a person who dies intestate is distributed in accordance with the state law on intestate succession.

Invasion of Privacy Subjecting the person or personality of someone to unwarranted or undesired publicity or exposure and giving rise to a legal cause of action for damages.

Joinder of Parties Where multiple plaintiffs or defendants are named in a proceeding.

Judge The person who guides a court proceeding to ensure impartiality and enforce the rules of evidence.

Judgment The final order of a court, based either on the jury's verdict or the judge's deliberations in a nonjury trial.

Judicial Notice The official recognition by a trial judge that an earlier legal decision or statute is applicable to the case under consideration.

Jury The individuals selected and sworn to hear the evidence and render a decision in a civil or criminal court action.

Law Rules that regulate human social conduct in a formally prescribed and legally binding manner. The two basic sources of law are legislative enactments, or statutes, and judicial decisions in litigated cases.

Lay Witness A person who testifies in court as to what was seen, heard, or otherwise observed, in contrast to an expert witness, who merely renders an *opinion* on some issue.

Legal Representative A person appointed by a court to prosecute or defend a legal action on behalf of someone not legally qualified to represent himself or herself in such action.

Legislative Enactment See *statute.*

Liability The state of being held legally responsible for harm caused another; normally assessed in money damages.

Liability Insurance A contract issued by a casualty insurance company to an individual under which the company, in return for a premium, agrees to defend all claims and pay all sums the policyholder is legally liable to pay third persons because of his or her negligent conduct.

Libel A false or malicious writing that is intended to defame or dishonor another person and published so that it will come to the attention of third parties.

Litigant Either party to a lawsuit.

Litigation A trial in court to determine legal issues, rights, and duties between the litigants.

Living Will A formal document executed by someone who chooses to die in dignity rather than be kept alive by artificial devices and procedures in the event of a terminal illness. Statutes spell out the circumstances in which the will is to become effective and how it applies to medical and nursing personnel.

Malice The intentional doing of a wrongful act without just cause or excuse, with an intent to injure another, or under circumstances that the law will imply an evil intent.

Malpractice Professional misconduct, improper discharge of duties, or failure to meet the standard of care expected of a reasonably prudent member of that profession in his or her dealings with clients or patients that causes harm to the latter.

Mature Minor or Emancipated Minor Generally, under state laws a person is considered a minor until the age of 18. However, both at common law and under some state laws a minor who is living away from home and is financially independent of his or her parents is considered an emancipated or mature minor. These individuals are allowed to act as if they were adults, and some state laws specifically permit such persons to give a valid consent to medical treatment for pregnancy, abortion, alcohol or drug abuse, and venereal disease without parental consent.

Negligence   The failure to act as an ordinary prudent person would act in the given circumstances; applies to the acts of laypersons and professionals.

Nuncupative Will   An oral will made by a person *in extremis* and deemed valid in some states if made before a sufficient number of witnesses and reduced to writing as soon as possible.

Nursing Diagnosis   Evaluation by the nurse of the totality of factors that may influence the patient's recovery. A good nursing diagnosis will identify the patient's specific nursing needs, define goals for improving the patient's care, and provide the physician with data necessary to make adjustments in treatment.

Personal Immunity   Immunity against being sued in a civil action, granted by law to certain classes of persons such as nurses employed by the federal government.

Personal Liability Rule   The legal doctrine that holds that every person is legally responsible for his or her own tortious conduct.

Plaintiff   The complaining party in a civil suit.

Practical Nurse   A nurse who has passed minimum standards of training and education established by a state before being licensed to perform selected nursing acts, and then only under the direction of a physician, dentist, or RN. The licensed practical nurse (LPN) is not authorized to supervise, manage a nursing unit, or teach.

Precedent   A rule of law decided by the court in a prior lawsuit that serves as legal authority in subsequent similar cases.

Preponderance of the Evidence   Sufficient credible evidence to convince a court or jury that the essential allegations made are more probably true than not.

Private-Duty Nurse   A registered professional nurse who independently contracts to give bedside nursing care to one specific patient.

Privileged Communication   See *confidential communication.*

Probate   The judicial proceeding in which a purported last will is held to be either valid or invalid.

Professional Nurse   A nurse who has passed minimum standards of education and training established by a state before being licensed to render nursing care, for pay, to persons in need of such care. Also referred to as a registered nurse or RN.

Proximate Cause   The act or event that, unbroken by any efficient intervening act or event, is the immediate cause of harm or injury and without which such harm or injury would not have occurred.

Proximately   Close, in point of time, to a preceding event such as a negligent act.

Reasonable Care   With respect to nurses, that degree of care normally exercised by other reasonably prudent nurses of comparable skill and learning under the same or similar circumstances.

Res Ipsa Loquitur   Literally, "the thing speaks for itself." A legal doctrine applicable to cases in which the defendant had exclusive control of the instrumentality or events that produced the patient's injury, which injury ordinarily could not have occurred without negligent conduct. When this rule is held applicable in a given case, the plaintiff's normal burden of proving the defendant's negligence is dismissed and the defendant instead has the burden of proving his or her freedom from negligence.

Respondeat Superior   "Let the master answer." The legal doctrine that holds the employer responsible for the negligent acts of his or her servants or employees while acting within the scope of employment.

Right-to-Die Law   A law that upholds a patient's right to choose death by refusing extraordinary treatment. Also referred to as a natural death law or living will law.

Right to Privacy   The right of every individual to be left alone or to be free from unwanted publicity. It includes the right to seclusion, the right not to have one's name or likeness appropriated for commercial purposes, and the right not to have personal information about oneself made public. If one's privacy is invaded without authorization, the law recognizes a legal right to recover damages in tort from the wrongdoer.

Sovereign Immunity   See *governmental immunity.*

Standard of Care   The legal criteria against which a defendant's conduct is compared in order to determine if such conduct amounts to negligence. In general, it consists of those acts performed or omitted that an ordinary, reasonably prudent nurse would have performed or omitted to perform under the same or similar circumstances.

Standing Orders   Medical orders written by a doctor that instruct nurses what treatment should be rendered under given circumstances when the doctor is not present.

Stare Decisis   Literally, "Let the decision stand." The legal principle indicating that courts should apply the rulings in previous cases to subsequent cases involving similar facts and legal questions.

Statute (Statutory Law)   An enactment by a legislative body having the force and effect of law. A formalized law, as opposed to judge-made common (decisional) law.

Statute of Limitations   Laws that set forth the length of time within which a person may file a specific type of lawsuit.

Subpoena   A court order requiring a person to appear in court and give testimony in a civil or criminal action.

Subpoena Duces Tecum   A subpoena that commands a person to appear in court and bring with him or her specific documents named in the subpoena.

Suit   A court proceeding in which one party seeks damages or the vindication of some legal claim or right; synonymous with lawsuit.

Summons   A document that gives official notification to a defendant that a suit has been filed against him or her, requiring the defendant to respond (answer) within a stated period of time.

Testator   A person who makes a will.

Tort   A civil wrong, either intentional or unintentional, giving rise to a legal claim for redress or money damages.

Tortfeasor   One who commits a tort; a wrongdoer whose actions give rise to a civil suit for money damages.

Verdict   The formal declaration of a jury's decision in a civil or criminal case.

Will   A legal declaration of a person's intentions concerning the disposition of his or her property after death; also called last will and testament.

Witness   One who is called to give testimony in a legal proceeding, either civil or criminal.

INDEX

THE NURSE'S LIABILITY FOR MALPRACTICE
A Programmed Course
ELI P. BERNZWEIG, J.D.
Mosby Year–Book, Inc.

This mask is provided for your use in covering the answers to the questions in the text. To gain maximum benefit from this programmed course, do not reveal the answer to a question until you have checked the response that you think is correct.

THE NURSE'S LIABILITY FOR MALPRACTICE
A Programmed Course
ELI P. BERNZWEIG, J.D.
Mosby Year–Book, Inc.

This mask is provided for your use in covering the answers to the questions in the text. To gain maximum benefit from this programmed course, do not reveal the answer to a question until you have checked the response that you think is correct.